■ Research Ethics Consultation

# Research Ethics Consultation

*A Casebook*

Marion Danis, MD
Emily Largent, BSN, RN
Christine Grady, RN, PhD
David Wendler, PhD
Sara Chandros Hull, PhD
Seema Shah, JD
Joseph Millum, PhD
Benjamin Berkman, JD, MPH
*Department of Bioethics*
*Clinical Center, National Institutes of Health*

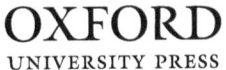

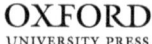

Oxford University Press, Inc., publishes works that further
Oxford University's objective of excellence
in research, scholarship, and education.

Oxford   New York
Auckland   Cape Town   Dar es Salaam   Hong Kong   Karachi   Kuala Lumpur   Madrid
Melbourne   Mexico City   Nairobi   New Delhi   Shanghai   Taipei   Toronto

With offices in
Argentina   Austria   Brazil   Chile   Czech Republic   France   Greece   Guatemala
Hungary   Italy   Japan   Poland   Portugal   Singapore   South Korea   Switzerland
Thailand   Turkey   Ukraine   Vietnam

Copyright © 2012 Oxford University Press

Published by Oxford University Press, Inc.
198 Madison Avenue, New York, New York 10016
www.oup.com

Oxford is a registered trademark of Oxford University Press
All rights reserved. No part of this publication may be reproduced, stored in a retrieval system,
or transmitted, in any form or by any means, electronic, mechanical, photocopying, recording,
or otherwise, without the prior permission of Oxford University Press.

___

Library of Congress Cataloging-in-Publication Data

Clinical research consultation : a casebook / Marion Danis . . . [et al.].
    p.; cm.
Includes bibliographical references.
ISBN 978-0-19-979803-2 (alk. paper)
1. Medical ethics consultation–Case studies. I. Danis, Marion.
[DNLM: 1. Ethics Consultation–Case Reports. 2. Ethics, Research–Case Reports. W 20.55.E7]
R724.C527 2012
174.2–dc23                                                                                  2011027685

___

The opinions expressed are those of the authors and do not reflect the position or policy
of the National Institutes of Health, the Public Health Service, or the Department of
Health and Human Services.

# ACKNOWLEDGMENTS

We greatly appreciate the support for and trust in our consultation service extended by the National Institutes of Health research community. We especially thank all of the requestors who kindly agreed to inclusion of their consultation requests in this book. Some requestors provided us with further insights about the consultations in which they were involved and about what happened after the consultation, for which we are grateful. We also wish to thank John Gallin, the director of the NIH Clinical Center; Zeke Emanuel who encouraged the creation of the electronic database that made this book possible; Catherine Yao, who carefully and cheerfully assisted us in reviewing the consultation database and selecting the cases presented herein; all members—past and present—of the Bioethics Consultation Service; and our friends and colleagues in the Department of Bioethics, particularly Alan Wertheimer who provided invaluable feedback on an earlier draft, Ben Chan who shared his expertise on evaluation of ethics consultation, and Catie Gliwa who offered meticulous revisions as we finalized the book.

# CONTENTS

| | | |
|---|---|---|
| *Foreword* | | xi |
| Introduction | | 1 |
| 1 | Starting Research | 21 |
| | Consult 1.1: Assessing Social Value | 24 |
| | Consult 1.2: Assessing Social Value for Local Populations | 28 |
| | Consult 1.3: Assessing Scientific Validity | 32 |
| | Consult 1.4: Placebo-Controlled Trials | 35 |
| | Consult 1.5: Addressing Ethical Issues in International Research | 37 |
| | Consult 1.6: Designing an Ethical Screening Process | 41 |
| | Consult 1.7: Reconciling Different Judgments Reached by Multiple Institutional Review Boards | 44 |
| 2 | Enrolling Research Participants | 49 |
| | Consult 2.1: Use of Nonmedical Criteria in Determinations of Study Inclusion or Exclusion | 53 |
| | Consult 2.2: Exclusion of an Individual Based on a New Comorbidity | 57 |
| | Consult 2.3: Enrolling Staff Members in Clinical Studies | 59 |
| | Consult 2.4: Identification of Potential Study Participants Through Publicly Available Records | 62 |
| | Consult 2.5: Enrollment of Research Participants in Multiple Protocols | 66 |
| | Consult 2.6: Obtaining Informed Consent from Individuals Who Are Blind, Illiterate, or Do Not Understand the Language in Which Consent Documents are Written | 69 |
| | Consult 2.7: Assessing whether Study Procedures are Coercive or Unduly Influential | 72 |
| 3 | Protecting Research Participants | 78 |
| | Consult 3.1: Justification of Research Risks | 81 |
| | Consult 3.2: Evaluation of Evolving Risks | 83 |
| | Consult 3.3: Respecting Participant Preferences While Minimizing Risk | 87 |

Consult 3.4: Addressing Medical Error 90
Consult 3.5: Reconciling Confidentiality and the
          Duty to Warn 92
Consult 3.6: Risks to Third Parties 97

4  Conducting Research with Vulnerable Populations 100
Consult 4.1: Exposing Children to Risk When There
          is no Prospect of Direct Benefit 105
Consult 4.2: Informing a Minor of His Diagnosis 107
Consult 4.3: Assignment of a Surrogate Decision
          Maker by a Cognitively Impaired
          Research Participant 110
Consult 4.4: Consent for Research in an Emergency 113
Consult 4.5: Research with the Terminally Ill 116
Consult 4.6: Caring for the Economically Disadvantaged 118

5  Balancing Clinical Research and Clinical Care 122
Consult 5.1: Fulfilling Ancillary Care Obligations 125
Consult 5.2: Disclosure of Incidental Findings 129
Consult 5.3: Obligations to Individuals Tangentially
          Related to Research 134
Consult 5.4: Withholding Care for Reasons
          of Scientific Validity 138
Consult 5.5: Meeting Clinical Needs without
          Compromising Scientific Validity 141
Consult 5.6: Access to Experimental Drugs
          Outside a Study Protocol 145
Consult 5.7: Noncompliance 147

6  Navigating Interpersonal Difficulties 157
Consult 6.1: Obligations to Prevent Harm and
          Protect Confidentiality 160
Consult 6.2: Excluding a Noncompliant Participant from
          a Study with the Prospect of Direct Benefit 164
Consult 6.3: Excluding a Noncompliant Participant
          from a Study with No Prospect of Benefit 166
Consult 6.4: Discharging an At-Risk Participant 168
Consult 6.5: Futile Care 171
Consult 6.6: Conflict Between the Research Team
          and Family Members 174
Consult 6.7: Conflict Between the Research
          Team and Surrogate Decision Maker 176
Consult 6.8: Respecting Medical Beliefs 182

| | | |
|---|---|---|
| 7 | Ending Research | 185 |
| | Consult 7.1: Study Discharge after Violation of Rules | 189 |
| | Consult 7.2: Discharge to Less Optimal Care | 192 |
| | Consult 7.3: Managing Participant's Post-trial Expectations | 196 |
| | Consult 7.4: Fulfilling Post-trial Obligations to Uninsured Participants | 199 |
| | Consult 7.5: Planning for Post-trial Consequences of Trial Intervention | 202 |
| | Consult 7.6: Addressing a Request for Withdrawal of Tissue Samples | 205 |
| | Consult 7.7: Questions about Discontinuation of a Trial by the Data Safety Monitoring Board | 208 |
| | Consult 7.8: Assigning Authorship | 212 |
| | Appendices | 219 |
| | Appendix 1 Consultations Organized by Subject Matter | 219 |
| | Appendix 2 Evaluation of the Clincal Center Bioethics Consultation Service | 220 |
| | Appendix 3 Clinical Center Policy M77-2: Informed Consent | 225 |
| | Appendix 4 Clinical Center Policy M92-7: Advance Directives | 237 |
| | Appendix 5 NIH Advance Directive for Health Care and Medical Research Participation | 242 |
| | Appendix 6 Clinical Center Policy M87-4: Research Involving Adults Who Are or May Be unable to Consent | 245 |
| | Appendix 7 Selected Publications Inspired or Informed by the Work of the Bioethics Consultation Service | 249 |
| | Index | 251 |

# ■ FOREWORD

This volume systematically organizes and utilizes the rich experiences of the Bioethics Consultation Service at the National Institutes of Health (NIH) Clinical Center and draws on the multidisciplinary skills and insights of its members, all of whom have spent considerable time thinking about, writing about, and practicing research ethics consultation. The result is a casebook that explores the diversity, complexities, and nuances of ethical questions and dilemmas faced during the course of clinical and translational research. The use of actual cases provides a tangible grounding for investigators, institutional review board (IRB) members, bioethics consultants, and others interested in enduring—as well as emerging—issues in bioethics. Perhaps most important, the use of actual cases challenges readers to explore how difficult ethical questions might be approached and resolved in practice.

The Clinical Center is the largest research hospital in the United States. Such a medical facility, where every patient is a research participant or is being considered for enrollment in a study, offers an extraordinary opportunity to examine the many interesting ethical questions that arise throughout the course of clinical research. Questions arise during the early stages of study design and extend through the dissemination of findings; they span the translational pathway from "first in human" trials to community-engaged research. I had the privilege to work at the NIH from 1998 to 2006 as an investigator, clinician, IRB chair, and ethics consultant. In that time, I also had the pleasure of befriending and collaborating with many of the authors of this book. The joy of being a member of the Consultation Service was that the ethical questions were often challenging; the consultants routinely engaged one another about ongoing consults, frequently differed in their perspectives on the issue at hand, and always engaged in careful deliberation to arrive at and provide reasonable advice. The consultation process was therefore both stimulating and rewarding.

There are lessons for academic health centers to glean from the research ethics deliberations at the NIH Clinical Center, and this book comes at an opportune time. Since 2006, the extramural NIH funding for the Clinical and Translational Science Awards (CTSA)—which replaced the decades-old Clinical Research Center (CRC)—now provides the infrastructure at academic health centers across the United States to conduct research with an explicit goal of bringing research advances into the clinical and population settings. More than three-quarters of CTSAs have initiated a research ethics consultation service. It is likely that the number of research-focused ethics consultation services and their utilization will continue to grow both within the CTSA context and beyond. As director of the University of Washington CTSA's Bioethics Consult Service, and the chair of the Consultation Working Group for the CTSA Consortium Clinical Research Ethics Key Function Committee, I appreciate how valuable it is to learn from the reflections and analyses offered here.

Readers who are familiar with bioethics consultation in the clinical setting will appreciate that clinical ethics committees and bioethics consultation services are the predominant approach for providing ethical advice for families, clinicians, and those responsible for clinical oversight, although their specific roles and relationships often vary between institutions. In the research context, a more explicit and systematic method of institutional oversight, based on federal regulations and using the IRB system, has become the standard mechanism to guide researchers facing ethical dilemmas. In this context, research ethics consultation services occupy complementary and overlapping roles with IRBs. At the NIH Clinical Center—or at any academic health center—one can therefore legitimately ask what value is added to the institution and to the research enterprise by a having a research-focused ethics consultation service rather than solely relying on the IRB to provide ethical guidance. At least two important contributions should be acknowledged.

First, there is value from having a consultation service available to provide a timely, explicit, and effective mechanism to engage stakeholders in deliberative and sustained conversation about ethical issues. In many cases, these issues will still need to be considered by the IRB responsible for the ethical and regulatory oversight of the study, but the consultation process can offer an analytic framework for the various stakeholders to better accomplish their mission: socially valuable, ethically conducted research. Occasionally, it is the IRB itself that will request this advice, either because it seeks additional expertise or to obtain an independent assessment. Some questions are more fine-grained than those typically addressed by IRBs, for example, they might focus on whether a particular participant comprehends a study or has the capacity to consent; or they may come from dilemmas faced by participants themselves, such as whether to share results with family members. Other questions are typically outside the typical scope of IRB review of a research protocol, such as initial discussions about study design strategies or questions about the impact of a manuscript's title on a community.

Second, through the work of a research ethics consultation service, there is the opportunity to generate a body of scholarship: the communication of ideas, insights, and experiences from which others can learn or to which they can respond critically. This casebook is itself an example of a consultation service's value added benefit—a point reinforced by the appendix, which lists diverse articles influenced or inspired by consultations. Such collaborative scholarship may contribute to institutional knowledge, but ideally it will also be shared with the larger research community to advance bioethics and ethical research.

Many clinical investigators conduct their research in clinical research centers where the scientific environment is like that at the NIH Clinical Center: diverse researchers, ethics consultants, IRB members, and institutional officials are aligned in wanting to promote ethical clinical and translational research. Together, colleagues face interesting and challenging ethical issues, and to quote Sam Spade, "It's not always easy to know what to do." This book offers the insights of an experienced group of research ethics consultants who have struggled to figure out what to do. I believe their insights and experiences will provide a firm foundation as all of us who aim to conduct ethically sound clinical research learn how to do it better.

*Benjamin S. Wilfond, MD*
*Director, Treuman Katz Center for Pediatric Bioethics,*
*Seattle Children's Hospital*
*Professor and Chief, Division of Bioethics,*
*Department of Pediatrics, University of*
*Washington School of Medicine*

# ■ Introduction

A focus on scandals and crises has historically dominated thinking about clinical research ethics. Although this has resulted in meaningful advances within the field, focusing primarily on egregious, unethical behavior fails to illuminate fully the interesting and important ethical questions faced by well-intentioned researchers conducting routine clinical research. Ethical challenges are common in determining appropriate research design and methodologies, recruiting and enrolling research participants, analyzing data, and reporting results. Even in a carefully and ethically designed and conducted clinical study, ethical challenges can arise from unexpected findings, a shifting medical or social context, or the activities of individual participants. They raise questions that can be difficult to address for many reasons: complexity of the facts of a case or the relevant concepts; lack of consensus within the clinical research community on what is ethically acceptable; regulatory ambiguity; uncertainty about risks, outcomes, and benefits; and sometimes stark differences in values held by the various stakeholders in a conflict.

Many people are involved in making sure that clinical research is ethical; this includes sponsors and regulators, institutional review boards (IRBs) and other independent reviewers, investigators, and research teams. Increasingly, however, the formal practice of ethics consultation—long familiar in clinical settings—has gained recognition as a distinct and valuable way to facilitate resolution of complex ethical issues in the research context.[1] Although there is no widely shared definition, we define clinical research ethics consultation as a service provided by a team of consultants to assist clinical researchers, IRB members, research participants, and others involved in the research enterprise in understanding and addressing ethical issues raised by clinical research. Because they engage with individuals involved in all facets of clinical research, clinical research ethics consultants enjoy a unique perspective on clinical research. In addition to providing a practically oriented service, they are in a position to identify and to prompt discussion of many important—and some underexplored—topics in research ethics.

This book shares the experiences of the Clinical Center Bioethics Consultation Service (hereafter, the "Consultation Service") at the National Institutes of Health (NIH). The Consultation Service has provided clinical research ethics consultation to the NIH community for more than a decade. Over the years, requests for ethics consultation have challenged our consultants to engage with theory and think conceptually about ethical questions while producing practical recommendations. For readers interested in clinical research ethics, the consultation reports and commentaries assembled here highlight many challenging cases and thought-provoking ethical issues. For readers with a particular interest in clinical research ethics consultation, the cases also offer insights into the Consultation Service's philosophy and methodology. We offer this book as a resource to anyone interested in research ethics, those engaged in research themselves, and those who endeavor to learn about and practice research ethics consultation.

The purpose of this introductory chapter is fivefold: first, to explain in more detail our motivations for assembling this volume; second, to provide a brief history of bioethics at the NIH; third, to describe how the Consultation Service functions; fourth, to consider some of the controversies that arise in the practice of clinical research ethics consultation and to discuss how our service addresses them; and fifth, to provide an overview of the book's organization and structure.

## ■ MOTIVATIONS FOR THIS PROJECT

Medical progress requires experimentation involving human participants.[2] Clinical research is the systematic investigation of human biology, health, or illness involving human subjects.[3] This includes research on identifiable human material or identifiable data as well as on persons.[4] Researchers and sponsors conduct clinical research in order to develop generalizable knowledge about prophylactic, diagnostic, and therapeutic procedures and to advance understanding of human health and the causes and courses of disease. Healthy volunteers and patient volunteers who participate in clinical research enable the attainment of socially valuable knowledge to benefit future patients. The benefits of clinical research for society have been significant, yet clinical research continues to pose profound ethical questions for all involved.[5]

Regulatory and ethical standards aim to minimize the possibility that the benefits or burdens of research are unfairly distributed or that clinical research is otherwise unacceptable.[6] In the United States, the federal regulations governing research outline subject protections in accordance with the widely shared ethical principles of respect for persons, beneficence, and justice that were outlined in the Belmont Report.[7] These regulations establish the minimum standard by which IRBs must judge the acceptability of research. Additionally, ethical soundness may be evaluated in light of codes of research ethics such as the Nuremberg Code, the Declaration of Helsinki, and the International Ethical Guidelines for Biomedical Research Involving Human Subjects, or in light of ethical frameworks proposed in the research ethics literature.[8]

Even when clinical research is conducted thoughtfully, in accordance with these regulations, guidelines, and frameworks, many important ethical questions are not easily addressed. Ethical issues often arise in situations that are conceptually and factually complex. As a result, the available guidance does not always neatly fit. In any case, application of available guidance requires judgment and care, and regulations, guidelines, and ethical frameworks may leave room for interpretation or offer conflicting guidance. In fact, broadly contentious ethical debates persist within the clinical research community. There is ongoing disagreement about the ethics of conducting research in developing countries,[9] using placebos,[10] deceiving study participants,[11] and involving children in research[12] to offer selected examples. In a rapidly evolving field like clinical research, regulatory and other guidelines are limited in their ability to anticipate all situations, and novel questions may confront clinicians before relevant guidance has been crafted. Furthermore, much of the existing guidance was developed in response to specific events or historic abuses and therefore leaves many "everyday" questions unaddressed. Some cases discussed in this volume highlight the complexities of applying formal guidance to real-world circumstances. Other cases offer analysis of emerging ethical questions or challenge conventional wisdom and may help advance thinking about conceptual issues that are hotly debated in the literature. This book may therefore serve as an important resource to those interested in research ethics.

Given the increasing interest in clinical research ethics consultation, we also aim to provide insight into the practical and conceptual aspects of this work. A significant proportion of researchers, sponsors, research participants, and others involved in clinical research anticipate and encounter ethical concerns and dilemmas.[13] Until recently, however, the utility of a clinical research ethics consultation service to support these individuals has been largely overlooked, and few ethicists have formally practiced research ethics consultation.[14] The launch of the NIH Clinical and Translational Science Awards (CTSA) program in 2006 bolstered growing interest in clinical research ethics consultation by requiring all applicants to address how they will handle ethical concerns raised by research. The belated attention to clinical research ethics consultation means there has been little discussion of how clinical research ethics consultants might translate conceptual ethics principles into meaningful, actionable advice, and many substantive and procedural questions remain unanswered.

The questions and challenges faced by the Consultation Service as it has evolved over a decade mirror in many ways those challenges encountered by the wider research community. As a contribution to the many active discussions regarding research ethics and to the specific discussions regarding research ethics consultation, we offer this collection of ethics consultation reports. Since 1999, the Consultation Service has maintained an electronic database that has recorded over 1,000 consultation reports and facilitated systematic review of our experiences. In addition to raising conceptually interesting and dynamic issues in research ethics, the selected consultation reports highlight the skills and knowledge needed to begin addressing these issues through research ethics consultation; illustrate how clinical research ethics consultants formulate their analyses and recommendations; and show how an active consultation service can enhance the quality of the clinical research endeavor. Though the assembled cases include specific details, the analyses and themes are germane to issues that arise in the routine conduct of research, are common to many clinical research settings, and are likely to be encountered by many clinical researchers and clinical research ethicists.

In presenting the cases here, we acknowledge that there are not always uniquely acceptable solutions to the questions and dilemmas with which we are confronted. At times, reasonable people may disagree with the analyses presented. Even members of the Consultation Service do not always agree with one another. We hope that our analyses spark further dialogue, bring more light to bear on interesting and important topics, and prompt reflection on the unique contributions to be made by clinical research ethics consultants.

## BIOETHICS AT THE NATIONAL INSTITUTES OF HEALTH

The mission of the NIH is "science in pursuit of fundamental knowledge about the nature and behavior of living systems and the application of that knowledge to extend healthy life and reduce the burdens of illness and disability."[15] To this end, the NIH is comprised of 27 institutes and centers (see Table I.1) and had a budget of $30.5 billion in fiscal year 2009.[16] Although coordination and collaboration

TABLE I.1. *Institutes and Centers of the National Institutes of Health*

| | |
|---|---|
| CC | NIH Clinical Center |
| CIT | Center for Information Technology |
| CSR | Center for Scientific Review |
| FIC | John E. Fogarty International Center for Advanced Study in the Health Sciences |
| NCATS | National Center for Advancing Translational Sciences |
| NCCAM | National Center for Complementary and Alternative Medicine |
| NCI | National Cancer Institute |
| NEI | National Eye Institute |
| NHGRI | National Human Genome Institute |
| NHLBI | National Heart Lung and Blood Institute |
| NIA | National Institute on Aging |
| NIAAA | The National Institute on Alcohol Abuse And Alcoholism |
| NIAID | National Institute of Allergy and Infectious Diseases |
| NIAMS | National Institute of Arthritis and Musculoskeletal and Skin Diseases |
| NIBIB | National Institute of Biomedical Imaging and Bioengineering |
| NICHD | Eunice Kennedy Shriver National Institute of Child Health and Human Development |
| NIDA | National Institute on Drug Abuse |
| NIDCD | National Institute of Dental and Cranio-facial Diseases |
| NIDCR | National Institute of Dental and Craniofacial Research |
| NIDDK | National Institute of Diabetes and Digestive and Kidney Diseases |
| NIEHS | National Institute of Environmental Health Sciences |
| NIGMS | National Institute of General Medical Sciences |
| NIMH | National Institute of Mental Health |
| NIMHD | National Institute of Minority Health and Health Disparities |
| NINDS | National Institute of Neurological Disorders and Stroke |
| NINR | National Institute of Nursing Research |
| NLM | National Library of Medicine |

*Source:* National Institutes of Health, "Institutes, Centers, and Offices," available at: http://www.nih.gov/icd/, accessed on February 3, 2012.

exist between the institutes and centers, each one is separately funded and has its own scope, programs, administration, research agendas, and training priorities.[17]

The NIH Clinical Center, located in Bethesda, Maryland, is the nation's largest hospital devoted entirely to clinical research. It is where NIH investigators—from across all institutes—admit research participants for inpatient services and see them in the outpatient clinic. Since it opened in 1953, more than 350,000 healthy and patient volunteers from around the country and the world have participated in the research conducted at the Clinical Center. Approximately 1,500 clinical research studies are in progress at the Clinical Center at any given time. About half of these are Phase I, II, or III tests of new drugs or medical treatments; the rest are long-term natural history studies of diseases and other studies of pathophysiology (see Tables I.2 and I.3).[18]

TABLE I.2. *Types of Clinical Trials*

**Treatment trials** test new treatments, new combinations of drugs, or new approaches to surgery or radiation therapy.

**Prevention trials** look for better ways to prevent a disease in people who have never had the disease or to prevent the disease from returning. Better approaches may include medicines, vaccines, or lifestyle changes, among other things.

**Diagnostic trials** determine better tests or procedures for diagnosing a particular disease or condition.

**Screening trials** test the best way to detect certain diseases or health conditions.

**Quality of life trials** (or supportive care trials) explore and measure ways to improve the comfort and quality of life of people with a chronic illness.

**Natural history trials** describe and measure the effects of disease progression or the recovery process. They establish a baseline for assessing the effectiveness of interventions.

**Pathophysiology trials** examine the functional changes that accompany a particular disease or syndrome.

*Sources*: National Institutes of Health, "How Does Clinical Research Work? Available at: http://clinicalresearch.nih.gov/how.html, accessed on November 19, 2009.
J. Logemann, "Natural History Studies: Their Critical Role," *Dysphagia* 12, no. 4 (1997): 194–195.

TABLE I.3. *Phases of Clinical Trials*

Clinical trials are conducted in "phases." The trials at each phase have a different purpose and help researchers answer different questions.

**Phase I trials**—Researchers test an experimental drug or treatment in a small group of people (20–80) for the first time. The purpose is to evaluate its safety and identify side effects.

**Phase II trials**—The experimental drug or treatment is administered to a larger group of people (100–300) to determine its effectiveness and to further evaluate its safety.

**Phase III trials**—The experimental drug or treatment is administered to large groups of people (1,000–3,000) to confirm its effectiveness, monitor side effects, compare it with standard or equivalent treatments, and collect information that will allow the experimental drug or treatment to be used safely.

**Phase IV trials**—After a drug is licensed (approved by the FDA) or treatment is launched, researchers track its safety, seeking more information about a drug or treatment's risks, benefits, and optimal use. These long-term studies involving large groups of participants continue to see if any unexpected side effects occur in a small percentage of individuals.

*Source*: http://clinicalresearch.nih.gov/how.html

The Department of Bioethics was formed in 1996 as a department within the Clinical Center. It replaced a preexisting Bioethics Program in the Office of the Clinical Center Director. The Department has authority and responsibility for bioethics within the Clinical Center and reports directly to the Director of the Clinical Center. However, because the Clinical Center's mission is to support clinical research conducted by other institutes, the Department of Bioethics' mission includes supporting the work of those institutes as well. In full, the mission of the Department of Bioethics reads:

> The Department of Bioethics is a center for research, training, and service related to bioethical issues. The Department conducts conceptual, empirical, and policy-related research into bioethical issues; offers comprehensive training to future bioethicists and educational programs for biomedical researchers and clinical providers; and provides high quality ethics consultation services to clinicians, patients, and families of the NIH's Clinical Center and advice to the NIH IRBs on ethical conduct of research protocols.[19]

Although this book focuses on the activities of the Consultation Service, some ancillary responsibilities assumed by the Department of Bioethics also bear mentioning. These responsibilities include serving on IRBs and joining clinical rounds; providing education and classes on the ethical conduct of clinical research; presenting Ethics Grand Rounds on interesting topics that have arisen in ethics consultation or on issues that have been identified as institutional gaps in ethics knowledge; and assisting with institutional policy development and quality improvement when ethical dilemmas may be involved. Each of these activities indirectly promotes utilization of the Consultation Service by building ethics capacity, raising the profile of the Department, addressing at the policy level issues raised by consultations that are likely to recur, and/or building relationships based on professional respect and trust. For example, a researcher who attended Grand Rounds conducted by the Department of Bioethics told us during a subsequent consultation: "After seeing that, I thought, 'Why wrestle with this alone? They do it all the time.'"

## ■ THE CLINICAL CENTER BIOETHICS CONSULTATION SERVICE

Ethics consultation is a primary service function of the Department of Bioethics. Here, we describe the philosophy and function of the Consultation Service as background for reading the remainder of the book.

### Our Philosophy

The Consultation Service commits itself to providing an opportunity for people to talk through clinical research and clinical care issues with a supportive group that understands the nature of the practical issues.[20] The belief that ethics consultation should provide an open space for deliberation about ethical issues guides the Consultation Service.[21] Fundamental to this philosophy is the view that all who come to the table deserve to be heard, regardless of their knowledge of the bioethics literature or their position in the institutional hierarchy. The Consultation Service's practices embody this commitment to openness and inclusivity. Anyone who works at the NIH or participates in research at the NIH Clinical Center can request a consultation. When a consult meeting is arranged, the requestor is encouraged to bring all who might have a stake in the issue at hand to the meeting unless there are good reasons to do otherwise. We attempt to ensure that everyone in attendance has the opportunity to speak about his or her concerns and to share his or her perspective.

## Our Role

The Consultation Service's primary goal is to assist researchers, research teams, research participants, and other individuals affiliated with the NIH intramural research program in the identification and analysis of ethical issues that arise in the course of conducting clinical research—from the conception of a research question, throughout recruitment and enrollment of research participants, data collection, and even beyond a study's completion. Through active listening, clarification of communication, careful articulation and analysis of the ethical question(s), and thoughtful development of ethical recommendations, our consultants enable requestors to better resolve the ethical issues at hand.

Requests for Consultation Service assistance reflect the variety of ethical questions that confront researchers and others involved in clinical research.[22] Historically, a third to half of consultation requests we have received in a given year have been related exclusively to research. Take, for instance, the general requirement that ethical research, with some exceptions, requires informed consent. Our Consultation Service has received many requests about translating this rule into practice. How should consent be handled if the research participant cannot read, cannot sign his or her name, or cannot speak the same language as the investigator (see *Consult 2.6*)? If the research involves a participant with dementing illness or cognitive impairment, we often help assess whether the potential participant is able to consent to research, and if not, whether a surrogate may and can consent on his or her behalf (see *Consult 4.3*). Occasionally, members of the Consultation Service monitor assent and dissent of vulnerable research participants and teach researchers and participants about research advanced directives. The remaining consultation requests arise within the research context but are more clinically oriented. For example, a research team may have ethical concerns about end-of-life decision making for a research participant (see *Consults 6.5* and *6.6*) or question an ethical obligation to provide clinically indicated care to research participants (see *Consults 5.1, 5.5, and 7.5*).

The roles of our research ethics consultants are varied, yet there are boundaries and limits to the roles consultants might assume. In particular, our consultants do not provide legal advice, which is more appropriate to the Office of General Counsel; nor do they serve as a proxy for institutional risk management, which is under the purview of the Office of Management Assessment. We are also distinct from the Office of Scientific Integrity, which handles questions about appropriate authorship and professional conduct. Though areas of overlapping interest and cooperation may be identified by consultation requests (see *Consult 7.8*), the primary responsibilities of the Consultation Service and these offices are distinct. Additionally, the Consultation Service does not police violations of policy or ethical standards. Policing would negatively impact the role of the Consultation Service as a trusted and nonpunitive source of advice. If we are called with a request to address misconduct or illegal activities, we usually refer the requestor to the offices intended and better prepared to confront these situations. Only in a particularly troublesome case, were the requestor to choose not to report an illegal practice, would we feel compelled to report it ourselves.

At the NIH, clinical research ethics consultation is performed exclusively by the Consultation Service rather than by the many IRBs who oversee research. Although the delegation of these responsibilities differs at other institutions, we find this division of labor appropriate. IRBs are oversight bodies; their main goal is protection of research participants, and the majority of human subjects research protocols must have IRB approval before they proceed.[23] Clinical research ethics consultation, unlike IRB review, is voluntary and advisory. Though this separation exists, IRBs occasionally work with the Consultation Service to address important questions that arise while reviewing research (see *Consults 2.4* and *2.7*). Some members of the Consultation Service are also voting members of NIH IRBs and recuse themselves from IRB review when these roles conflict.

## Our Consultants

Our Consultation Service is comprised of three categories of individuals: senior ethicists who are faculty in the Department of Bioethics (hereafter, "attendings"), trainees who are in the bioethics training fellowship (hereafter, "fellows"), and members of the Clinical Center Ethics Committee. Consultation Service attendings and fellows have backgrounds in medicine, nursing, law, philosophy, health policy, and the social sciences. The Ethics Committee is comprised of clinical investigators from various NIH institutes and centers as well as physicians, nurses, social workers, a lawyer from the NIH Office of General Counsel, the directors of the Department of Spiritual Ministry and the Department of Social Work, the Clinical Center patient representative, and several community members. Involving the Ethics Committee allows the Consultation Service to encourage deliberation among peers, to promote research ethics education within the NIH community, and to engage the research community (members of which serve on the Ethics Committee on a rotating basis) in the consultation process.

## Our Skills and Knowledge

The Consultation Service shares a belief with other ethics consultants that effective ethics consultation demands ethical assessment skills, process skills, and interpersonal skills.[24] Ethical assessment skills allow consultants to identify and analyze the ethical issues that emerge within a particular consultation. Assessment also entails identifying which issues more appropriately relate to some other discipline (e.g., medical or legal) rather than being of ethical import. Process skills include information gathering, facilitation of discussion, advocating on behalf of interested parties, and building support for an ethically acceptable plan. Interpersonal skills—such as the ability to communicate interest, respect, empathy, and cultural sensitivity—promote trust and collegiality.

Many knowledge areas identified in the literature as relevant to clinical ethics consultation are also relevant to effective clinical research ethics consultation. Like their clinically oriented peers, research ethics consultants must possess knowledge of moral reasoning and ethical theory; grasp bioethical issues and concepts; and understand institutional policies, laws, and professional codes of ethics relevant to consultation. Research ethics consultants, however, require additional knowledge of the scientific process and norms of research culture, commonly used clinical research methods, the terminology of biomedical research, and the social and historical context of clinical research to be effective.[25] Research ethics consultants must also be versed in the regulations and codes that govern research and be familiar with the research ethics literature. The cases selected for inclusion in this book reflect the ways in which the Consultation Service has continuously drawn on these knowledge areas in the course of providing consultation.

Rarely will any individual be expert in all areas relevant to identifying, analyzing, and resolving ethical issues related to clinical research. As discussed previously, the Consultation Service includes individuals with diverse educational and professional backgrounds and, therefore, with complementary competencies. We value this diversity and our resultant ability to bring a multidisciplinary focus to our consultations. When a consultation raises a novel question or one requiring a specific expertise, it is not unusual for the attending or fellow on call to solicit advice from other members of the Consultation Service, the Department of Bioethics, the Ethics Committee, or the wider NIH community who can bring particular expertise to bear on the case analysis.

## ■ THE CLINICAL CENTER BIOETHICS CONSULTATION SERVICE PROCESS

The Consultation Service staff has made efforts to standardize the consultation process in order to ensure consistently high-quality responses to the requests we receive. Our process typically involves four stages: intake, case review, preparation and dissemination of the report, and evaluation. Some consultation reports within this book illustrate variations on the process or highlight important issues about process, and we provide further information about our processes in those consults.

### Intake

One attending member of the Consultation Service and one fellow from the Department of Bioethics are on call at all times. Requests for consultation may come to their attention in any one of several ways: via a call to the Department seeking assistance, through the requestor's placement of an order in the electronic medical record, through a page to the fellow on call by the Clinical Center page operator, by referral from the inpatient clinical rounds conducted by research teams, or as the result of a request for guidance directed to a member of the Department. Consult requests are voluntary and requestor initiated. After speaking with the requestor about the reason for consultation, the fellow collaborates with the attending to determine the most effective way to address the ethical question(s).

### Case Review

Some questions can be resolved immediately over the telephone. If not, a first meeting is typically held within 24 hours or at the earliest convenience of the requestor. If an investigator calls from one of the nursing units needing to determine whether a research participant is capable of consenting to research (or, in lieu of that, capable of choosing a surrogate decision maker on his or her behalf to consent to research), the Consultation Service attending and fellow may be at the individual's bedside within the hour. At the other extreme, if a person with a disease process known to cause cognitive impairment is being considered for enrollment in a protocol and is traveling a long distance to the NIH, an assessment of the ability to give consent may be scheduled weeks in advance. Similarly, a meeting may be delayed to ensure availability of as many members of the research team as possible or to allow the members of the Consultation Service sufficient time to complete necessary background research and literature reviews.

In the majority of cases, the attending and fellow perform consultations. Whenever possible, members of the Ethics Committee receive an invitation to join. On exceptional occasions, a consultation is held during the monthly Ethics Committee meeting in order to involve the entire committee in consultation. More complicated cases may demand particular expertise or benefit from multiple perspectives, thus leading to the involvement of additional members of the Department of Bioethics or experts in a particular area (e.g., legal counsel). Whenever appropriate, research participants, family members, surrogate decision makers, and others involved in the study participant's care (e.g., nurses, chaplains, or social workers) are invited to participate in the consultation process.

Consultation meetings are typically led by the attending ethics consultant. The structure of the discussion focuses first on clarifying the requestor's key questions and concerns and what he or she hopes to get out of the consultation. Next, the requestor is asked to present the facts of the case, and the Consultation Service team may ask questions to clarify or learn more. Only then does an analysis of the case begin. This analysis entails a dialogue among the requestor and members of the Consultation Service team. The preferences of the research participant, surrogate, and health care team members are elicited. The ethical principles and values that are pertinent to the question at hand are discussed among the group. Options and recommendations are explored at the meeting. Occasionally, a second meeting and more extended conversations are pursued to allow further consideration of the issues. Typically, following any meeting with a consult requestor, the Consultation Service team debriefs to review how the meeting went, to resolve any discrepant impressions or assessments, and to discuss what to include in the consultation report. The content of all these discussions is kept confidential.

## Preparation and Dissemination of the Consultation Report

Following the consultation meeting, the fellow and attending prepare a consultation report with input from other members of the Consultation Service who may have participated. The report is a vehicle for documenting the discussion that occurred during the meeting, presenting additional ethical analysis, and outlining recommendations. While recommendation for writing ethics consultation chart notes, based on experience at several institutions, have been published by several bioethicists (26, 27), no regulatory or professional body has set standards for documentation of ethics consultation.[26] Members of the Consultation Service have, however, found standardized documentation to be useful. Our consultation reports share a common structure that includes the reason for the consultation request, background information, and the process followed during the consultation, and concludes with the analysis and recommendations. Occasionally, a draft of the consultation report is sent to the requestor to ensure that the background facts or summary of the ethical analysis are presented accurately from his or her perspective. Following completion of the case report, it is *(1)* submitted to the consultation requestor, *(2)* included in the research participant's medical record, if applicable, and (3) added to the Consultation Service's secure electronic database.

## Evaluation

The Consultation Service continuously strives to improve the quality of the clinical research ethics consultation services offered to the NIH community (see Appendix). This is done, in part, through ongoing evaluation of consultations. There are three primary methods of evaluation. First, each requestor is asked to fill out a feedback form. Second, at the monthly meeting of the Clinical Center Ethics Committee, the chief of the Consultation Service presents a report that summarizes the number and nature of consultations from the previous month, and one or more of the consultations is discussed in detail for educational and evaluative purposes. Third, once a year, the chief of the Consultation Service in conjunction with a fellow makes a presentation to the Ethics Committee from the Department of Bioethics. This presentation focuses on the total number of consult requests for the year, trends in consultation requests, and a summary of the feedback received from requestors. This allows for insightful discussions about how to improve the Consultation Service and meet the evolving needs of the Clinical Center community.

## ■ UNRESOLVED QUESTIONS IN THE PRACTICE OF RESEARCH ETHICS CONSULTATION

A number of questions persist in the practice of clinical research ethics consultation. In this section, we identify four of these challenging questions and offer our current practices in resolving them. Readers will see that these themes run throughout the consults discussed in this casebook.

## Who Should Define the Scope of the Consultation Question?

When a requestor calls to request a clinical research ethics consultation, the Consultation Service occasionally identifies additional ethical concerns that may exceed the scope of the original ethical query. For example, a requestor may ask about the appropriateness of enrolling a particular individual in a study protocol. In exploring this question, the ethics team may realize that some aspect of enrollment is likely to cause recurring concerns that would best be addressed by revising the protocol (see *Consult 3.2*). Or a clinical research team may request a consultation to discuss one facet of study design, and in the course of discussion, the Consultation Service perceives other aspects of the study design to be ethically problematic. In such situations, a delicate balance must be struck. On the one hand, a key goal of the Consultation Service is promotion of ethical decision making in the broadest sense. On the other hand, another key goal of the Consultation Service is promotion of clinical research ethics consultation services, and the literature documents that those considering ethics consultation often hesitate because they worry about opening Pandora's box once they seek advice.[27]

When approaching situations like these, Consultation Service ethicists find it important to appreciate that even thoughtful and well-intentioned requestors may not initially realize that the case at hand has such implications. To promote ethical research, consultants should raise the broader ethical questions they have identified in the meeting with the requestor and document them in the consultation report so that the requestor has a written record for reflection. Unless the Consultation Service team believes the broader concerns are pressing or the requestor wishes to expand the scope of the consultation to include the new questions, it often makes the most sense to focus recommendations as much as possible on the initial request rather than imposing additional ethical recommendations.

## How Should Consultants Handle Conflicts between Regulations or Policies and Their Analysis?

The Consultation Service routinely works with requestors to identify and apply the regulations relevant to their ethical questions. On rare occasions, consultants may wonder whether the regulations pertaining to the situation at hand provide optimal guidance for how to achieve the most ethically sound resolution. In such circumstances, our consultants may provide analysis and recommendations that go beyond the regulations or allow for a certain interpretation of a regulation or policy. The Consultation Service has been asked, for example, to consider the ethics of using stored samples from deceased research participants in research to which the individuals did not consent—or actively opposed—while living. The consultants worked with legal counsel to better understand what the regulations permitted.[28] Ultimately, their analysis acknowledged that although the regulations would allow these stored samples to be used for research, the *ethical* recommendation was to respect the decedent's stated wishes regarding research participation. If the conflict between the regulations and the ethicist's advice truly cannot be resolved, one approach is to specify in the consult report what the regulations require while acknowledging the conflict.

Occasionally, institutional policy plays a role in ethical issues or dilemmas for researchers.[29] Although ethicists may find it difficult to criticize institutional policy or advocate for restraint of the research endeavor in their capacity as employees, the Consultation Service believes that the most ethically sound policies protect the research endeavor in the long term. Doing nothing to foster institutional change would seem to ignore ethical obligations to facilitate an organizational culture that is receptive to the identification and resolution of ethical conflicts. When ethical analysis raises concerns about policy, our practice is to have the ethics consultant speak to the Ethics Committee about the possibility of working with institutional leadership to revise policy (see *Consult 5.2*). Some of our consultations have resulted in revisions to policies like the HIV-testing consent policy and a policy on research with adults who are or may be unable to consent (See Clinical Center Policy M87-4 in Appendix 6).

## How Should Requests for Anonymous Consultations Be Handled?

At times, the Consultation Service receives requests for anonymous or confidential consultations. Oftentimes, these cases involve a junior investigator, a nurse, or a social worker who fears retribution from the lead investigator or another authority figure for raising ethical questions about research. Similarly, research participants may come to the Consultation Service with a question but fear being removed from research they feel is in their medical best interests (see *Consult 5.6*). Fear of retaliation from seeking ethics consultation is common.[30]

In cases such as these, the approach of the Consultation Service is to determine why a requestor wants the consultation to remain anonymous. This is not only informative for the consultant; it may provide an opportunity to allay the requestor's fears or correct misperceptions about the consultation process. Consultants inform requestors that ethics consultations are kept confidential, are intended to identify and discuss approaches to resolve problems rather than punitive mechanisms, and the end results are not dictates but recommendations to help the requestor better address their ethical question. If a requestor continues to desire an anonymous consultation, we respect this wish.

When respecting a request for anonymity, our policy is to inform the requestor that, in doing so, we can only provide limited advice because we are not hearing a full description of the ethical question from all interested parties. Nonetheless, we strive to equip the requestor with analytic tools and strategies to handle the situation independently. Under these circumstances, we do not place a consult report in the medical record, even if it would be standard practice. This approach is predicated on the view that one of the most valuable aspects of ethics consultation is the provision of an opportunity for those whose voices might not otherwise be heard to participate in ethical discussion.

## Should Study Participants Be Included in Consultations?

Ethics consultants differ in their views about a requirement to notify patients or study participants whose circumstances or behaviors have precipitated a request for ethics consultation. Advocates of procedural fairness support the formation of transparent, consistent processes for including research participants and their surrogates in ethical consultation relevant to their participation in research.[31]

The Consultation Service generally supports the inclusion of research participants and surrogates in consultations. However, the important goal of ensuring procedural fairness must sometimes be balanced against other relevant considerations. For example, a researcher may contact the Consultation Service proactively to strategize about the fairest way to handle a situation and avoid a possible conflict with a study participant (see *Consult 6.3*). We offer such proactive consultation because studies from the clinical setting show that proactive consultation can reduce conflict and improve clinical outcomes.[32] Additionally, ethics consultants are not the sole purveyors of ethical reasoning and behavior. Although we encourage the involvement of all stakeholders in consults, the Consultation Service willingly discusses ethical quandaries with researchers and others so that they can then manage them independently. Ethical reasoning is part of a professional clinician's or clinical investigator's capabilities, and an important function of the consulting ethicist is to foster these capabilities. When a consult does not include the affected research participant, we always remind requestors that we are available as the situation unfolds for further meetings that include the participant and/or his or her surrogates.

## THE CONSULTATIONS IN THIS BOOK

All the consultation reports included in this volume are from actual NIH cases. Within the text, each consultation is introduced with a "Reason for Consultation" explaining the ethical issue that prompted the request for a consultation and a "Narrative" providing the relevant background information. Seeing the question and background presented in this way allows the reader to engage in his or her own ethical analysis before reading the analysis offered by the Consultation Service.

The "Analysis and Recommendations" come directly from actual consultation reports. Limited edits have been made to enhance readability and to remove or modify any information that would identify the requestors. However, the essence of the analyses and recommendations remains unchanged. Readers will note that the write-ups differ in style and tense from one to the next, sometimes dramatically. This is a reflection of diverse authorship: case reports are primarily written by the bioethics fellow and attending on call. The variations in diction and syntax may help readers compare the effectiveness of different writing styles in communicating with ethics consult requestors.

Following each consultation report, we provide an "Authors' Commentary." This commentary can address matters such as the following: Are there additional issues that could or should have been explored in the consultation report? Might the Consultation Service have offered different advice upon further reflection? What variations of this case are commonly seen? Have ethical guidelines or views in the literature changed since the case was decided? What lessons can be learned from the case? In some cases, readers will also be provided with information about how the case was ultimately resolved. In addition to highlighting interesting and important ethical issues in clinical research, these commentaries serve to illustrate the controversial nature of some of the issues addressed and emphasize the fact that many ethics consultations require analysis of issues on which people can reasonably disagree.

The consultation reports are best understood as an analysis and recommendations for a particular requestor at a particular point in time. In some consult reports in this book, the ethical questions and dilemmas were not immediately resolved by clinical research ethics consultation. This book includes cases in which the relevant details of the situation, and therefore the ethical analysis, evolved over time (see *Consults 1.3* and *6.7*). These consultations illustrate that the ethics consultation process should be dynamic and receptive to new facts as they emerge. Relevant new considerations sometimes become apparent after a consultation report has been prepared, and in cases like these, the Consultation Service has been willing to modify its analysis as needed.

## Consent and Confidentiality

Either the consult requestor or someone in the requestor's stead approved the inclusion of each consultation report in this book. If the consult requestor could not be located, another authorized individual from the initial requestor's study protocol, IRB, research branch, or institute gave approval. Details—including names, diagnoses, demographic characteristics of the requestors and others mentioned in the report, and the identity of various IRBs or institutes—have been removed or altered to protect the privacy and confidentiality of involved study participants, investigators, NIH centers, institutes, collaborators, and other interested parties in ways deemed irrelevant to the ethical analysis. Actual names of persons, in particular, have been replaced with fictitious names. Notably, there is one consult relating to the depiction of research in the media for which the requestor and other involved parties consented to an unaltered presentation of their consultation; this exception is indicated in the text.

## Organization of the Book

Ethical dilemmas may be confronted at all stages of clinical research—when designing a study, while conducting it, and after the study is over. We have divided this volume into seven chapters thematically addressing ethical challenges that arise as clinical research progresses:

- Starting Research—Researchers may anticipate ethical dilemmas even before research has started. These quandaries may be about the trial

specifically or broadly related to the anticipated social value of the research. This chapter presents a collection of cases highlighting ethical issues in study design, determination of social value, use of placebos, and selection of an acceptable study population.
- Enrolling Research Participants—Studies are approved by IRBs with a set of inclusion and exclusion criteria, but under some circumstances, even with these criteria as guidance, decisions to enroll or not enroll an individual can cause ethical concern. This chapter presents a collection of cases that discuss screening, informed consent, exclusion criteria, considerations against enrollment, and enrollment of participants in multiple protocols.
- Protecting Research Participants—In ethical research, all individuals must be protected and their welfare respected and promoted. This chapter presents a collection of cases highlighting confidentiality, dealing with adverse events, and evaluating research risks.
- Conducting Research with Vulnerable Populations—Conducting research with particularly vulnerable populations is a frequent source of ethical concern. Two frequent concerns are the acceptability of studying a vulnerable population and how to establish sufficient protections for vulnerable participants. This chapter presents a collection of cases focused on evaluation of the acceptability of research risks, capacity assessment, and identification of surrogate decision makers.
- Balancing Clinical Care with Clinical Research—Research protocols often include some aspect of clinical care or enroll individuals for whom medical needs become apparent in the course of research. This chapter presents a collection of consultations that examine conflicts between research and care, the extent of the obligation to provide ancillary care during research, the management of incidental findings that may have been unanticipated, and the therapeutic misconception.
- Navigating Interpersonal Difficulties—Interpersonal issues can complicate clinical research. Ethical disagreements may arise between members of a research team or in the course of working with individual research participants. This chapter presents a collection of consultations that deal with noncompliance, research participants and family members who are confrontational or possibly dangerous to other research participants or staff, and discharging individuals against medical advice.
- Ending Research—Many ethical questions remain at the end of a trial and after its conclusion. Ethical concerns may also arise if a decision must be made to end a particular research participant's enrollment before a protocol has come to an end or to end a study prematurely out of concern for subject safety. This chapter presents a collection of cases dealing with decisions to end the research participation of particular individuals or stop an entire study, post-trial obligations, and authorship.

Sorting consultation reports into these distinct sections was difficult at times because clinical research ethics consultations are often complicated and include of a number of ethical issues simultaneously. In choosing where to place each consultation, we focused on the central ethical question and the content of the Analysis and Recommendations. Because there is significant overlap, an Appendix sorts cases by additional features (e.g., pediatric or international research) that may be of particular interest to readers.

## CONCLUSION

We hope this book will be a useful resource to those who want to learn about clinical research ethics, are interested in practicing clinical research ethics consultation, or are committed to the ethical conduct of clinical research. We anticipate that the quandaries that led to the consultations shared here will interest those involved in clinical research, and that the analyses will be of value to those who encounter similar questions. While we do not necessarily expect agreement with all the analyses and recommendations, we trust that they will serve to stimulate further deliberation about research ethics and the philosophies, methodologies, knowledge, and skills necessary to addressing ethical questions and controversies in the conduct of clinical research.

## NOTES

1. E. Fox, S. Myers, and R. Pearlman, "Ethics Consultation in United States Hospitals: A National Survey," *The American Journal of Bioethics* 7, no. 2 (2007): 13–25.

M. Cho, S. Tobin, H. Greely, J. McCormick, A. Boyce, and D. Magnus, "Strangers at the Benchside: Research Ethics Consultation," *American Journal of Bioethics* 8, no. 3 (2008): 4–13.

I. de Melo-Martin, L. I. Palmer, and J. J. Fins, "Viewpoint: Developing a Research Ethics Consultation Service to Foster Responsive and Responsible Clinical Research," *Academic Medicine* 82, no. 9 (2007): 900–904, 910.1097/ACM.1090b1013e318132f318130ee.

2. World Medical Association, *The Declaration of Helsinki: Ethical Principles for Medical Research Involving Human Subjects*; 2008.

3. Nuremburg Military Tribunal, from U.S. v. Karl Brandt, et al, *The Nuremburg Code*, available at: http://ohsr.od.nih.gov/guidelines/nuremberg.html.

U.S. Department of Health and Human Services. *Protections of Human Subjects*, 45 CFR §46; 1991.

4. United States Department of Health and Human Services, National Institutes of Health, Office for Human Research Protections, The Common Rule, Title 45 (Public Welfare), Code of Federal Regulations, Part 46 (Protection of Human Subjects), Subparts A-D; 2001.

5. A. Wertheimer, *Exploitation* (Princeton, NJ: Princeton University Press, 1996).

L. DeCastro, "Exploitation in the Use of Human Subjects for Medical Experimentation," *Bioethics* 9 (1995): 259–268.

6. E. J. Emanuel, D. Wendler, and C. Grady, "What Makes Clinical Research Ethical?" *Journal of the American Medical Association* 283, no. 20 (2000): 2701–2711.

7. United States Department of Health and Human Services, National Institutes of Health, Office for Human Research Protections, *The Common Rule, Title 45 (Public Welfare), Code of Federal Regulations, Part 46 (Protection of Human Subjects), Subparts A-D*; 2001.

The National Commission for the Protection of Human Subjects of Biomedical and Behavioral Research, *The Belmont Report: Ethical Principles and Guidelines for the Protection of Human Subjects of Research* (Washington, DC: Department of Health, Education, and Welfare, 1979).

8. The National Commission for the Protection of Human Subjects of Biomedical and Behavioral Research, *The Belmont Report: Ethical Principles and Guidelines for the Protection of Human Subjects of Research* (Washington, DC: Department of Health, Education, and Welfare, 1979).

Nuremburg Military Tribunal, from U.S. v. Karl Brandt, et al., *The Nuremburg Code*, available at: http://ohsr.od.nih.gov/guidelines/nuremberg.html.

World Medical Association, *The Declaration of Helsinki: Ethical Principles for Medical Research Involving Human Subjects*, 2008.

The Council for International Organizations of Medical Sciences (CIOMS) in collaboration with the World Health Organization (WHO), *The International Ethical Guidelines for Biomedical Research Involving Human Subjects*, 2002.

E. J. Emanuel, D. Wendler, and C. Grady, "What Makes Clinical Research Ethical?" *Journal of the American Medical Association* 283, no. 20 (2000): 2701–2711.

9. D. Wendler, E. Emanuel, and R. Lie, "The Standard Care Debate: Can Research in Developing Countries Be Both Ethical and Responsive to Those Countries' Health Needs?" *American Journal of Public Health* 94, no. 6 (2004): 923–928.

H. Varmus and D. Satcher, "Ethical Complexities of Conducting Research in Developing Countries," *New England Journal of Medicine* 337, no. 14 (1997): 1003–1005.

10. F. Miller, "The Debate over Placebo-Controlled Trials," *PLoS Medicine* 2, no. 6 (2005): e157.

F. Miller and D. Wendler, "Placebo Research and the Spirit of Informed Consent," *Psychosomatic Medicine* 67, no. 4 (2005): 678.

The Council for International Organizations of Medical Sciences (CIOMS) in collaboration with the World Health Organization (WHO), *The International Ethical Guidelines for Biomedical Research Involving Human Subjects*, 2002.

World Medical Association, *The Declaration of Helsinki: Ethical Principles for Medical Research Involving Human Subjects*, 2008.

11. F. Miller, J. Gluck, and D. Wendler, "Debriefing and Accountability in Deceptive Research," *Kennedy Institute of Ethics Journal* 18, no. 3 (2008): 235–251.

12. D. Coleman, "The Legal Ethics of Pediatric Research," *Duke Law Journal* 57, no. 517 (2007).

P. Litton, "Non-Beneficial Pediatric Research and the Best Interests Standard: A Legal and Ethical Reconciliation," *Yale Journal of Health Policy, Law, and Ethics* 8 (2008): 359.

13. J. McCormick, A. Boyce, and M. Cho, "Biomedical Scientists' Perceptions of Ethical and Social Implications: Is There a Role for Research Ethics Consultation?" *PLoS ONE* 4, no. 3 (2009): e4659.

14. I. de Melo-Martin, L. I. Palmer, and J. J. Fins, "Viewpoint: Developing a Research Ethics Consultation Service to Foster Responsive and Responsible Clinical Research," *Academic Medicine* 82, no. 9 (2007): 900–904, 910.1097/ACM.1090b1013e318132f318130ee.

15. National Institutes of Health, "About NIH," July 21, 2009, available at: http://www.nih.gov/about/, accessed on August 12, 2008.

16. NIH Office of Budget, "NIH History of Congressional Appropriations, Fiscal Years 2000–2009," available at: http://officeofbudget.od.nih.gov/pdfs/FY10/Copy%20of%20Apphisic.pdf, accessed on December 3, 2009.

17. E. Emanuel, "The Blossoming of Bioethics at the NIH," *Kennedy Institute of Ethics Journal* 8, no. 4 (1998): 455–466.

18. National Institutes of Health, NIH Clinical Center, available at: http://clinicalresearch.nih.gov/clincenter.html, accessed on November 19, 2009.

19. NIH Clinical Center, The Department of Bioethics, available at: http://www.bioethics.nih.gov/home/index.shtml, accessed on November 20, 2009.

20. J. W. Ross, J.W. Glaser, D. Rasinski-Gregory, J.M. Gibson, and C. Bayley "Case Consultation and Review: Matching Skills and Expectations." In *Health Care Ethics Committees: The Next Generation*, . (Chicago: American Hospital Association), 91–107.

21. M. Walker, "Keeping Moral Space Open: New Images of Ethics Consulting," *The Hastings Center Report* March-April (1993): 33–40.

22. G. DuVal, G. Gensler, and M. Danis, "Ethical Dilemmas Encountered by Clinical Researchers," *The Journal of Clinical Ethics* 16, no. 3 (2005): 267–276.

23. United States Department of Health and Human Services, National Institutes of Health, Office for Human Research Protections, The Common Rule, Title 45 (Public Welfare), Code of Federal Regulations, Part 46 (Protection of Human Subjects), Subparts A-D, 2001.

24. M. Aulisio, R. Arnold, and S. Youngner, "Health Care Ethics Consultation: Nature, Goals, and Competencies," *Annals of Internal Medicine* 133, no. 1 (2000): 59–69.

American Society for Bioethics and Humanities Clinical Ethics Task Force, *Improving Competencies in Clinical Ethics Consultation: An Education Guide* (Glenview, IL: ASBH, 2009).

25. M. Cho, S. Tobin, H. Greely, J. McCormick, A. Boyce, and D. Magnus, "Strangers at the Benchside: Research Ethics Consultation," *American Journal of Bioethics* 8, no. 3 (2008): 4–13.

26. K. A. Bramstedt, A. R. Jonsen, W. S. Andereck, J. W. McGaughey, and A. B. Neidich, "Optimising the Documentation Practices of an Ethics Consultation Service," *Journal of Medical Ethics*, 35, no. 1 (2009): 47–50.

N.N. Dubler, C.B. Lieberman. Chapter 6: How to Write a Bioethics Mediation Chart Note. In Bioethics Mediation: A Guide to Shaping Shared Solutions. Revised and Expanded Edition. (2011) Vanderbilt University Press.

27. G. DuVal, B. Clarridge, G. Gensler, and M. Danis, "A National Survey of U.S. Internists' Experiences with Ethical Dilemmas and Ethics Consultation," *Journal of General Internal Medicine* 19 (2004): 251–258.

28. K.A. Berkowitz, N.N. Dubler. Chapter 9. Approaches to Ethics Consultation (p 142) in Handbook for Health Care Ethics Committees, L.F. Post, J. Blustein, N.N. Dubler, Eds. (2007). Johns Hopkins University Press.

29. D. Resnik, "Research Ethics Consultation at the National Institute of Environmental Health Sciences," *American Journal of Bioethics* 8, no. 3 (2008): 40–46.

30. M. Danis, A. Farrar, C. Grady, et al., "Does Fear of Retaliation Deter Requests for Ethics Consultation?" *Medicine, Health Care, and Philosophy* 11 (2008): 27–34.

31. S. Wolf, "Toward a Theory of Process," *Law, Medicine, and Health Care* 20, no. 4 (1992): 278–290.

32. L. J. Schneiderman, H. D. Teetzel, D. O. Dugan, J. Blustein, R. Cranford, K. B. Briggs, G. I. Komatsu, P. Goodman-Crews, F. Cohn, and E. W.Young, "Effect of Ethics Consultations on Nonbeneficial Life-Sustaining Treatments in the Intensive Care Setting: A Randomized Controlled Trial," *Journal of the American Medical Association* 290 (2003): 1166–1172.

F. Cohn, W. Rudman, L. J. Schneiderman, and E. Waldman, "Proactive Ethics Consultation in the ICU: A Comparison of Value Perceived by Healthcare Professionals and Recipients," *Journal of Clinical Ethics* 18 (2007): 140–147.

# 1 Starting Research

When planning a research study, thoughtful investigators may foresee important ethical issues likely to arise during the conduct of the research or even after its completion. This chapter explores ethics consultations arising at the start of research. In particular, the chapter will focus on questions regarding social value, scientific validity, study design, and institutional review board (IRB) review of research.

Research has social value when it attempts to answer a scientific question that has the potential to advance health and well-being.[1] Ensuring that a study has sufficient social value promotes the responsible use of limited social resources and helps to justify exposing human beings to research-related risks. Research without sufficient social value might include a risky study of a clinical phenomenon that is of little consequence or lacks broader significance. If research results are unlikely to be useful, a study lacks social value and may be unethical to conduct. *Consult 1.1* addressed whether the uncertain—and potentially limited—social value of a study was nonetheless sufficient to justify exposing participants to risk. The study in question was designed to examine how individuals infected with the human immunodeficiency virus (HIV) would respond to a smallpox vaccine. The concern was that if the risk of individuals with HIV becoming infected with smallpox, through an outbreak or bioterrorist attack, was negligible or purely theoretical, the social value of the study might be too low to justify the risks.

There are many interesting but unresolved questions about determining the social value of research, including what legitimately counts as social value. Does social value include only the generalizable knowledge produced by research? Furthermore, must there be local social value for a study to be ethical? Commentators disagree on whether research has sufficient social value if it does not address an important research question for the host country or community (where the research is carried out), but rather contributes to other important goals like training young researchers, building capacity for future research, or developing useful infrastructure.[2,3] At the time *Consult 1.2* arose, notwithstanding the many open questions about social value, there was considerable agreement in the literature that research must produce knowledge that has value for the population or community involved. The widely endorsed ethical requirement that research should produce generalizable knowledge that responds to the health needs or priorities of the host community is often referred to as "responsiveness."[4] *Consult 1.2* posed an interesting challenge for responsiveness. The question was whether it would be ethical to conduct an early phase study of a malaria vaccine designed for people who live in malaria-endemic regions with healthy volunteers in Baltimore, a nonendemic region. This consult raised questions about whether responsiveness should only apply to developing country settings, what its goals are, and how these goals can best be achieved. By stimulating our thinking about a widely accepted ethical requirement for research, this consult motivated us to conduct further conceptual research in this area.[5]

Ethical research must also be scientifically valid and methodologically rigorous—that is, carefully designed to answer the question of interest. Scientific validity requires that methods are feasible, well-tailored to the questions and objectives of the research, adequately powered, and inclusive of a robust plan for data analysis.[6] Research that lacks scientific rigor will be unlikely to achieve its aims, and research participants may therefore be exposed to risk for no reason. The use of scarce public funds for research on studies that lack scientific validity is similarly problematic. In *Consult 1.3*, a researcher asked the Consultation Service whether it would be ethical to conduct research on a journalist's cells so that the journalist could write about research and the experience of being a research participant for a public audience. This consult raises the interesting question of whether there are other types of social value that might justify research and its risks, even if it is not being done in order to answer a broader scientific question.

The need for a methodologically rigorous study design can sometimes come into conflict with other ethical considerations, such as the balance of risks and potential benefits. *Consult 1.4* presented a situation in which an investigator asked whether it would be ethically acceptable to employ a blinded, placebo-controlled study design that included using "sham" intravenous lines (IVs) with saline for half of the children enrolled. There is general agreement that experimental interventions should be tested against an established or proven effective intervention when one exists.[7] It is also relatively uncontroversial to use a placebo if the risks of placebo use are trivial, or when there is scientifically compelling reason to use placebo and the placebo will not cause "serious or irreversible harm."[8] Accordingly, this case required balancing the scientific need for a placebo control against the risks, and determining whether the risks of administering an invasive placebo to some pediatric research participants in this particular study could be justified.

In situations where there is no standard of care to which the experimental intervention could be compared, there may be few good alternatives to placebo use. When there are existing treatments that have been proven to be effective, one critical step in ethical study design is determining to what the experimental intervention should be compared. It can be difficult to decide which standard of care is the right comparator for a number of reasons. Practice in different places can vary considerably and may not be evidence based, which makes it challenging to define the standard of care simply by referencing what physicians commonly use or do.[9] Even when it is clear what the best proven therapy is, that therapy may not be available everywhere that research is conducted, and there may be discrepancies in the standards of care around the world as a result of global economic disparities. Therefore, even interventions that are recognized as the best proven standard of care around the world may be out of reach for many people. When this is the case, comparing the experimental treatment against the best proven treatment may provide data that are simply irrelevant for the local context.

For these reasons and others, research in developing countries has proven to be a source of considerable controversy. In *Consult 1.5*, the consult requestor planned to conduct research in Uganda but was unfamiliar with the special ethical considerations that are unique to international research. The Consultation Service provided comprehensive guidance about issues raised in international research ethics that were relevant to the study in question. This consult touched on issues ranging from how to address concerns about stigma from HIV testing to whether the community should be involved in deciding what benefits of research should be shared.

Finally, the requirement for independent ethics review, such as that provided by IRBs in the United States, helps assure that ethical issues—including but not limited to the ones identified earlier—are addressed adequately in research protocols. Determining how an ethics consultation service should function in relation to the IRB is sometimes challenging. As discussed earlier, the ethics consultation service can assist investigators in thinking about ethical aspects of study design prior to IRB review. Ethics consultation also can be effective in the midst of IRB review; for example, when an IRB approves a protocol with stipulations or does not approve (i.e., puts on hold or "tables") a protocol for specific reasons, and an investigator requests assistance from a consultation service to address the required revisions. *Consult 1.6* addressed concerns that emerged from an IRB's initial review—and tabling—of a protocol that proposed to enroll a vulnerable adult population. The consultation service helped the research team develop a clearer justification for the proposed design of the study, and a more sensitive approach to eligibility screening to help reduce the associated risk of psychosocial harm to potential subjects, that were ultimately acceptable to the IRB.

Interaction between researchers and ethicists after IRB review is completed can be more complicated, given that the role of the consultation service is only advisory, whereas the IRB's role is defined by federal regulations in the United States. Moreover, the federal regulations do not include a right to appeal (or a process for appealing) IRB determinations, which means that they are generally binding. When a researcher disagrees with an IRB's determination regarding the acceptability of a protocol, however, he or she can provide the IRB with additional and/or amended information and request reconsideration. Accordingly, another role for the Consultation Service in relation to IRBs can be to serve researchers as a sounding board and help develop a well-reasoned argument for reconsideration by IRBs when it might be warranted.

Some variability among different IRBs' assessments can legitimately be expected because IRBs are given discretion in interpreting and applying federal, state, and local regulations and guidance. However, a lack of uniformity in ethical review can be problematic, especially if it leads to inadequate protections for some study participants. Variability across IRBs has been documented in a number of different contexts, including in IRBs' assessments of the risk levels and potential benefits of various procedures; requirements for informed consent and assent; and process-related metrics such as length of time from submission to approval or judgments about whether a study merits expedited or full IRB review.[10,11] Within the context of a single, multisite trial, such variability can be especially problematic when it leads to differential treatment of participants or complications in implementing the research plan at the different sites. These problems have led to a proposal to revise the Common Rule to allow more streamlined review of multisite research.[12] *Consult 1.7* addressed a lack of consensus about the appropriate standard of care for the provision of anesthesia during magnetic resonance imaging (MRI) in children and about the relative risk level of each procedure. The consult involved a seven-site clinical trial in which the different IRBs disagreed about whether conscious sedation or general anesthesia and endotracheal intubation (GETA) was safer for infants on the study undergoing MRI. The role of the consult team was to help the researchers explore options for reconciling IRB judgments rendered at the various sites.

## CONSULT 1.1: ASSESSING SOCIAL VALUE

### Reason for Consult

Dr. Dorothy Klein, an investigator, asked the Consultation Service the following question: Is it ethical to test the safety and efficacy of smallpox vaccination in people living with HIV with relatively intact immune systems, if the research is being done in anticipation of a smallpox attack?

### Narrative

In the wake of the September 11th terrorist attacks, the U.S. government began preparing for the possibility of a smallpox attack by bioterrorists by developing a program of smallpox vaccination.

Dr. Klein explained that some data about the risks associated with smallpox vaccination exist from the previous routine use of this vaccine in the United States and other countries. Existing data demonstrate that most people develop mild reactions to the vaccine, but some people experience more serious and even life-threatening conditions. Those believed most likely to experience side effects include people with weakened immune systems such as individuals who are infected with HIV, recipients of a vital organ transplant, under treatment for cancer, or taking immunosuppressive drugs. The current recommendation is that individuals with any of these conditions not be vaccinated against smallpox.

Dr. Klein's team proposes a new smallpox vaccine study based on the argument that HIV-infected individuals are not a homogenous group and thus may not be uniformly susceptible to adverse responses to the vaccine. The investigators are interested in determining whether HIV-infected individuals who are at the healthier end of the spectrum could be safely vaccinated. A healthy person's CD4 count can vary from 500 to more than 1,000. HIV progresses to acquired immunodeficiency syndrome (AIDS) when an infected person's CD4 count becomes less than 200.

The research team has therefore written a protocol to assess the safety and immunogenicity of a particular smallpox vaccine in HIV-infected individuals with stable disease. For example, to be eligible, individuals must be on highly active retroviral therapy, with CD4 counts greater than $350/\text{mm}^3$, and no history of opportunistic infections.

A meeting was held with three attending members of the Consultation Service, three consulting members of the Bioethics Department, and Dr. Klein's team. Dr. Klein and a colleague also attended a full Ethics Committee meeting for a further discussion.

## Analysis and Recommendations

The present risk of smallpox attack is unknown. There is some concern that the risk of an attack is too small or uncertain to justify the predictable risks of the vaccine for HIV-infected individuals. Given that the government is planning to implement a smallpox vaccination program at this time, however, the uncertain likelihood of a smallpox attack does not automatically make the research devoid of utility and therefore unethical.

### *Ethical Arguments in Favor of the Research*

1) The research has social value because of its ability to inform vaccination policy. The research may help determine the following:

   I. Whether people infected with HIV face a high enough additional risk from the vaccine that individuals should be screened for HIV prior to vaccination.

II. Whether some HIV-infected individuals should be allowed to choose vaccination.

III. In the absence of screening, how to best treat HIV-infected individuals who are unaware of their HIV status and are inadvertently vaccinated.

2) The research also has social value because of its ability to inform policy about the response to a smallpox attack. It may help determine how to best protect HIV-infected individuals in the event of an attack.

In both cases, the study's potential social value stems from the idea that when policy is grounded in scientific evidence it tends to (1) better respond to human health needs; (2) use resources more efficiently; and (3) more fairly treat populations with unique needs. In particular, fairness in including a population that is generally excluded from research and finding needed information about that group seems to have been a driving force behind the study.

## Ethical Arguments Against the Research

1) The social value is limited by the fact that the study may not be definitive enough to guide policy.

Some concern has been expressed that the statistical power of the proposed study will not allow the study to achieve its goals. In general, it is agreed that ethical research requires methodology and statistical power adequate for achieving an interpretable answer to the question posed. However, the nature of research is such that often a series of small studies need to be undertaken in order to answer a question that ultimately could influence public policy, which suggests that this study has value as a part of a larger project.

2) The social value is limited by the uncertainty of a smallpox attack.

Since the possibility of an attack is uncertain (and, according to some, quite low), excluding HIV-infected individuals from vaccination does not put them at immediate risk of harm. According to this argument, the increased fairness and efficiency of a science-based vaccination policy may not be sufficient to justify the risks of vaccination in the context of the study without a known risk of smallpox.

3) The risks might not be sufficiently minimized.

There may be an alternative way of answering some of the questions that minimizes risks and/or makes benefits accrue more directly to research participants. For example, one possibility is a retrospective study of vaccinated HIV-infected health care workers who were not aware of their status (or did not reveal it) at the time of vaccination.

Members of the Consultation Service recommend that the following considerations be taken into account when assessing the ethics of this study:

1) Concern about bioterrorism has increased dramatically during the past year. How to best respond to the possibility of bioterrorism is a complicated question both scientifically and ethically. If public health interventions are being planned, it is wise to consider how they will impact different populations in the community, particularly vulnerable groups.
2) Because there are a growing number of individuals in the population who are immunocompromised—whether due to infections, treatment regimens for autoimmune diseases, cancers, or transplantation procedures—and because plans to vaccinate the population against smallpox are proceeding, research that gradually and systematically explores the safety of vaccines in HIV-infected and immunocompromised individuals seems prudent and important.
3) The likelihood of generating sufficient data to learn about the risks associated with vaccination for HIV-infected individuals through observational studies of vaccination in the population is small when the immunization policy involves exclusion of individuals who are known to be infected.
4) With regard to timing, it is preferable to conduct studies before some standard approach of exclusion is adopted and becomes well entrenched without an evidence base to justify it.
5) Finally, some have recommended that the investigators seek the opinions of representatives of the HIV-positive community. While having the support of the relevant community does not inherently mean that a study is ethical, it seems important to determine how representatives of the HIV-positive community view the study's potential for social value and the acceptability of the study's risks.

## Authors' Commentary

This consult came to the Consultation Service in early 2002 when smallpox was viewed as a credible threat. Fortunately, in the years following this case, the threat of a smallpox attack has not materialized. Despite the shifting security issues that affect us today, this consultation raises questions that are still pertinent. As unique and specific as the consideration of enrolling HIV-infected individuals in a smallpox vaccine study may seem, it belongs to a class of ethical questions that are unlikely to fade away.

The most challenging question posed by this consult is how to weigh the uncertainty of a future attack against the very real risks of an intervention being tested to combat it. Assessing the social value of this research might be more difficult than it is for most other kinds of research, because whether an attack occurs depends on the activities of only a few bad actors. As antibioterrorism research increases, it may be important to involve the national security community in setting priorities for this category of research. This may enable classified information to be used to inform judgments about social value, and research and intelligence efforts to be better coordinated.

More recently, a related case was brought to the Consultation Service involving the question of whether pregnant women should be included in research on public health measures to combat an anthrax attack. These cases teach us that, in the effort to anticipate and counter bioterrorist threats, it will be very important to consider measures that will also be useful for vulnerable or underresearched groups in society. The needed public health response will likely challenge the long-standing exclusion of certain groups from research—including pregnant women, children, and HIV-infected individuals—because of concerns about vulnerability. Moreover, it is clear from these cases that as bioterrorism and the responses to it evolve, further ethical analysis of biodefense research is needed and may become increasingly important in the future.

## CONSULT 1.2: ASSESSING SOCIAL VALUE FOR LOCAL POPULATIONS

### Reason for Consult

Dr. Edward Ng, an investigator, requested a consult to discuss a study he is designing. He has several questions, including the following: What is an appropriate study population for Phase I (first in human) malaria vaccine trials? Is it ethically acceptable to enroll individuals in the United States? In Mali?

### Narrative

Malaria is a serious and potentially fatal disease caused by a parasite that is transmitted by mosquitoes. Individuals infected with malaria typically suffer from high fevers, chills, and flulike symptoms. Cerebral malaria causes changes in mental status and coma and is fatal in about 20% of all cases.[13] A global eradication program in the 1950s and 1960s succeeded in eliminating malaria risk in most developed countries, but malaria remains a significant cause of morbidity and mortality around the world. In 2006, 247 million people were infected with malaria, and 1 million people died from it.[14]

Seeking to address this important problem, investigators—including Dr. Ng—have developed several potential malaria vaccines, also known as "candidate vaccines." The furthest advanced are intended to prevent serious disease progression in already infected infants and adults. If proven effective, these vaccines will benefit in countries like Mali, where malaria is prevalent. Dr. Ng explained to the Consultation Service team, however, that these candidate vaccines are not expected to prevent infection with malaria and are therefore not likely to be of medical benefit to American travelers or military personnel.

Dr. Ng and his fellow researchers are planning to conduct early phase research into a malaria vaccine in the United States but are unsure whether it is ethical to expose research participants in the United States to risk if the study has no value for their community. In particular, this study may contradict the Declaration of Helsinki's requirement that medical research is ethically permissible only if it has the potential to benefit the population being studied in the research.

## Analysis and Recommendations

### Enrolling Research Participants in the United States

1) Risks to individuals

The investigators believe that new vaccines pose a lower risk of severe adverse effects than other novel drugs, with anaphylactic shock being the most likely—though still extremely rare—serious risk. All agreed that risks to potential participants are not greater than those in other Phase I trials regularly conducted in the United States.

2) Principled permissibility

The Declaration of Helsinki (2000) states: "Medical research is only justifiable if there is a reasonable likelihood that the populations in which the research is carried out stand to benefit from the results of the research." The ethics consult team acknowledges that some bioethicists might interpret this guideline as prohibiting testing of a malaria vaccine in the United States because malaria is not endemic here. Many bioethicists, however, would accept such trials in principle, on the grounds that the concerns about unfair background conditions and possible exploitation of individuals and communities in developing country settings that prompted development of the guideline do not apply to this case. U.S. participants should be told that the aim of the study is to develop a vaccine for malaria endemic regions, and they should be able to freely decide whether to enroll.

3) Relevance of adverse events data to the target population

Pointing to data from a prior Phase I malaria vaccine trial in which Australian adults exhibited much higher rates of adverse reactions than adults and children from Papua New Guinea, the investigators raised the concern that Americans may experience different reactions to the vaccine than the target population in Mali. Such results could forestall further development and testing of a vaccine that might be safe and effective for the intended population, or facilitate the development of a vaccine that would not be useful for the target population. While these would be unintended and unfortunate consequences of testing with a U.S. sample, it does not render use of American participants unethical per se (assuming the chance of this is sufficiently low such that the study still has value). Indeed, if a Phase I trial is deemed unacceptable in Mali (see later), testing with a U.S. population would provide the greatest opportunity for continued development of a safe and effective malaria vaccine candidate.

## Enrolling Research Participants in Mali

1) Responsiveness to the health needs of the target population

Responsiveness to the health needs and/or health priorities of the community in which research is conducted is a widely endorsed ethical requirement. The idea is that research should have local social value by virtue of asking scientific questions that address important problems for the communities that are burdened by research participation. For instance, CIOMS Guideline 10 declares: "Before undertaking research in a population or community with limited resources, the sponsor and the investigator must make every effort to ensure that the research is responsive to the health needs and the priorities of the population or community in which it is to be carried out . . . ." Development of a vaccine is clearly responsive to the health needs of the general Malian population.

2) Safety of participants

One researcher expressed the fear that, in case of rare complications, individuals would be at greater risk of death in Mali than in the United States. However, all investigators agreed that the most likely adverse event is anaphylactic shock, which could likely be treated adequately in Mali's major medical centers, where the trial would be conducted.

3) Acceptability to target population

It is not clear, however, that such trials would be considered acceptable by the IRB or by other individuals in Mali. One investigator pointed out that the Malian IRB is highly reluctant to permit research if the studied intervention has not been previously tested in Europe or the United States and that Mali hosted its first Phase I trial in 2002 following a year of extensive discussions.

The Consultation Service recommends that, in principle, it is ethically permissible to conduct a Phase I malaria vaccine trial in either the United States and Mali or both, but researchers would need to ensure that Malians find such a trial acceptable before proceeding.

## Authors' Commentary

This consultation touched upon an area of considerable controversy: whether local social value of the generalizable knowledge produced by the study is a necessary condition of research. The guidance cited in this report has changed since the consultation was written. The World Medical Association, which authored the Declaration of Helsinki, has clarified its stance, both broadening the requirement that research have local social value in some respects and making it more restrictive in others. The 2008 version of the Declaration of Helsinki now provides that "Medical research involving a disadvantaged or vulnerable population or community is only justified if the research is responsive to the health needs and priorities of this population or community and if there is a reasonable likelihood that this population or community stands to benefit from the results of the research."[15] Thus, this clarification requires that ethical research be both responsive to health needs and priorities and that the products of the research are made reasonably available to the local community. However, because the requirement is limited to research with disadvantaged or vulnerable populations, it is not interpreted to apply to healthy volunteers in developed countries. Therefore, the analysis in *Consult 1.2* is supported by the new version of the Declaration of Helsinki. Although there are clearly populations in developed countries that should be considered disadvantaged or vulnerable, it is also true that worries about exploitation may be most salient for research hosted by communities in developing countries.

This particular study prompted discussion in the bioethics literature as an interesting challenge to the responsiveness requirement. Interestingly enough, Ruth Macklin has argued that the insistence of the African country on having early phase research conducted in the United States would not be reason enough to make an exception to the responsiveness requirement—the African country would have to offer a justification, and it could not just require that residents of the United States bear the burdens of early phase research.[16] Additionally, a debate taking pro and con positions on this case was included in a casebook written by members of the Department of Bioethics.[17]

This consult also led to conceptual work and to the publication of several articles by members of the Department of Bioethics on the responsiveness requirement. The fact that the ethical guidelines in the literature stated that responsiveness should apply to research conducted in developing countries (and not developed ones) spurred our department to think about the fundamental basis for this requirement. More specifically, we have examined what justifies the responsiveness requirement, whether responsiveness is a necessary requirement for ethical research, and what effects the requirement might have on the interests of developing countries.[18] Through the workings of the Consultation Service, we are sometimes faced with questions or issues that are unsettled or that challenge conventional wisdom. These questions provide an opportunity for further research and contributions to the literature.

## ■ CONSULT 1.3: ASSESSING SCIENTIFIC VALIDITY

### Reason for Consult

Dr. Catherine Allen, a National Institutes of Health (NIH) program director, requested a consultation to determine whether it is ethically acceptable to test a journalist's cells so that the journalist can write about the research in a forthcoming book.

### Narrative, Part I

Dr. Bok's lab, which is in Dr. Allen's program, studies genetic mutations that are caused by toxic exposures. Dr. Allen was approached by a well-respected scientific journalist, Mr. David Duncan, who was interested in having his own cells tested as part of a book he is writing about genetic mutations.

In its initial meeting with Drs. Allen and Bok and a lawyer from the NIH Office of General Counsel, the Consultation Service recognized that examining the journalist's DNA could be part of an interesting journalistic story. The tests, however, would not be of scientific value to Dr. Bok's lab.

### Analysis and Recommendations, Part I

The consult team identified the following concerns:

1) *Use of federal resources:* Since the results of the test are not likely to be of research value, performing the tests could appear to be a misuse of federal resources.
2) *Fairness:* In addition to the journalist, many individuals may want Dr. Bok to perform tests on their cells. To comply with Mr. Duncan's request while rejecting other, similar requests would be unfair. Thus, by performing the tests, Dr. Bok may set a precedent that would make it difficult for him to reject similar requests in the future.
3) *Danger of misleading readers:* Because Dr. Bok's line of research is at a very preliminary stage, the consult team was concerned that it would be difficult to present the results in a way that is accessible to the public without suggesting that the results are *(1)* reliable and *(2)* have practical

significance. This is of special concern, given the fact that many different parties are interested in the significance of genetic mutations.

These concerns led to an initial recommendation that it would be advisable to decline Mr. Duncan's request. If, however, Dr. Bok decided to go ahead with Mr. Duncan's request, the consult team suggested that he give consideration to some further issues, including the following:

1) *Understanding of results:* Dr. Bok should address concerns about the public being misled by the reported results of the test.
2) *IRB review:* According to Title 45 CFR part 46, the tests that would be performed on the journalist do not constitute research, and so they might not require IRB approval. However, if Dr. Bok performs the tests on the journalist, he should receive an exemption from the NIH Office of Human Subjects Research for conducting the tests without IRB review.
3) *Clinical Laboratory Improvement Amendments (CLIA) Requirements*: The Centers for Medicare & Medicaid Services (CMS) regulate all laboratory testing performed on humans in the United States through the CLIA requirements. If Dr. Bok performs the tests, he would need to make sure that he does not violate CLIA regulations.

## Narrative, Part II

Following the initial consultation on this issue, Mr. Duncan (the journalist) and Dr. Bok (the investigator) requested a second ethics consultation meeting to revisit the question of whether it would be acceptable to test Mr. Duncan's cells so that he can write about the experience. In the follow-up meeting, Dr. Bok talked about the current tendency among some policy makers to use cell-based toxicology testing as a basis for public policy decisions. Dr. Bok explained that he believes this is premature because the science is not advanced enough to draw any conclusions about clinical toxicity. He sees educational value in Mr. Duncan's work if it accurately portrays the current limits of the science.

Mr. Duncan, who was not a part of the first meeting with the Consultation Service, expressed desire to report on Dr. Bok's research in his forthcoming book. Given Mr. Duncan's demonstrated ability to make science accessible to lay readers and the importance of Dr. Bok's work, the book potentially holds considerable educational value for the public and for policy makers.

## Analysis and Recommendations, Part II

The Consultation Service recommends that the potential educational value in cooperating with Mr. Duncan may be a legitimate reason for granting the request—as long as several concerns, described next, are adequately addressed.

NB: The Consultation Service was careful to express no opinion about any of the legal issues raised by Mr. Duncan's request. Further discussion with the Office of Legal Council may be warranted.

1) Dr. Bok has not yet decided whether, if he complies with Mr. Duncan's request, he will include Mr. Duncan's cells in his dataset. He is working with a predefined population, and adding a data point now may threaten the validity of his results. If Dr. Bok ultimately decides to include Mr. Duncan in his dataset—or foresees any other possible future research applications for Mr. Duncan's cells or test results—Dr. Bok should consult with his IRB and consider submitting a protocol before proceeding.
2) If, instead, Dr. Bok sees testing Mr. Duncan's cells as having purely educational value, then he has to decide whether the potential educational value of the test does in fact justify the expenditure of federal resources. He should consult with his institute director before arriving at this decision.
3) A concern about fairness was raised in the original consult meeting. This concern was largely alleviated given that Mr. Duncan's request ultimately hinged on its potential educational value, rather than his access to personal test results.
4) If Mr. Duncan misinterprets the results of the test or presents those results in a way that invites misinterpretations, the potential educational value of complying with his request would not be realized. Dr. Bok should develop a written agreement with Mr. Duncan to help assure that Mr. Duncan's book will not misrepresent his research, for example, an agreement that Mr. Duncan would not publish without Dr. Bok's approval.
5) Given the interest of policy makers in Dr. Bok's toxicology research and the publicity that may arise from Mr. Duncan's publication, Dr. Bok should discuss any decision to work with Mr. Duncan with his institute's policy office.

## Authors' Commentary

This consultation unfolded over two separate meetings with the Consultation Service, and the ultimate conclusion was different than the one from the initial meeting. This two-part consultation exemplifies how the consultative process can be iterative and how a clinical research ethics consultation service should be open to reconsidering its recommendations under certain circumstances. The initial session took place with the scientific team exclusively, and the subsequent meeting took place with the journalist present. The Consultation Service team's consequent change of view provides a vivid example of the impact of having all the relevant voices at the table during research ethics consultations.

The consult team concluded with the assessment that while the tests to be conducted on the journalist's cells were generally of little scientific value, it would still be helpful to provide some general guidelines to the researcher regarding how to proceed if he should decide to include the results of his experimentation with the journalist's cells in his dataset. What began as a discussion about the appropriateness of an activity of limited research value grew into a discussion of the potential for important public benefit from the activity in question. Interestingly, the consult team was originally concerned that allowing the journalist's cells to be tested—and providing Mr. Duncan with the results—could inappropriately promote the notion that individual test results from this research are beneficial. Over the course of the consult, however, the team came to appreciate that the journalist's participation actually had the potential to help correct the public's overestimation of the benefits of the research conducted by Dr. Bok—a surprising result. This outcome suggests that social value may sometimes be derived from aspects of research that go beyond the data that are collected, at least in some limited cases. Mr. Duncan ultimately published his book, in which he described the experience of his genetic testing at the NIH, in 2009.[19]

## ■ CONSULT 1.4: PLACEBO-CONTROLLED TRIALS

### Reason for Consult

Dr. Geeta Persad, a fellow working on a research team, contacted the Consultation Service asking whether it is ethical to use a sham intravenous (IV) and saline infusion as a placebo control in a pediatric study.

### Narrative

In her conversation with the ethics team, Dr. Persad explained that she is studying young children with a rare skeletal disorder that causes extreme growth deficiency. In the proposed study, children would receive the study drug or be in a control group for 1 year to assess improvements in growth, increases in bone density, decreases in bone pain, and overall function. The study drug must be given intravenously.

During the process of designing the study, a question arose about whether the study team should consider performing a "sham IV" infusion of an inert saline solution—that is, a placebo—to ensure that the control group would undergo procedures that are comparable to participants in the other arm of the study. Placebos are commonly equated with sugar pills, the administration of which involves relatively little risk. However, because the study drug in this case is administered via an IV infusion, a placebo comparison would require administering the inert comparison substance (saline) in the same way—via an

IV line. Administering a placebo via an IV line is invasive and involves risks to participants that would need to be balanced against the potential scientific benefits of using a placebo in the control arm. Notably, the effects of the drug are apparent on X-ray: unlike the proposed placebo, with each infusion of the study drug, distinct transverse lines appear on the X-rays taken of the children's bones. The children's parents have already been told that they will be allowed to see X-rays taken as part of the research. The members of Dr. Persad's team all agreed that it will be difficult to maintain a true blind.

## Analysis and Recommendations

To be optimally effective, a placebo control requires that the study participants, their parents, and the research staff be blinded to whether the treatment being administered contains the active study intervention or the inert (placebo) substances. In this particular study, however, the effects of the study drug would be readily apparent on X-ray. Given that parents had already been told that they will be able to see the X-rays, it will be infeasible to blind the children, their families, or the investigators.

The Consultation Service team concluded that unless the blind could be made reasonably secure, its scientific purpose would be lost. Accordingly, exposing children to the risks associated with a sham IV could not be ethically justified. At the conclusion of the ethics consultation, Dr. Persad and the other researchers seemed to be leaning against placebo control.

## Authors' Commentary

In this consult, the characteristic of the study drug that rendered the placebo control ineffective (its visibility on X-ray) obviated the need for further discussion of the ethics of using a "sham IV" placebo control. If it had been practically feasible to carry out the blinding in this study, additional questions about the relative risks and potential benefits of the proposed "sham IV" infusion, and whether the sham was justified in the context of using growth and bone density as "hard" endpoints—questions that would ultimately need to be decided by an IRB—would have required further attention in this consultation. This is especially true because the protocol is a pediatric research protocol, and the federal regulations governing pediatric research place limits on the amount of net risk that children may be exposed to in research.[20] Evaluation of the risks of placebo use in children under the regulations is not straightforward.[21] Furthermore, the ethics of the use of invasive sham interventions is ethically controversial. This consult and other studies proposed at the NIH spurred conceptual work on this issue by members of the Department of Bioethics.[22]

# CONSULT 1.5: ADDRESSING ETHICAL ISSUES IN INTERNATIONAL RESEARCH

## Reason for Consult

Dr. Shimon Tanaka is preparing a protocol to study the prevalence of pulmonary hypertension associated with sickle cell disease in Uganda and requests a consult regarding ethical issues to consider when conducting international research in a developing country.

## Narrative

Dr. Tanaka explained that the goal of his study is to determine the prevalence of pulmonary hypertension associated with sickle cell disease (SCD) and the influence of common infectious diseases on the prevalence of pulmonary hypertension in a population in Uganda. This will be a cross-sectional study of 600 Ugandan males and females over the age of 10. Half of the research participants will have SCD, and the other half, who will not have SCD, will serve as controls. A medical history, physical, and echocardiogram will be performed. Blood will be drawn to confirm the diagnosis of SCD and to test for comorbidities such as HIV, hepatitis B and C, and a number of parasitic infections, including malaria, schistosomiasis, and hookworm. In addition, the protocol aims to look for genetic polymorphisms (variations) that may predispose sickle cell patients to pulmonary hypertension.

Dr. Tanaka requested an ethics consult to review the proposed research with particular attention to important issues in international collaborative research, including benefit sharing and responsiveness to host country health needs and priorities. Because several members of the Clinical Center Department of Bioethics have expertise in international research ethics, two additional attendings from the Consultation Service with relevant expertise participated in this consult.

## Analysis and Recommendations

During the consult meeting, members of the ethics and research teams discussed several ethical considerations in the context of international research.

First, there is widespread concern about the potential for researchers from wealthy countries like the United States to exploit the circumstances of poorer communities. To address this concern, further description of the possible benefits of this study and the value to Uganda of determining the prevalence of pulmonary hypertension would be helpful. This could include describing the current standard of care for treating SCD and associated pulmonary hypertension in Uganda; the reasons for conducting the study in this particular community; any plans for further collaboration with the community, including the possibility of subsequent treatment studies; any plans for training Ugandan physicians in the treatment of SCD or pulmonary hypertension; as well as plans to develop other capacity through training or resources. We suggest consulting with community representatives about the possible benefits and value of this study to Uganda to ensure that they regard those benefits as appropriate and sufficient.

Second, participants will be tested for and potentially diagnosed with HIV, hepatitis B and C, malaria, schistosomiasis, and hookworm. To evaluate study risks and benefits to participants in Uganda, a careful description of how individuals who test positive for these infections will be managed (e.g., referred or treated) is important. Will or could treatment for any of these infections be provided through the study, such as for schistosomiasis, hookworm, or malaria? What arrangements have been made for referring individuals to treatment protocols in Uganda, especially for HIV and hepatitis B and C? How will results be given to participants? Where will the testing be done?

Third, in the current draft of the protocol, due to recognition of stigma and cultural taboos regarding HIV in Uganda, HIV testing is described as voluntary, and "anonymous" testing is planned for those who decline HIV testing. We discussed the ethical and possible legal difficulties of doing HIV testing on those who decline to be tested. To illustrate: to participate in the study, a subject's blood must be tested for HIV, but declining to know results poses ethical dilemmas for the investigative team. The team would know that some subjects need treatment despite their disinterest in test results, and concern would be raised for their sexual partners.

In light of these considerations, we suggested instead that HIV testing be an integral part of the protocol. HIV testing is not only important to the study's scientific objectives but also allows for appropriate HIV-related treatment and care for the tested individual. Because all research participation is voluntary, individuals who do not want to be tested for HIV can choose not to participate in the study. The investigators should become familiar with Ugandan cultural, legal, and religious norms and expectations regarding reporting of HIV and partner notification. The protocol should describe and justify what they plan to do in this regard.

Fourth, the current draft protocol proposes to enroll individuals over the age of 12. Clearer justification for including children of this age is warranted. In addition, assuming this study does not have the potential for direct benefit, investigators will need the assent of children deemed capable. With regard to that requirement, the Consultation Service suggested that further thought be given to the definition of adult and child in this community, how children will be enrolled, how they will determine which children are capable of assent, how assent will be obtained, and how test results (e.g., HIV positive results) will be shared with the children and their families.

Fifth, it was suggested that in addition to IRB and Research Ethics Committee (REC) review, Dr. Tanaka should investigate any legal and regulatory requirements for foreign-sponsored research in Uganda.

Sixth, as the current protocol includes testing for genetic polymorphisms, we suggested careful description of the consent process for genetic testing and any plans for sharing results with participants, as well as plans for managing the genetic samples, including the extent to which identifiers will be retained, where the samples will be stored, and who will have access to them.

In summary, the Consultation Service's recommendations are as follows:

- To give careful consideration to the following issues and discuss the decisions made in the protocol:
  - What benefits the study will provide to the host community
  - How ancillary care for individuals who test positive for infectious diseases will be managed, including whether individuals will receive test results and treatment
  - What the consent process for genetic testing, plans for sharing results with participants, and details about sample collection and storage will be
  - Whether and how to enroll children in the research
- To consult with the community about whether the benefits of the research are appropriate and sufficient
- To make HIV testing required for study participants and develop a plan regarding reporting of HIV and partner notification that is consistent with local laws and practices
- To investigate and comply with local laws governing research

Based on this discussion, the investigators planned to make revisions to the protocol prior to submission for scientific review and IRB review.

## Authors' Commentary

This consult was fairly unique in that the requestor chose to seek out expertise regarding quite a broad array of questions in international research ethics. International research ethics is a complex and evolving area of bioethics that is thought to involve unique ethical concerns due to asymmetries of power and differences in the medical needs and access to health care of developed and developing world populations. Fortunately, several members of the Consultation Service had relevant expertise in this subfield and worked collaboratively to advise the requestor. Because bioethics covers a diverse range of issues, our consultation service sometimes goes outside of the Clinical Center Department of Bioethics to consult with other bioethicists who have expertise in the relevant subfield. Consulting with other bioethicists within the service or beyond can be a useful way for ethics consultation services to cover a wide range of issues responsibly.

Many of the issues that arise in international research ethics are not unique to the international context and may also arise in domestic research. Concerns about the exploitation of developing country populations, however, are especially salient in international research. It is widely accepted that one way to address concerns of exploitation is to ensure that participants and host communities receive a share of the benefits of research. Prominent ethical guidelines recommend that the research respond to the host country's health needs and priorities and that the products of the research or the knowledge generated be made reasonably available to the host community.[23] Several members of the Department of Bioethics have argued that this "reasonable availability requirement" can require too much in some cases or too little in others.[24] For instance, if reasonable availability had been applied to this consult, it would suggest that the researcher should share knowledge generated by the research, but he would not be obligated to offer any additional benefits, like building capacity or providing health care, to the community.

The Consultation Service recommended that the researchers consider other potential benefits for the host community and consult with the community to see whether these benefits are appropriate and sufficient. This recommendation reflects a view held by the consult team that has been published as the Fair Benefits framework. The Fair Benefits framework holds that participants and host communities involved in research should receive a fair share of the risks, burdens, and benefits of research in comparison with sponsors and researchers.[25]

It is interesting to question whether the ethics team should have informed the requestor about the division between those who argue for reasonable availability and those who endorse the Fair Benefits framework. In most cases, how much to inform consult requestors about debates internal to bioethics will require a judgment call. Some consult requestors may be ethically sophisticated and interested in hearing about these debates—or perhaps even in engaging in them. At the same time, some consult requestors may have an interest in obtaining clear advice from experts with well-considered views and limited interest in hearing the more complex picture of the range of views within the field. How much information to give requestors about debates like these should be decided on a case-by-case basis. If, however, the view held by the consultant is an idiosyncratic or unpublished view, or is clearly a minority position within the field, then it may be incumbent upon the consultant to place his or her view in context.

In the 7 years since this consult was written, views regarding benefit sharing have moved forward. Some commentators have criticized the Fair Benefits framework. Among other arguments, commentators have suggested the framework is not specific enough about what communities are owed and fails to consider how background injustice might affect interactions between people from developed and developing countries.[26] One of these critics has recently developed an alternative account of benefit sharing,[27] which has attracted criticism of its own.[28] While researchers, sponsors, and communities struggle with these decisions, the debate within the international research ethics community over what is owed to research participants and communities in multinational research will likely continue.

## CONSULT 1.6: DESIGNING AN ETHICAL SCREENING PROCESS

### Reason for Consult

Ms. Camilla Quentin, a social scientist, asked for assistance addressing the IRB's concerns regarding a protocol that she is helping to design.

### Narrative

Ms. Quentin is advising a graduate student, Ms. Kuami Sanjay. Both women have questions about Ms. Sanjay's dissertation project, which is a qualitative study on how asymptomatic individuals with positive genetic test results for Huntington disease (HD) psychologically cope with their status. HD is a neurodegenerative genetic disorder. Ms. Sanjay expects most, but not all, of the research participants to be recruited from an HD center at an academic medical institution in a different state. One to two additional sites, which have not yet been identified, will be required to ensure a sufficient number of participants. The proposed format of the study includes a brief telephone screen, and for those who qualify, an hour-long telephone interview.

The academic medical center's IRB recently tabled the protocol, and Ms. Quentin requested assistance in addressing some of the IRB's concerns. In particular, the IRB's concerns included the following: *(1)* adequate planning for adverse events; *(2)* clarifying the inclusion/exclusion criteria; *(3)* determining how to inform prospective subjects that they do not qualify for the study without having to tell them that they are symptomatic for HD over the phone; and *(4)* the validity of relying on self-reports to determine whether someone is asymptomatic.

During the consultation, Ms. Sanjay explained that what matters for the scientific purposes of the study is that the subjects *believe* themselves to be asymptomatic rather than *actually* being asymptomatic.

## Analysis and Recommendations

If Ms. Sanjay is correct that what matters is that subjects *believe* themselves to be asymptomatic, relying on self-reported asymptomatic status would not threaten the scientific validity of the study. For the same reason, it may not be necessary to verify the genetic test results. In addition to concerns about scientific validity, however, there is an ethical concern that subjects be competent to provide valid informed consent.

The Consultation Service recommends that the inclusion criteria be amended to require both:

1) That research participants believe themselves to be asymptomatic for HD (by self-report)
2) That research participants are capable of consenting to research participation

The latter criterion will require the investigators to develop a way to screen for neurological/psychiatric symptoms (whether caused by HD or not) that would render valid consent impossible. This screening can, perhaps, be incorporated into the informed consent process. For example, the IRB suggested distributing informational materials about the study in written form in advance of the screening interview. During the screening interview, the researchers could ask questions about the protocol to ascertain capacity (e.g., Does the participant know that enrollment is voluntary? Does he or she know what the risks and benefits of participating are?). These recommendations fully address issues (2) and (4) raised by the IRB.

These recommendations also appear to largely address issue (3), as there will no longer be a need to inform potential subjects if they are symptomatic. If they do not qualify for participation in the study, it would be either because they already believed themselves to be symptomatic or because they were unable to provide valid informed consent. The consult team noted, however, that issue (3) is not entirely addressed, as some excluded volunteers could infer that they are likely to be symptomatic for HD.

With regard to the IRB's questions (1) and (3), the consult team recommends that, if feasible, all recruiting be done through HD centers. This should further reduce the possibility of potential subjects learning that they are symptomatic for HD as a result of failing the screening interview, as presumably patients being monitored by HD centers are likely to know if they are symptomatic. This should also reduce, but not eliminate, the risk of adverse events.

The investigators still need to develop a detailed plan to identify and deal with adverse events. Ideas discussed during the consultation include the following:

A. Identifying in advance ways to recognize distress/discomfort over the phone

B. Being prepared to provide specific mental health resources for referral (recruiting exclusively through HD centers can also be of help here, because the subjects would presumably already have functioning support networks in place to which they could be directed should the need arise)
C. Preparing a contingency plan for possible emergencies, for example, acute suicidal ideation
D. Asking questions at the end of the main interview to assess levels of distress
E. Following up over the phone 1–2 days after the interview

The consult team offered to review the changes made by the investigators prior to the protocol's resubmission to the IRB.

## Authors' Commentary

This consultation helped the research team respond to the IRB's very appropriate concerns in a way that ultimately led to the protocol being approved and to the research being conducted successfully and without any reported adverse events. The Consultation Service's recommendations were straightforward and relatively manageable for incorporation into this graduate student dissertation project. A key factor in the success of this consult was the fact that it was scientifically acceptable for the research team to rely on the participants' *perceived* asymptomatic status via self-report. If the study aims had instead required objective verification of participants' asymptomatic status, the approach described in this consult would have been insufficient. More rigorous screening requirements would have entailed rendering clinical judgments about the presence or absence of HD symptoms, either by the members of the research team or perhaps by clinical staff at the sites from which participants were being recruited. Such judgments would be difficult to carry out via telephone screening alone, and they would also run the risk of revealing information that was at odds with a participant's own perceptions. This, in turn, would have required a plan for determining whether and how best to disclose such findings to subjects with adequate counseling to help minimize psychosocial harms associated with learning about the onset of symptoms. These requirements might also have made it more difficult to recruit a sufficient number of participants for the study and required resources that exceeded what a graduate dissertation could be expected to support. If that had been the case, the consultation service would have been in the more difficult position of suggesting that the research team substantially alter its study aims or design, given that the requirements to conduct the proposed study ethically could not be met.

## CONSULT 1.7: RECONCILING DIFFERENT JUDGMENTS REACHED BY MULTIPLE INSTITUTIONAL REVIEW BOARDS

### Reason for Consult

Dr. Pamela Nelson, an investigator, asked for assistance in determining how a disagreement among different IRBs reviewing a multicenter study might be ethically resolved.

### Narrative

Dr. Nelson is participating in a multicenter study measuring the effectiveness of a new cardiac medication in infants. One of the study's secondary endpoints is measured by cardiac MRI. Initially, the MRI was to be done under conscious sedation, which is standard clinical practice at most of the study centers. This protocol was reviewed and approved by all of the local IRBs.

As Dr. Nelson described it, during protocol implementation, the clinical practice at one of the study sites changed. This site now requires general anesthesia and endotracheal intubation (GETA) for infants undergoing MRIs. After much discussion, the study protocol was amended to require GETA at all of the sites.

Although the investigators and anesthesiologists from all seven centers were communicating about the issue and were all willing to use GETA, the local IRBs disagreed about its use in this study. During IRB review of the protocol amendment, three IRBs approved the change requiring GETA at all of the sites, and four did not. The reason that some IRBs gave for not approving the change was that the MRI is not part of standard clinical care, and GETA constitutes more than minimal risk with no direct benefit to the child.

### Analysis and Recommendations

Diverse opinions among IRBs are inevitable and sometimes legitimate. A range of opinion about the risk of clinical procedures can be due to differences in the level of experience and expertise in the use of procedures at different institutions, the interpretation of the medical literature regarding these procedures, and/or the ethical judgments about how to assign levels of risk in pediatric research. At this time, there is no consensus in the literature about the appropriate standard of care for the provision of anesthesia during MRI in children.

Given the many acceptable reasons for differing opinions, the ethics consult team recommends that the protocol be modified so that either conscious sedation or GETA be acceptable in the protocol, provided that the resulting variability would not affect the primary outcome of the study. Each institution can then choose the approach it deems preferable. Because the standard of care may change during the course of the study, institutions might change their preferred approach over time.

It is suggested that the different centers plan a secondary analysis as part of the existing study to test the relative safety of conscious sedation and general anesthesia for infants with cardiac anomalies who are undergoing cardiac MRIs. This would not entail any change in the study design and could provide highly valuable information, given the lack of data and consensus about the preferred type of anesthesia.

## Authors' Commentary

This consultation examined what should be done in the face of differing IRB judgments about the risks of a procedure in a multisite trial. Some of the problems associated with variability in IRBs' judgments may soon be addressed through a 2011 proposal to revise the U.S. Common Rule, which includes a potential mandate that all domestic sites in a multisite study rely upon a single IRB as their IRB of record for that study.[29] However, this consult request came to the Consultation Service in 2004, a time at which multi-IRB review was the standard for multisite research, and at which there was also an evolving consensus about the comparative risks of and optimal procedures for administering sedation and/or analgesia to children to achieve immobilization during MRI procedures.[30] The ethics consult team concluded that the variability in IRB judgments was both appropriate and understandable in this context, and that the protocol should, accordingly, be revised to accommodate both the sedative and anesthetic procedures. Because sedation- and anesthesia-related outcomes are dependent, at least in part, on the level of training and experience of the medical staff, as well as on site-specific practices, supporting each center's ability to select its preferred approach was likely to enhance the overall safety of performing these potentially risky procedures in children.

Presumably, although the consult report does not discuss this question directly, the use of different sedation/anesthetic methods at the various sites would not undermine the study's ability to compare the effectiveness of the new cardiac medication across the sites. At the very least, a suggestion to provide a secondary analysis would provide an opportunity to examine differences between the two approaches in the context of this drug study. Research on the risk of sedation and anesthesia continues to emerge,[31] and the American Academy of Pediatrics continues to refine guidance on its use in children for diagnostic procedures.[32]

Although this consult pointed to equivocal data in the literature about the comparative risks of sedation and anesthesia in children, it did not directly address the question of whether either of these approaches involved greater than minimal research risks to children without the prospect of direct benefit. The regulations governing research with children permit IRBs to approve nonbeneficial research in two categories: *(1)* research that poses minimal risk and *(2)* research that poses a minor increase over minimal risk and offers the potential to develop important generalizable knowledge about the research participants' disorder or condition.[33]

We can also assume from the information provided in the consult report that the IRBs judged that the approach they were willing to approve (conscious sedation or GETA) posed at most only a minor increase over minimal risk to participants. Yet four of the IRBs that reviewed this multisite study did not approve the use of GETA because they felt it posed greater than (and, presumably, more than a minor increment over) minimal risk to children that could not be justified because these were research rather than clinically indicated MRIs. A study conducted by the NIH Department of Bioethics provides further evidence that IRB chairs are divided over the risks posed by MRIs in children, even without sedation (9% of IRB chairs considered an MRI without sedation to be greater than a minor increase over minimal risk), and there appear to be persistent differences in IRB judgments about the risk levels of common procedures.[34] These differences may be more or less well supported by the available data, and a more systematic approach is certainly needed.[35]

Ultimately, this consult helped the investigators develop a plan for revising their study protocol to give all sites a choice about which procedure to implement. In doing so, it avoided calling into question the IRBs' evaluations of the risk level and the balance of risks and benefits. In seeking advice on whether the choice of anesthesia made sense, the requestor made the case that there was disagreement among the community about the safest approach for infants. The variation among IRBs reflected that lack of consensus. Because of the Consultation Service's limited advisory role, it generally has no standing to contest or override any IRB determination (although a consultation service can provide an IRB with advice directly if solicited e.g., by the IRB chair). Arguably, even under a different set of facts where the IRB's judgment departed from a settled view in the community, the consult team might simply provide the researchers with guidance on how to present a case to the IRB for reconsideration, being careful not to usurp the IRB's federally mandated charge. However, the scope of the ethics consultation role would be more challenging to determine if, for example, there was a concern that the IRB was not applying the pediatric regulations appropriately.

## ■ NOTES

1. E. J. Emanuel, D. Wendler, and C. Grady, "What Makes Clinical Research Ethical?" *Journal of the American Medical Association* 283 (2000): 2701–2711.

2. A. J. London and J. Kimmelman, "Justice in Translation: From Bench to Bedside in the Developing World," *Lancet* 372, no. 9632 (2008): 82–85.

3. C. Grady, "Ethics of International Research: What Does Responsiveness Mean?" *Virtual Mentor* 8 (2006): 235–240, available at: http://virtualmentor.ama-assn.org/2006/04/pfor2-0604.html, accessed on January 29, 2009.

4. National Bioethics Advisory Commission, "Ethical and Policy Issues in International Research: Clinical Trials in Developing Countries," National Bioethics Advisory Commission, Bethesda (2001), available at: http://bioethics.georgetown.edu/nbac/pubs.html, accessed on January 29, 2009; Council for International Organizations of Medical Sciences (CIOMS), "International Ethical Guidelines for Biomedical Research Involving Human Subjects," CIOMS, Geneva (2002), available at: http://www.cioms.ch/frame_guidelines_nov_2002.htm, accessed on January 29, 2009; World Medical Association General Assembly, World Medical Association Declaration of Helsinki, *Ethical Principles for Medical Research Involving Human Subjects*, 2008; A. J. London, Responsiveness to Host Community Health Needs. In *The Oxford Textbook of Clinical Research Ethics*, ed. E. J. Emanuel (Oxford: Oxford University Press, 2008), 737–744.

5. R. Wolitz, E. Emanuel, and S. Shah, "Rethinking the Responsiveness Requirement for Research in Developing Countries," *Lancet* 374, no. 9692 (2009): 847–849.

6. E. J. Emanuel, D. Wendler, and C. Grady, "What Makes Clinical Research Ethical?" *Journal of the American Medical Association* 283 (2000): 2701–2711.

7. Council for International Organizations of Medical Sciences (CIOMS), *International Ethical Guidelines for Biomedical Research Involving Human Subjects*, CIOMS, Geneva (2002), available at: http://www.cioms.ch/frame_guidelines_nov_2002.htm, accessed on January 29, 2009; World Medical Association General Assembly, World Medical Association Declaration of Helsinki, *Ethical Principles for Medical Research Involving Human Subjects*, 2008.

8. CIOMS 2002.

9. F. G. Miller and H. J. Silverman, "The Ethical Relevance of the Standard of Care in the Design of Clinical Trials," *American Journal of Respiratory and Critical Care Medicine* 169 (2004): 562–564.

10. H. Silverman, S. C. Hull, and J. Sugarman, "Variability among Institutional Review Boards' Decisions within the Context of a Multicenter Trial," *Critical Care Medicine* 29, no. 2 (2001): 235–241.

11. R. McWilliams et al., "Problematic Variation in Local Institutional Review of a Multicenter Genetic Epidemiology Study," *Journal of the American Medical Association* 290, no. 3 (2003): 360–366.

12. "Advanced Notice of Proposed Rule Making," 76 *Federal Register* 44512, July 26, 2011.

13. A. A. Omari and P. Garner, "Malaria: Severe, Life-Threatening," *Clinical Evidence* (Online), July 1, 2007, at 913.

14. Available at: http://www.who.int/mediacentre/factsheets/fs094/en/index.html

15. Declaration of Helsinki, 2008.

16. R. Macklin, *Double Standards in Medical Research in Developing Countries* (New York: Cambridge University Press, 2004), 26–27.

17. J. V. Lavery, C. Grady, E. R. Wahl, and E. J. Emanuel, *Ethical Issues in Biomedical Research: A Casebook* (New York: Oxford University Press, 2007), see Case 11.

18. See, e.g., R. Wolitz, E. Emanuel, and S. Shah, "Rethinking the Responsiveness Requirement for International Research," *Lancet* 374, no. 9692 (2009): 847–849; C. Grady, "Ethics of International Research: What Does Responsiveness Mean?" *Virtual Mentor* 8 (2006): 235–240.

19. D. Duncan, *Experimental Man: What One Man's Body Reveals about His Future, Your Health, and Our Toxic World* (Hoboken, NJ: Wiley, 2009). Both the author and consult requestor granted permission for this citation to be included here.

20. 45 C.F.R. 46 (Subpart D).

21. F. G. Miller, D. Wendler, and B. Wilfond, "When Do the Federal Regulations Allow Placebo-Controlled Trials in Children?" *Journal of Pediatrics* 142, no. 2 (2003): 102–107.

22. F. G. Miller and D. Wendler, "The Ethics of Sham Invasive Intervention Trials," *Clinical Trials* 6, no. 5: 401–402; S. Horng and F. G. Miller, "Ethical Framework for the Use of Sham Procedures in Clinical Trials," *Critical Care Medicine* 31, no. 3 (Suppl. 2003): S126–S130; S. Horng and F. G. Miller, "Is Placebo Surgery Unethical?" *New England Journal of Medicine* 347, no. 2 (2002): 137–139.

23. Council for International Organizations of Medical Sciences, World Health Organization, *International Ethical Guidelines for Biomedical Research Involving Human Subjects* (2002); World Medical Association, Declaration of Helsinki (2008).

24. Participants in the 2001 Conference on Ethical Aspects of Research in Developing Countries, "Moral Standards for Research in Developing Countries: From 'Reasonable Availability' to 'Fair Benefits,'" *Hastings Center Report* 34, no. 3 (2004): 17–27.

25. Ibid.

26. A. J. London and K. J. Zollman, "Research at the Auction Block: Problems for the Fair Benefits Approach to International Research," *Hastings Center Report* 40, no. 4 (2010): 34–45; A. Ballantyne, "'Fair Benefits' Accounts of Exploitation Require a Normative Principle of Fairness: Response to Gbadegesin and Wendler, and Emanuel et al.," *Bioethics* 22, no. 4 (2008): 239–244.

27. A. J. Ballantyne, "How to Do Research Fairly in an Unjust World," *American Journal of Bioethics* 10 (2010): 26–35.

28. A. Wertheimer, J. Millum, and G. O. Schafer, "Why Adopt a Maximin Theory of Exploitation?" *American Journal of Bioethics* 10 (2010): 38–39 (2010); C. MacDonald and N. Walton, "The Perverse Consequences of a Proposed Global Tax on Research," *American Journal of Bioethics* 10, no. 6 (2010): 46.

29. Advanced Notice of Proposed Rule Making. 76 *Federal Register* 44512, July 26, 2011.

30. See e.g., S. Malviya et al.,"Sedation and General Anaesthesia in Children Undergoing MRI and CT: Adverse Events and Outcomes," *British Journal of Anaesthesia* 84, no. 6 (2000): 743–748.

31. G. Serafini and N. Zadra, "Anaesthesia for MRI in the Paediatric Patient," *Current Opinion in Anaesthesiology* 21, no. 4 (2008): 499–503; A. A. Shorrab, A. D. Demian, and M. M. Atallah, "Multidrug Intravenous Anesthesia for Children Undergoing MRI: A Comparison with General Anesthesia," *Paediatric Anaesthesia* 17, no. 12 (2007): 1187–1193.

32. American Academy of Pediatrics, "Guidelines for Monitoring and Management of Pediatric Patients during and after Sedation for Diagnostic and Therapeutic Procedures: An Update," *Pediatrics* 118, no. 6 (2006): 2587–2602.

33. 45 C.F.R. 46.404, 406.

34. S. Shah, A. Whittle, B. Wilfond, G. Gensler, and D. Wendler, "How Do Institutional Review Boards Apply the Federal Risk and Benefit Standards for Pediatric Research?" *Journal of the American Medical Association* 291, no. 4 (2004): 476–482.

35. A. Rid, E. J. Emanuel, and D. Wendler, "Evaluating the Risks of Clinical Research," *Journal of the American Medical Association* 304, no. 13 (2010): 1472–1479.

# 2 Enrolling Research Participants

Clinical research aims to advance our understanding of human health and illness and to identify tools for the safe and effective clinical application of interventions to prevent or treat illness. This advancement of biomedical knowledge would not be possible without the willingness of individuals and groups to serve as study participants. Attention to the ethical selection, recruitment, and enrollment of research participants is fundamental to avoiding exploitation, maximizing the value of research, minimizing harms, and demonstrating respect for the groups and individuals who take part in research.[1] The cases in this chapter illustrate complex challenges that can arise when determining who should be included in the study population, considering the ethical acceptability of reasons to exclude some individuals or groups, and designing recruitment and enrollment strategies.

The process of enrolling research participants begins with identifying the appropriate study population. Both for reasons of science and fairness, the careful identification and selection of research participants is important. The clinical relevance of research findings depends on the extent to which the research sample is similar to the clinical population of interest. Therefore, inclusion of representative individuals is scientifically important in order to maximize the value, generalizability, and usefulness of data. At the same time, fairness requires an equitable distribution of the burdens *and* benefits of research within the scientifically appropriate subject pool. Although much of the existing guidance and literature focuses on shielding research participants from risks (a topic explored further in Chapter 3: Protecting Research Participants and Chapter 4: Conducting Research with Vulnerable Populations), excluding individuals or groups from research in order to protect them can also be problematic, as it may limit their access to interventions with some prospect of immediate benefit and may also impair clinicians' ability to apply research findings to similar others.[2] For example, if research on treatment for lung cancer always excludes people infected with HIV, physicians have no evidence base for safely and effectively treating lung cancer in the setting of HIV.[3]

Research protocols delineate specific inclusion and exclusion criteria outlining who can and cannot participate in a study based on considerations of science and fairness. Sometimes, however, investigators face concerns about including or excluding individuals for reasons that are not captured by the specified inclusion and exclusion criteria, or they face situations that would have been difficult to anticipate in advance. Often these concerns are more social than medical in nature. Investigators may be concerned about whether they should include or exclude otherwise scientifically eligible individuals or groups in a study because of poverty, country of origin, or other demographic characteristics. This was the main issue in *Consult 2.1*, in which a treatment for aplastic anemia was being studied as an alternative to bone marrow transplant, which is the standard of care. The investigators wondered whether it was ethically acceptable to enroll individuals who, because they could not afford it, had not received the standard of care. This consult raised the question of how to balance access and protection: the investigators wanted to offer potentially beneficial research interventions to individuals with aplastic anemia without taking unfair advantage of their lack of access to medical care. This case also raised the possibility of exclusion as discrimination, a topic that needs further exploration.

Ethical challenges related to balancing access and protection arise for groups of research participants but also for individual participants, as was the case in *Consult 2.2*. In this consultation, an individual who was otherwise eligible and interested in participating in a Phase I cancer study had a recently diagnosed comorbid psychiatric condition for which he was receiving treatment. Psychiatric disorders were not listed as an exclusion criterion for the cancer study, and there was no clear scientific or safety reason to exclude *all* potential participants with mental disorders. Nonetheless, because this individual's psychotic break was both recent and new, the team worried about the potential impact of the research on his safety and the potential impact of his mental health on his ability to adhere to the study protocol. Multiple requests for bioethics consultation have included questions about whether it is ethically acceptable to exclude a potential research participant solely in light of expectations that he or she will have difficulty complying with study requirements. Several consultations of this nature are presented in Chapter 6: Navigating Interpersonal Difficulties.

In addition to protecting research participants through thoughtful elaboration of inclusion and exclusion requirements, questions emerge regarding what additional safeguards are appropriate when vulnerable persons may be enrolled in research. At issue in *Consult 2.3* was whether and how members of the research staff might ethically be included in a study. This particular consultation concerned NIH employees participating as healthy volunteers in vaccine studies, but the Consultation Service has received other requests to analyze the ethical implications of having employees participate in studies related to an illness or condition they have. Employees are not vulnerable in the way children or the cognitively impaired might be. Vulnerability, however, can be understood in different ways. For example, in the case of employees, their asymmetrical relationship with their employer or their financial dependence might make it hard for them to refuse to participate in research.[4] As a result, employees might be vulnerable to coercion or to exploitation. On the other hand, researchers and staff are often deeply interested in the scientific questions being investigated, highly motivated to participate in the research endeavor, and likely to have a better understanding of what enrolling entails than a layperson would. This consult challenged the bioethics consultants to consider protections relevant to the specific strengths and vulnerabilities of employees enrolling as research participants.

When planning a study and preparing a protocol for submission to the institutional review board (IRB), an investigator identifies the population to be studied and proposes methods for recruitment. For research teams, there are many vexing practical and ethical issues related to recruitment. Unfortunately, more than one in five trials sponsored by the National Cancer Institute fail to enroll a single participant, and only half reach the minimum sample size needed for a meaningful result.[5] Yet, despite the importance of enrolling a sufficient number of research participants, ethical considerations may limit recruitment options. Little has been written about the ethics of different recruitment methods, yet IRBs do sometimes disapprove or stipulate changes in proposed recruitment methods. One review showed, for example, that almost half of 117 U.S. IRBs had policies related to incentive payments for recruitment, with 28% prohibiting them.[6] In *Consult 2.4*, an IRB was concerned that a proposed recruitment method, identifying potential research participants through public records, might cause unnecessary distress for prospective participants and violate their privacy. Interestingly, this case involved evaluating the recruitment method itself—before the individuals were actually participants—as a research risk that had to be justified by the value and importance of the study question. This consult also illustrates the fact that a research ethics consultation service can have value as an independent entity providing assistance to an IRB while recognizing that any final decision is in the domain of the IRB.[7] Notably, the IRB had previously rejected the proposed recruitment method and requested assistance from the Consultation Service when asked by the research team to review and reconsider its decision.

Finding research participants can be problematic for investigators and can considerably impede the progress of research. In our experience, investigators sometimes recruit individuals who are already participating in another study. They may recruit from their own or from colleagues' studies. This strategy is appealing because barriers to identifying participants with the relevant characteristics may be more easily overcome, and individuals participating in a study have already demonstrated an interest in research. For example, an investigator may recruit participants for an imaging study from another imaging study at the National Institutes of Health (NIH). At times, participants themselves volunteer for multiple studies. Enrollment in multiple research studies can be a natural byproduct of the investigator–research participant relationship and offer benefits to both parties. Some individuals with HIV, for example, have been coming to the NIH over several decades to participate in HIV/AIDS research and have enrolled in numerous trials. Yet enrollment in multiple studies—especially simultaneous enrollment—also holds the potential to raise serious concerns regarding safety and burden to the participants and possibly threatens the integrity of the data collected in some or all of the studies.[8] In *Consult 2.5*, an investigator asked the Consultation Service to analyze the ethics of individuals participating in multiple protocols and to consider the possibility of developing an institutional policy.

With few exceptions, once participants have been recruited for clinical research, they are asked to give informed consent before research can begin. Informed consent is generally understood to include four elements: *(1)* a potential research participant's capacity to consent, *(2)* disclosure of study information to the potential participant, *(3)* comprehension of the information by the potential participant, and *(4)* a voluntary choice about participation. Informed consent is central to ethical research and receives considerable attention in regulatory guidance and ethical guidelines. Yet, in practice, there are multiple challenges to obtaining valid, informed, and voluntary consent.[9] For example, research participants may lack the capacity to give informed consent, a situation discussed in Chapter 4: Conducting Research with Vulnerable Populations. Individuals participating in research may have a mistaken belief—also known as a therapeutic misconception—that procedures intended solely for research have been selected for their medical benefit, which is discussed in Chapter 5: Balancing Clinical Research and Clinical Care. In this chapter, *Consult 2.6* presents challenges to informed consent posed by the inability of participants to read a consent form either because they are blind, illiterate, or speak a language other than the one used in the informed consent document and participant materials.

Many research ethics guidelines and the federal regulations warn against the possibility of coercion or undue influence when recruiting and enrolling research participants.[10] These topics have received considerable mention within the research ethics literature, but they have not been clearly or consistently defined.[11] Coercion is usually understood as a threat to make a person worse off if he or she does not do what is demanded.[12] A classic example is the robber who says, "Your money or your life." A person is unduly induced or influenced when his or her judgment about accepting research risk is distorted in response to a sufficiently attractive offer.[13] For instance, an individual who is very risk averse may agree to participate in a risky study he or she would not otherwise enroll in because the researchers offer a substantial financial incentive.

Not uncommonly, investigators offer incentives for enrollment in the form of payment or provision of health care. Controversy persists about the ethically appropriate level and type of incentives in the context of different kinds of research. IRBs and others often worry about the possibility of coercion and undue influence in relation to offers of payment, gifts, or medical care.[14]

When individuals or groups might be vulnerable to coercion or undue influence, the regulations require additional safeguards to protect their rights and welfare.[15] The regulations give investigators and IRBs considerable discretion about inclusion criteria and application of appropriate protections to mitigate vulnerability. *Consult 2.7* raised these issues. As part of a proposed research study, a free hysterectomy would be offered to women in need of one. Not offered as an incentive to enroll, the hysterectomy was necessary to answer the scientific question; nonetheless, the IRB asked for input from the Consultation Service after some of its members raised concerns that some women who might not otherwise enroll would participate because of the free hysterectomy.

## ■ CONSULT 2.1: USE OF NONMEDICAL CRITERIA IN DETERMINATIONS OF STUDY INCLUSION OR EXCLUSION

### Reason for Consult

A principal investigator approached an ethicist from the Department of Bioethics during clinical rounds and requested a consultation to ask, "Is it ethical to enroll children who lack access to standard care in my study?"

### Narrative

For children with aplastic anemia (a blood disorder in which the body's bone marrow does not make enough new blood cells), especially those with severe neutropenia (an abnormally low number of white blood cells), bone marrow transplantation with minimal delay is the preferred treatment in order to avoid complications from excessive transfusions and infections and thereby improve survival. For some children, however, bone marrow transplantation may not be an option. The investigator explained to the Consultation Service that reasons for this include the following: they do not have a suitable match; their parents decline bone marrow transplantation (e.g., on religious grounds); or, in some cases, because bone marrow transplantation is unaffordable. Immunosuppressive therapy is the treatment of choice for patients who are not candidates for bone marrow transplantation.

The proposed protocol has been designed by the research team to evaluate immunosuppressive drugs in the treatment of pediatric patients with diagnoses of aplastic anemia and severe neutropenia. The research question is: Do the possible benefits of immunosuppressive drugs outweigh the risks involved in forgoing or delaying a bone marrow transplant? The protocol has been written such that bone marrow transplantation will ultimately be offered to those children who do not respond to the immunosuppressive drugs.

Since a large percentage of children who are not candidates for bone marrow transplant are those whose families lack the means to pay for transplantation, the study may rely in part on enrollment of children who lack such means. This may include uninsured children from the United States as well as children from developing countries. The research team is not planning to actively target individuals in the developing world for recruitment, nor indigent patients in the United States. The investigator requested this consult on behalf of the team, which is merely wondering at present whether indigent children who present themselves as potential research participants may ethically be enrolled.

Given that bone marrow transplantation is the preferred treatment for aplastic anemia but is not available in the developing world or to the domestic indigent, would it be ethically acceptable to include children from other countries and indigent children from the United States in a protocol testing immunosuppressive therapy as an alternative treatment and to offer them a transplant as a backup treatment in case immunosuppression fails?

## Analysis and Recommendations

In evaluating the ethics of this proposed protocol, it appears that there is a valuable scientific question. The proposed study design of assigning everyone to immunosuppressive drugs and using bone marrow transplant as a backup will allow the investigator to answer the question in a rigorous way and minimize risks to participants. The Consultation Service initially questioned why the investigator had not chosen a randomized design of immunosuppressive drugs versus transplantation, but the investigator and his team said there would not be an adequate number of participants to do the study in this way.

The researchers wondered whether the availability of a transplant for those participants who fail to respond to immunosuppressive therapy would constitute an undue inducement. The availability of bone marrow transplantation as a backup for those who do not respond to immunosuppressive therapy is not seen as an undue inducement precisely because it is a backup only for those who do not respond.

The major ethical concern, therefore, regards the selection of research participants. Poor individuals, both from the United States and elsewhere, although not specifically targeted for selection, are likely to make up a percentage of the subject pool because of lack of access to transplantation. In the present case, knowing that the experimental treatment would be too expensive to be widely available in the communities from which the participants are selected might also raise worries about possible exploitation.

The Consultation Service attending suggested that recruitment efforts should not target poor populations but need not necessarily exclude them. To exclude these individuals from the protocol would have the perverse effect of discriminating against them for economic reasons, and denying the possible benefits of research participation to precisely the population with the fewest options for treatment. Even if the proposed treatment turns out to be statistically less effective than bone marrow transplant, it still may be better than the alternative, which, realistically, may be no treatment at all in some cases.

It was further recommended that eligibility criteria for the proposed study should be carefully thought through and specified to minimize risks to participants. Specific eligibility criteria related to the prospective participants' social situation might appropriately be included. In addition, investigators must make it extremely clear to participants beforehand what the NIH can and cannot do for them and what their other options are (for example, by informing them of possible resources for obtaining a transplant elsewhere). The Department of Bioethics and the Consultation Service would be happy to help in crafting language or strategies if that would be helpful.

## Authors' Commentary

To guide clinical practice with informative and relevant research findings, the NIH and the U.S. Food and Drug Administration (FDA) now require that historically excluded "vulnerable" populations (such as pregnant women, children, and minorities) be included in clinical research unless there are compelling scientific and ethical grounds for their exclusion.[16] Aplastic anemia can develop at any age, though it is most common in younger people and, therefore, there was good scientific reason to enroll children in the proposed study. In some cases, exclusion may be ethically important to avoid harm to persons at particular risk or who are particularly vulnerable in some way.[17] The goal of this consult was to determine whether that was the case here. Finding the right balance between inclusion and exclusion is a continuous challenge in clinical research.[18] In this consultation, the ethics consultants identified the ethical tension that can arise between concern for protecting indigent groups from exploitation and undue influence on the one hand and, on the other, not denying them access to interventions that could offer direct medical benefits and which they want.

While the consultation report only briefly states that the protocol does not pose worries about exploitation or undue inducement, it is worth examining these issues to a larger extent here. Morally problematic exploitation involves one party taking unfair advantage of another party.[19] Exploitation has several features: it requires that the exploiter benefit from the interaction; it does not preclude the possibility that the exploited party may benefit too; the exploited party may even give consent. The fact that a party is vulnerable is not sufficient to be considered exploitation. Exploitation mainly concerns taking an unfair advantage that leads to an unfair outcome as judged by some normative standard. A full rationale for these criteria cannot be provided here, but the reader can find a useful, more extensive analysis of the concept of exploitation and the application of this analysis in the work of Alan Wertheimer. Wertheimer argues that it is not necessarily morally problematic for one party—such as a researcher—to exploit an unfair situation, such as the poor conditions in a developing country where he might easily enroll study participants. In making this claim, Wertheimer contends that taking advantage of an unfair situation is different from taking unfair advantage. We should note that others disagree with this contention.[20]

The investigator requesting this consult worried about taking advantage of a situation in which children who lack access to treatment participate in research in order to obtain medically indicated care. Enrolling research participants who do not have access to a particular therapy for economic reasons is not inherently exploitative when judged against a societal background of unequal access to desired treatment. As argued by Pace et al.,[21] while it is morally inappropriate specifically to target poor individuals for research *because* they may be more willing, more convenient, or less costly than others, it is also inappropriate and unfair to exclude them or erect barriers to their participation without a good scientific reason for doing so. Some individuals may welcome the opportunity to participate in a research study that offers a reasonable risk/benefit ratio, which this trial arguably did. In cases such as this, it is important to determine whether the proposed study would satisfy the ethical requirement of fair subject selection. Three major requirements are necessary for selection of research participants to be deemed "fair": *(1)* participants should be chosen on the basis of the study's scientific goals; *(2)* participants should be chosen so as to minimize the risks and enhance benefits to individual participants and society; and *(3)* distribution of the benefits and burdens of research should be fair. Further discussion of this issue is included in Chapter 5: Balancing Clinical Research and Clinical Care.

Undue inducement is a concern that an offer is so attractive that it might lead individuals to participate in research to which they have strong objections.[22] The worry is that the offer—be it money, medical care, or other appealing goods—could distort a potential research participant's reasoning about enrollment and increase the likelihood of enrolling in excessively risky research. A number of conceptual arguments as well as empirical data have further examined when this concern is warranted and how it can be mitigated. Grant and Sugarman have argued that incentives become problematic when combined with other factors, particularly when the prospective research participant is in a dependent relationship with the researcher; the risks are particularly high; the research is degrading; or the incentive is particularly large such that it overrides a strongly held or principled aversion to the research.[23] Emanuel has argued that the protection from high-risk research is best accomplished by the IRB review process rather than by minimizing payment.[24] It has also been argued that payment may engender better understanding of research since the offer of payment is likely to disabuse study participants of any expectation that the research is for their medical benefit.[25] Interestingly, surveys in which individuals are offered various hypothetical levels of payment for enrollment in research do not indicate that higher payment excessively affects willingness to participate in research.[26]

The consultants in this case did not think that the availability of bone marrow transplant as a backup necessarily met the criteria for undue inducement. A study of immunosuppressive treatment does not appear to constitute "unreasonable" risk for individuals who do not have access to a bone marrow transplant or choose not to have one. In fact, identifying the risks and benefits associated with immunosuppressive treatment as an alternative to bone marrow transplantation was the research question. It was expected that, for some individuals, immunosuppressive treatment would obviate the need for a bone marrow transplant, which rendered research participation a reasonable clinical option. Further discussion of undue inducement and the complexities of determining when something might constitute undue inducement occurs later in this chapter in *Consult 2.7*.

## CONSULT 2.2: EXCLUSION OF AN INDIVIDUAL BASED ON A NEW COMORBIDITY

### Reason for Consult

Dr. Todd Jefferson requested a consultation to determine whether there are ethical reasons not to enroll Mr. Garcia in a Phase I (first in human) protocol in light of his recent psychotic break.

### Narrative

The Consultation Service attending and fellow on call, the psychiatrist overseeing Mr. Garcia's care, and Dr. Jefferson met to discuss Mr. Garcia's medical history. Dr. Jefferson explained to the research team that Mr. Garcia, a 63-year-old male, has a diagnosis of metastatic cancer. A month ago, he was admitted to the NIH Clinical Center for evaluation and possible enrollment in a Phase I study of an experimental chemotherapeutic regimen. After admission, but prior to enrolling in the study, he experienced periods of increasing confusion culminating in an acute psychotic break. He was started on haloperidol (an antipsychotic medication) with resolution of his symptoms, and he has remained on low-dose haloperidol since.

Later the same day, the Consultation Service attending and fellow on call met with Mr. Garcia and his daughter. Mr. Garcia appeared nervous but quite lucid and exhibited the capacity to make decisions for himself. He was able to describe what the protocol entailed, including details such as the name of the medication and the postintervention stay in the intensive care unit. He also described what he saw as alternatives to participating. He seemed to understand that this is an experimental intervention (although he was not clear about the meaning of "Phase I") and that the decision to participate is his. He said he feels lucky to have the opportunity to participate. He was aware that he may be monitored more closely than other research participants because of his recent psychotic episode. Nevertheless, he expressed a strong desire to participate in the study, and his daughter supported this desire.

## Analysis and Recommendations

Mr. Garcia had a reasonable understanding of the study details and clearly stated that it is his choice to participate. There does not appear to be any ethical reason why, with close monitoring of his clinical status, he should not be allowed to enroll in this Phase I protocol.

## Authors' Commentary

At the point of enrollment in a study, an investigator may have specific concerns that mental illness could threaten research participant safety by elevating research-related risks or diminish compliance during the course of participation, possibly threatening the scientific integrity of the data. These could be sufficient reasons to exclude a mentally ill individual. For example, a study designed to test the efficacy of a new drug may require participants to go off all other medications; this could be inadvisable for an individual with a history of schizophrenia that is well controlled by medication. Alternatively, the research team may simply be nervous about enrolling a participant with mental illness without being able to fully articulate the basis for their concern. The ability of clinicians and clinical investigators to predict whether participation in a study will be complicated by the comorbidity of a newly diagnosed mental illness is not very good.

While this consultation report does not disclose the precise nature of the investigator's concerns, an exploratory discussion with Dr. Jefferson might have made a valuable contribution. For example, the ethics consultant can explore with the investigator whether there are any specific procedures in the protocol—such as a stay in intensive care or administration of a medication that frequently causes delirium—that constitute additional risk for a prospective research participant who is potentially prone to psychotic episodes. Similarly, if the Phase I protocol in question is likely to involve long periods of susceptibility to infections during which it would be very inadvisable for a participant to withdraw from the study, this might be a reason to have reservations about enrollment at the outset.

Other factors relevant to the ethical analysis include the potential of the study to benefit the prospective research participant, the availability of alternatives to research participation, and the prospective participant's understanding and preferences regarding research participation. As occurred here, it is important to include the prospective mentally ill research participant—or the appropriate surrogate decision maker—as well as the research team in these discussions. In this case, the bioethics consultants might have pointed out that, by enrolling Mr. Garcia, the investigators would assume an obligation to monitor his well-being and may need to terminate his participation early if his mental condition deteriorates.

## CONSULT 2.3: ENROLLING STAFF MEMBERS IN CLINICAL STUDIES

### Reason for Consult

Dr. Jerome Beasley, a principal investigator, phoned the Department of Bioethics with the following inquiry: Should staff members be allowed to enroll in studies? If they are allowed to enroll, what kinds of protections or safeguards would be required? He was referred to the Consultation Service.

### Narrative

Dr. Beasley is conducting vaccine studies and needs healthy volunteers to enroll. Some members of his laboratory staff have volunteered to participate in these trials. There are two main points in favor of enrolling staff members who desire to volunteer: (1) it is difficult to recruit volunteers for these studies, and (2) staff participation demonstrates a willingness to assume the same risks that they are asking others to assume. According to Dr. Beasley, the anticipated medical risks to participants are low, involving only minor side effects and the collection of several blood samples.

The vaccine studies will be conducted at a single site on the NIH campus. Dr. Beasley explained that NIH investigators developed the vaccines, not outside manufacturers. Thus, the members of the research team will be conducting their own internal safety monitoring and doing all of the necessary lab work. Because of their long-term work in vaccine development, the participating staff members really want to volunteer for these studies.

### Analysis and Recommendations

Historically, auto-experimentation has received some praise, but there are good reasons to be cautious about enrolling oneself and members of one's research team in a clinical trial. Deciding whether to enroll team members will turn on weighing three categories of considerations:

(i) The reasons to enroll staff members
(ii) The reasons not to let them enroll
(iii) The extent to which safeguards can be used to minimize the associated ethical risks

## With Respect to Reasons to Enroll Staff Members:

- The primary reason to enroll staff members is the need for volunteers and the difficulty in recruiting. During our discussion, Dr. Beasley estimated that 2%–6% of research participants might come from his staff, but that the enrollment of staff actually improves recruitment of nonstaff volunteers because the staff members are more active in recruiting friends and family if they are participating. Therefore, the enrolled staff members and others they recruit could account for a significant percentage of the individuals needed to complete the study. Whether enrolling staff members will be required to recruit a sufficient number of participants should be assessed.

## With Respect to Reasons Not to Enroll Staff Members:

- First, there are concerns about possible bias due to conflicts of interest. Because research team members already have an interest in the potential success of the vaccines, they might consciously or unconsciously underreport adverse events or err in the opposite direction, knowing that they may be tempted to underreport. The possibility for bias in these single-site studies could be higher than for similar multiple-site trials, where data are coordinated by a central site; in the single-site studies, all data are being collected and analyzed here, possibly by team members who are also research participants.
- Second, there are confidentiality concerns. A volunteer's health condition may become known to members of the research team during preenrollment screening or during monitoring in the trial. Enrollees that suffer adverse events would also be known to their colleagues.
- Third, there are concerns about undue pressure to volunteer. Some members of the research team may feel pressured to participate by virtue of the participation of other team members and/or perceived expectations of their supervisors. This is a serious concern, especially with younger staff members who might feel pressure to be in the "good graces" of the principal investigators. Those in a position to evaluate others should not

consider a person's willingness to volunteer when evaluating his or her job performance.

## *With Respect to Safeguards:*

It may be that the reasons for allowing staff to enroll—the need to recruit volunteers, to demonstrate acceptance of risk, and to respect autonomous decision making of staff members—trump ethical concerns about staff enrollment, including possible bias, confidentiality, and pressure. However, there are safeguards that should be employed to ameliorate some of the risks associated with these three concerns.

- First, if staff members are allowed to enroll, their consent should be obtained by someone other than the research team. That independent person should ascertain whether the potential volunteer feels any pressure, either directly from a superior or even indirectly by an atmosphere in which fellow employees are discussing their participation in one of the trials.
- Second, because there is a risk that a volunteer's medical condition will become known to other members of the team, staff members must be informed of this risk before they consent to enroll. Unexpected clinical findings should be referred to a consultant for further evaluation.
- Third, if staff members are allowed to enroll, it is a good idea to limit the number of them that may join a particular study. This recommendation would be particularly applicable, based on fairness considerations, for a study for which there would likely be greater willingness by community members to volunteer (e.g., for a potential study for an H5N1 vaccine).

## Authors' Commentary

There is a long tradition of encouraging or even pressing employees and other subordinates to participate in research. Around 1900, Walter Reed was charged with identifying the cause of yellow fever. Members of his Yellow Fever Board—though not Reed himself—served as subjects in his research, in part because concerns about human experiments were running high. This approach was not without risks; two members of the Board, Jesse Lazear and Clara Maas, died in the course of the experiments.[27] As this consultation request illustrates, researchers and research staff continue through the present time to participate—or to desire to participate—in their own research, and this continues to raise ethical questions.

Subsequent to this consultation request and other similar inquiries about the ethical acceptability of enrolling staff members, the Consultation Service had a request from an IRB chair to aid in the development of an institutional policy that would systematically address the question of employee enrollment in research, particularly research conducted by an employee's supervisors or other superiors. In discussions aimed at developing such a policy, several points were emphasized, many of which echoed this consultation report. In general, it was thought that employees and members of their immediate families should not participate in research conducted within their own research unit or in research conducted by any of their direct supervisors. Exceptions, subject to approval by the relevant institute's clinical director and IRB, might be appropriate if the research *(1)* presents minimal risk and is unlikely to be influenced by the participant (i.e., the participant will not be in a position to bias the data by, for instance, underreporting symptoms), and/or *(2)* is of potential direct therapeutic benefit to the participant. Additionally, when a protocol includes subordinate employees, further safeguards would pertain: *(a)* subordinates may not be solicited directly; *(b)* consent should be obtained in a manner free from any appearance of coercion (e.g., not by the supervisor or peers working on the study); *(c)* the protocol should detail a plan to ensure that neither participation nor refusal to participate will have an effect, either beneficial or adverse, on the participant's employment or work situation; and *(d)* protections of participants' privacy and confidentiality should be delineated.[28]

## ■ CONSULT 2.4: IDENTIFICATION OF POTENTIAL STUDY PARTICIPANTS THROUGH PUBLICLY AVAILABLE RECORDS

### Reason for Consult

An IRB chair requested a bioethics consultation to determine whether a proposed recruitment method is ethically acceptable.

### Narrative

In a meeting with the Consultation Service and several members of the Ethics Committee, the IRB chair explained that the IRB had previously approved a study protocol including recruitment of individuals seen at local hospitals following a motor vehicle accident (MVA). Because recruitment had been poor using this method, the investigators returned to the IRB and asked to amend their protocol. They would like IRB approval to obtain the names and contact information of individuals involved in MVAs from publicly available police records and then call these individuals to ask whether they would like to enroll in the study. The local police department has already agreed to permit the investigators access to MVA records.

This amendment has been voted down by the IRB. Members of the IRB expressed at least two worries: *(1)* individuals might be upset, angry, or irritated that investigators had obtained their names by accessing police records; and (2) obtaining the police records is an unjustifiable intrusion into the privacy of individuals. The IRB did not feel that their concerns could be allayed merely by demonstrating that it was legally acceptable for the investigators to use the information from police records because their concerns are ethical, not legal.

The principal and associate investigators feel that the recruitment method is ethically acceptable and have therefore asked the IRB to reconsider their determination. In response, the IRB requested an ethics consult. The IRB members recognize that their past voting history could possibly inhibit their ability to look at this issue objectively, and they wanted additional opinions on the matter.

## Analysis and Recommendations

We suggest that the IRB contact the Office of General Counsel for clarification regarding whether the police records qualify as "publicly available."

The Consultation Service highlighted several considerations that might be kept in mind when the IRB next deliberates:

- People have varying views about what constitutes an intrusion of privacy. For example, some people might consider it an intrusion of privacy when a person knocks on the door of their home and asks for directions, but others would not. The IRB members should be aware that their views of privacy may or may not reflect the views of all members of the public. Some individuals may not consider acquisition of their names from police records to be an intrusion of privacy.
- Even if the recruitment method intrudes on privacy, the study may still be approvable, since there are both justifiable and unjustifiable intrusions. The benefits of the study should be weighed against the harms caused by any intrusion of privacy. The recruitment method may be justified if enough benefits result from the intrusion.
- Whether an intrusion of privacy is justifiable depends, in part, on the necessity of the intrusion. Presumably everyone would agree that if there were a way to conduct the study without intruding into anyone's privacy, the proposed recruitment method would not be justifiable. However, it may (or may not) be justifiable in this circumstance, given that all other reasonable recruitment methods have not yielded a sufficient number of research participants to power the study.
- The IRB is right to be concerned about the possibility that the recruitment method will upset, anger, or irritate individuals. It is possible, however, to become overly concerned with harms, especially minor ones. One possible viewpoint is that, while the recruitment method might produce upset, anger, or irritation, those reactions are minor and ephemeral, and

therefore of comparatively little concern when compared to the benefit that could be brought about by this study.
- The IRB might think about whether the proposed recruitment approach offers any ethical advantages over other methods (even if it also involves risks that the other methods do not). For example, it may be that a call from an unknown investigator puts less pressure on potential participants than a proposal put forward by a hospital worker.
- It might be useful to think about the morality of analogous recruitment methods. For example, in our meeting, it was pointed out that brain tissue banks access death records and then call a decedent's family members to ask whether samples of the deceased's brain tissue may be kept in a bank. The IRB might also investigate the recruitment methods used during other studies of this nature.
- It might be useful to compare this method to recruitment methods that the IRB has previously approved, including those that it has approved for this study. There may be no ethically relevant difference between some of them.
- Finally, the IRB should note one curious feature of this case. Normally, when an IRB deems a certain risk to be justified, it is (rightly) presuming that in addition to IRB approval, the risk will be agreed to during the informed consent process by the person who will experience the risk, and before the risk is experienced. But that is not the case here. In this case, the IRB must decide whether to allow a certain risk that will be experienced *before* informed consent to that risk has been obtained.

All six members of the Consultation Service team felt that the proposed recruitment method was ethically acceptable. The reasons varied, but it was generally agreed that the intrusions into privacy and the possibility of provoking untoward emotions were outweighed by the value of the study. This was true even though many members of the consult team were surprised to learn that MVA reports, including contact information for the people involved in the MVAs, are publicly available information. In addition, some members of the consult team were moved by the fact that this recruitment method has been used in other studies, reportedly without provoking strong negative reactions.

The question for the IRB is essentially about how to compare competing concerns: concerns for individual privacy and concerns for the advancement of scientific knowledge and social welfare. There is no mathematical formula for comparing competing concerns. When competing concerns are particularly unbalanced, it may be clear which concerns outweigh others. However, when the concerns are more closely balanced, reasonable people will disagree about which concerns are paramount, and therefore about which course of action is ethical. When an IRB member knows that reasonable people might disagree on the morality of an issue, how should he or she vote? There are several options:

1. One is to cast a vote based on one's own estimation, instinct, or guess about the relative weightings of the competing concerns, even though one recognizes that other reasonable individuals might weigh them differently.
2. Another would be to adopt the position that when the IRB member knows that reasonable individuals could disagree about how to weigh the competing concerns, the IRB member should vote to approve the protocol. This stance would reflect the view that the job of the IRB member is to vote down clearly unacceptable research, but to otherwise allow research to go forward.
3. A final option would be to adopt the position that when an IRB member knows that reasonable individuals could disagree about the morality of a course of action, the IRB member should vote not to allow the research. This stance would reflect the view that the job of the IRB member is to approve only clearly acceptable research, and otherwise to disallow the research.

## Authors' Commentary

In this case, the Consultation Service team found the proposed recruitment strategy acceptable, whereas the IRB initially had not. The ethics consultants dealt with this difference of opinions as tactfully as it could in the consultation report: by giving both the pros and cons of the recruitment method, explicitly expressing their own point of view, and acknowledging that reasonable people may disagree. The IRB is a regulatory body, and the Consultation Service is an advisory body. Hence, while offering their viewpoint, the bioethics consultants acknowledged that, ultimately, the decision to approve or disapprove the proposed protocol amendment rested entirely with the IRB. Subsequent to the consult, the IRB took several steps. Its members sought the opinion of NIH legal counsel and brought the protocol to the attention of their institute's clinical director. Ultimately, the amendment was approved, but few individuals enrolled, and the study eventually was closed.

A study conducted in New Zealand examined new automobile drivers and their likelihood of having traffic crash injuries; researchers identified newly licensed drivers through public records. This pilot study, in which participants gave researchers consent to access their traffic crash, conviction, as well as hospital admission records, was approved by the regional health ethics committee. Report of this study did not mention concerns about identifying participants through public records, suggesting that such a recruitment strategy was acceptable in that country.²⁹ This study and the consult report highlight the need for more research regarding what methods the public and other stakeholders in human subjects research find acceptable for identifying and recruiting potential study participants.

## ■ CONSULT 2.5: ENROLLMENT OF RESEARCH PARTICIPANTS IN MULTIPLE PROTOCOLS

### Reason for Consult

After attending an Ethics Committee meeting, Dr. Silvia Dali asked the Consultation Service for assistance identifying the ethical and scientific concerns stemming from the common practice of research participants enrolling in multiple protocols (simultaneously or sequentially).

### Narrative

Dr. Dali studies individuals with obesity and enrolls them in protocols in which she offers an intervention and examines its effects on weight control. She was prompted to ask for the Consultation Service's assistance after discovering that some of the participants in her current obesity study are enrolled in other research protocols—for example, trials of investigational weight-loss drugs—that are likely to affect her study and interfere with her research results.

This concern is not unique to Dr. Dali's research. Sometimes research participants enrolled in one NIH protocol are recruited to participate in additional protocols. They may be recruited by an investigator with whom they are already working; for instance, an individual may come to the NIH to participate in a natural history study and later be invited to join a treatment study. Or individuals may be recruited by other NIH investigators; adolescents participating in research at the NIH were, for example, recruited for an ongoing study of their motivations for participating in research. It is also possible for individuals to enroll independently in multiple protocols, sometimes—as happened to Dr. Dali—without telling researchers about other studies in which they are involved.

Dr. Dali met with two members of the Consultation Service as well as representatives from the NIH Office of Communications and the Patient Recruitment and Public Liaison Office. The topic was also discussed at an Ethics Committee meeting, which Dr. Dali attended.

### Issues Identified and Analysis

Participation in multiple protocols can be generally problematic:

1) *Such participation may lead to extensive amounts of compensation.* Some individuals have essentially made a career—or at least a steady part-time

job—out of participation in multiple protocols. This raises concerns that such participation as a whole can constitute undue inducement. However, if any given individual study provides an appropriate amount of compensation, the accumulation of such compensation should be similarly appropriate.

2) *Such participation might lead to risky amounts of procedures like blood draws and radiation exposure.* Though individual investigators are expected to consider the risks of enrollment in their protocols, and the IRB is expected to review this risk, an investigator who has no knowledge about the cumulative risks that may ensue from a volunteer enrolling in additional protocols obviously cannot protect the volunteer from those risks.

The NIH's Clinical Research Information System (CRIS) contains a list of all NIH protocols in which an individual is (or has been) enrolled. Currently, there is not a straightforward way in CRIS to easily access aggregate information about procedures to which an individual has been exposed, for example, the number of blood draws or X-rays. Additionally, if a participant is enrolled in a study outside of the NIH, it would not routinely be documented in CRIS. Knowledge about how much risk the individual has been exposed to relies on his or her self-report.

The strategy of simply asking prospective study participants whether they are already enrolled in other protocols can be ineffective when they have a financial or other incentive to lie; it is unclear how common such deception is. It is also likely that the strategy of asking potential participants about other research participation is underused due to investigators neglecting to consider the possibility of enrollment in additional protocols.

3) *Participation in multiple protocols might invalidate or distort the results of various protocols.* A research participant may, for example, be involved in both a weight-loss protocol and a vaccine trial; the investigators in the vaccine trial could erroneously conclude that weight loss is an effect of the vaccine trial. The members of the Ethics Committee agreed that enrollment in multiple protocols can jeopardize study results, particularly when one protocol is a longitudinal observational study and the second protocol is an interventional study.

A related concern also arose: that of investigators seeking to recruit individuals who are already enrolled in a study. This is primarily a problem when participation in multiple protocols would invalidate the science; the only way to responsibly enroll in the second protocol would be to drop from the initial protocol. This is a waste, both in terms of recruitment and of the time and resources of the dropped study. Recruitment of participants from one protocol into another should be discouraged in cases where the first protocol is jeopardized, so long as it does not undermine participants' right to withdraw from a study for whatever reason.

4) *Individuals might decide to cease participation in their original protocol if offered the chance to participate in what seems to them to be a better protocol, thereby undermining the soundness of the original protocol's data.*
5) *Research participants at the NIH might feel more reluctant than they otherwise would to turn down an investigator who requests their participation in a protocol because of their affiliation with the institution.*

## Recommendations

1) The electronic medical record should be modified to include all pertinent information on protocol participation, including research procedures and non-NIH study participation.
2) Questions about any other protocols in which individuals are involved should be included in the evaluation and enrollment process as a default, rather than the current ad hoc strategy. Screening questions about protocol participation could be added to the participant screening tool utilized by the Patient Recruitment and Public Liaison Office; this information could be entered into CRIS.
3) Require investigators to check CRIS for apparent protocol conflicts with prospective research participants and ask participants personally about clinical trial enrollment. Investigators could, at the same time, check to ensure there is not an excessive number of blood draws, excess radiation exposure, and so on. This requirement could be waived in studies where there are no possibilities of protocol incompatibility and no cumulatively risky procedures like blood draw and radiation exposure.
4) Officially discourage investigators from recruiting participants who are already enrolled in other studies when that would cause the participant to be dropped from the original study, while ensuring that participants' right to withdraw is not infringed.

## Authors' Commentary

The team that prepared this consultation report raised a number of concerns that may arise when individuals choose to participate in multiple protocols. They suggested that enrollment in multiple protocols be officially discouraged in situations that would require participants to be dropped from one protocol to enroll in another, or in any situation in which multiple protocol enrollment might reasonably be *expected* to jeopardize participant safety or undermine scientific validity. The authors of this volume agree that so long as participation in multiple protocols does not jeopardize the health of participants and does not interfere with any of the protocols scientifically, repeated participation can be ethically acceptable; they are less worried than the Consultation Service attending was at the time about excessive payment. To reduce the likelihood of problems, practical means should be available so that investigators can coordinate their efforts and access information from the electronic medical record regarding the full research participation history of prospective study participants.

The enrollment of individuals in numerous studies as a way of making a living is increasingly gaining attention both among the public and the research ethics community. Individuals who approach research participation as a job can be identified through sites like www.guineapigzero.com, "an occupational jobzine for people who are used as medical or pharmaceutical research subjects."[30] While some view so-called guinea-pigging as ethically problematic, disagreements persist within the research ethics community. The concerns that have been raised in relation to individuals making a career of research participation include, aside from undue inducement, concerns about commodification and degradation, coercion, and exploitation. Mikhail Valdman has presented a useful analysis of the worries that underlie the repeated participation and remuneration of research participants.[31] He sorts these worries and suggests that they fall into two domains: *(1)* concerns about the nature of what is being "sold," and *(2)* concerns about the conditions under which the transaction occurs. He argues that, while there may be worries about coercion, exploitation, or undue influence because research participants may be uninformed, impulsive, or desperate, so long as the interaction between investigators and research participants is consensual and mutually beneficial, these worries can be addressed. Valdman's analysis can serve as a useful guide for research ethics consultants as they examine the acceptability of the particular conditions surrounding cases of repeated participation in research.

The possible implications of participation in multiple protocols for participant safety and the integrity of the science raise the need for investigators and others to be aware of and sensitive to the ethical consequences of more than just their own research. It is mutually advantageous for investigators to be considerate of one another's research and not recruit study participants into new studies that interfere with ones in which they are already enrolled. Coordinating research participation in this way may require institutional policies, or minimally, institutional support.

## CONSULT 2.6: OBTAINING INFORMED CONSENT FROM INDIVIDUALS WHO ARE BLIND, ILLITERATE, OR DO NOT UNDERSTAND THE LANGUAGE IN WHICH CONSENT DOCUMENTS ARE WRITTEN

### Consult 2.6(a): Reason for Consult

Sybil Vaughn, a nurse, contacted the Consultation Service to determine how one might document consent for an individual who does not speak English and is illiterate in his native language.

## Narrative

Ms. Vaughn explained over the phone that Mr. Bruni, a prospective research participant, was transferred to the NIH this morning to be enrolled in an observational study. Though capable of giving consent, Mr. Bruni is reported to be illiterate and only speaks Italian. The principal investigator described the study to Mr. Bruni with the help of an interpreter. Mr. Bruni expressed interest in enrolling, and his sister, who came to the Clinical Center with him, supports this decision. The research team would now like to know how to obtain his informed consent so that Mr. Bruni can be enrolled in their study.

## Analysis and Recommendations

The fellow on call gave a copy of the Clinical Center policy on informed consent to the nurse and described the section of the policy related to non-English-speaking individuals. The policy requires translation of the informed consent document and the availability of an interpreter when there is an expected population of participants who do not speak English.

When there is no anticipation of a group of non-English participants, but a non-English-speaking individual becomes eligible and interested in enrolling, NIH policy requires an IRB-approved oral consent process with a qualified interpreter. A short written consent form is available in many languages online. The policy on informed consent also suggests an oral process for participants who are blind or illiterate as delineated by the regulations in 45 CFR 46. 117. The Consultation Service recommended that the principal investigator contact the IRB chair to describe Mr. Bruni's case and request approval of an oral consent process.

## Consult 2.6(b): Reason for Consult

Daryl Saunders, a nurse manager, called to determine what the requirements are for informed consent for someone who is blind.

## Narrative

Casey Wright, a blind research participant, is enrolled in several research protocols at the NIH and has been scheduled for an operative procedure later this week. The surgery is clinically indicated, not a research procedure.

Mr. Saunders called the Consultation Service and described his plan for obtaining informed consent: the surgeon will read the consent aloud to Mr. Wright, his father, and his wife. Mr. Saunders will also be present in the room to witness the consent process. Mr. Wright will then sign the consent form, should he elect to undergo the surgical procedure, and will be given a copy of the consent on tape.

## Analysis and Recommendations

The planned consent process is appropriate for the clinical procedure. It does not, however, meet federal standards for oral consent for research. Therefore, any samples collected during the procedure should not be used for research purposes without first obtaining oral consent consistent with the federal regulations.

## Authors' Commentary

Valid informed consent is generally thought to have four elements: a competent prospective participant (or surrogate); an exchange of information about the purpose and nature of a study; comprehension of the information; and a voluntary agreement to participate. The federal regulations go into greater detail regarding the content that should be disclosed and specify that informed consent documentation must include the following elements:

- A statement that the study involves research
- An explanation of the purposes of the research
- The expected duration of the subject's participation
- A description of the procedures to be followed
- Identification of any procedures that are experimental
- A description of any reasonably foreseeable risks or discomforts to the subject
- A description of any benefits to the subject or to others which may reasonably be expected from the research
- A disclosure of appropriate alternative procedures or courses of treatment, if any, that might be advantageous to the subject
- A statement describing the extent, if any, to which confidentiality of records identifying the subject will be maintained
- For research involving more than minimal risk, an explanation as to whether any compensation is offered, and an explanation as to whether any medical treatments are available, if injury occurs, and if so, what they consist of, or where further information may be obtained
- An explanation of whom to contact for answers to pertinent questions about the research and the research subject's rights, and whom to contact in the event of a research-related injury to the subject
- A statement that participation is voluntary, refusal to participate will involve no penalty or loss of benefits to which the subject is otherwise entitled, and the subject may discontinue participation at any time without penalty or loss of benefits, to which the subject is otherwise entitled

Even after a researcher or research team understands the ethical principles underlying informed consent and ensures that the aforementioned checklist is satisfied, many procedural details can require clarification. These two consultations exemplify many of the requests for assistance surrounding informed consent received by the Consultation Service. In these two cases, there did not appear to be concerns about the prospective participants' cognitive abilities or ability to grasp information. Cases of that nature can be found in Chapter 4: Conducting Research with Vulnerable Populations. Rather, the central ethical concern here was how to present the necessary information.

Since the goal of informed consent is to provide prospective participants with the information they need to make a decision about research participation, such information should always be in a language and format that the individuals can understand. As mentioned in the consultation report, according to NIH policy, when a study expects participants whose primary language is other than English, the investigator should have the written consent form translated into that language. If, as is often the case, a non-English population has not been anticipated, and a prospective participant considering enrollment does not speak English, the policy allows for an oral consent process in which the study details are presented through an interpreter. The participant is then asked to sign a short generic consent form in his or her native language. International participants from many countries are seen at the NIH; therefore, the short generic consent to research form has been translated into 30 different languages, including Spanish, Chinese, German, Urdu, Bengali, and Hindi, among others, and is available on the Clinical Center intranet.

Although a great deal of emphasis is often put on the written consent form in research, if a person cannot read the form because he or she cannot see it, cannot read at all, or can only read in another language, it is reasonable to offer the person comparable information orally. In the case of another language, the oral presentation should be facilitated by a qualified interpreter. In the first of these consults, the informed consent process was constrained both with regard to Mr. Bruni's ability to understand English and his ability to read in his native language. Such individuals often pose an underappreciated, doubly difficult problem with literacy. We recognize that many people who are illiterate may hesitate to admit or display their inability to read. Having a nonthreatening way of verbally assessing potential participants' understanding of the research in which they may possibly enroll addresses this issue.

## ■ CONSULT 2.7: ASSESSING WHETHER STUDY PROCEDURES ARE COERCIVE OR UNDULY INFLUENTIAL

### Reason for Consult

An IRB member approached the Consultation Service with the following questions: *(1)* Is the offer of a free hysterectomy coercive given that women will have to agree to participate in a clinical trial to receive it? *(2)* Does the device manufacturer stand to profit unjustifiably while U.S. taxpayers pay for the hysterectomies?

## Narrative

The IRB has been asked to approve a Phase I-II proof of concept study (an early investigation that aims to determine whether a new scientific idea or concept holds promise for further development and to obtain safety information simultaneously). The protocol is an investigation of a new device used to ablate benign uterine tumors that develop in the uterus. The ultimate goal of ablation is to avoid the need for hysterectomy, the standard treatment for uterine fibroids. The primary objective of this study is to gain information about the safety and the treatment capabilities of the device, not to measure the effectiveness of the device in reducing the need for hysterectomy. The NIH investigators and the device manufacturer have a Cooperative Research and Development Agreement (CRADA), a written agreement between a private company and a government agency to work together on a project.

Women who have uterine fibroids and are planning to have a hysterectomy will be referred to the investigators as possible research participants. Women who enroll will first go through the ablation procedure. Risks of the procedure include abdominal pain/cramping, nausea, minor skin burns, and leg or back pain. No more than 30 days after ablation, participants will undergo an abdominal hysterectomy. The investigators will then study the removed uterus to determine how well the fibroids were ablated. The risks and benefits to the participant are the direct consequences of the ablation and hysterectomy procedures. Participants will not be charged for these procedures, nor will they be paid any money.

The Consultation Service was given a copy of the protocol to review. The attending and fellow on call attended a meeting of the IRB in order to discuss the ethical questions raised by members of the IRB and make recommendations.

## Analysis and Recommendations

### *Is the Offer of a Free Hysterectomy a Coercive Offer?*

Because coercion is usually understood as a threat to make a person worse off if he or she does not do what is asked, the Consultation Service does not think the offer of a free hysterectomy is coercive.

Several members of the IRB expressed a worry that the offer of a free hysterectomy constitutes an undue inducement. Undue inducement is understood as an offer sufficiently attractive that it is capable of distorting an individual's judgment and leading him or her to accept unreasonable risks. In this case, the question is whether the offer of a free hysterectomy might distort potential participants' judgments about the risks of the experimental procedure and whether the risks are reasonable. The risks of the experimental procedure, as described earlier and in the protocol, are infrequent and mostly transient. On the basis of these risks alone, the Consultation Service was of the opinion that a reasonable person might choose to participate in the research with or without the hysterectomy. Therefore, offering a free hysterectomy is not undue inducement.

### Does the Device Manufacturer Stand to Profit Unjustifiably While U.S. Taxpayers Pay for the Hysterectomies?

If a study is valuable or worth doing, taxpayers can also benefit. Because the NIH mission is research to improve the health of the public, NIH conducts and supports research that has scientific, clinical, or social value. Pharmaceutical, device, and other companies collaborate on intramural NIH studies through CRADAs and provide funds for studies of their products. The amount of funding provided and how funds will be applied is decided by the parties involved under the technology transfer guidance. It is conceivable that through the CRADA, the company would or could contribute to the cost of the hysterectomies. To the extent that products are shown to be safe and effective through such research, the companies stand to profit.

Determining whether a study has value and is worth doing requires understanding the state of the science and evaluating the proposed scientific design. As we understand it, the goal of ablation is to avoid the need for hysterectomy. However, avoidance of hysterectomy is not an endpoint in this proposed study, as all participants will have a hysterectomy. Therefore, the risks to participants must be justified by the value of the knowledge that will be gained about the safety and treatment capabilities of the ablation device. Scientific review is needed in order to assess how valuable this knowledge would be. The Consultation Service supports the IRB's requirement that the protocol undergo scientific review.

We recommend the following:

1. The protocol should clarify who will decide when the hysterectomy takes place and on what grounds. At the moment, it simply states that all participants will get a hysterectomy "within a window of 30 days."
2. The protocol should specify how potential research participants will be referred, and whether the referrals will be internal or external to the NIH (or both). There are two reasons that this makes a difference.
    a. First, the risk/benefit profile for participants is more favorable for women who already plan to have a hysterectomy. Women recruited for

this study should have decided on a hysterectomy before they have contact with the study team to avoid the possibility of a real or perceived conflict of interest in which the team has the opportunity to convince a potential participant that she should have a hysterectomy.
   b. Second, women referred internally will already be participating in another NIH protocol and might feel pressure to enroll in this study in order to not jeopardize the benefits they are already receiving from NIH.
3. In general, the investigators should make clear to potential participants what their options are, and this should be delineated in the protocol and consent form. In particular, they should ensure that potential participants are committed to getting a hysterectomy. In addition, investigators should clearly inform the women that the planned abdominal hysterectomy is important to the research goals and will be planned even if the woman's symptoms might abate after the ablation in order to accurately assess the extent of ablation of the fibroid tissue without tissue distortion. Nonetheless, participants always retain the right to withdraw their consent. Finally, subjects should be told that vaginal hysterectomy is an option they might have if they do not enroll, and that the risks of this procedure are generally lower than the risks of abdominal hysterectomy, which is what will be done as part of the study.
4. The protocol and consent form should be changed so that they no longer state that getting the experimental procedure is a benefit for research participants. It is not a benefit, given that these women are going to have a hysterectomy anyway.

## Authors' Commentary

Two noteworthy features of this consultation bear mentioning. First, the request came from an IRB. As discussed in the Introduction, the IRB fills a regulatory role while the role of the Consultation Service is advisory. While these roles are distinct and decisions about the ethical acceptability of a trial ultimately fall to the IRB, beneficial collaborations can arise. Second, the consultation raised a question related to the proper use of public funds for the conduct of research. As discussed in Chapter 1: Starting Research, social value and scientific validity are necessary to ensure that scarce research resources are used ethically. This is likely why the IRB and ethics consultants agreed that scientific review is needed. The IRB expressed an additional concern, however, about public-private collaboration: federal funds may support research that results in private profits. The consultants correctly pointed out that such collaborations are not uncommon and are governed by technology transfer guidance, as was the case here.

The consultation team did not provide an ethical analysis of this practice, which can include, for example, concerns about the distribution of benefits and investigators' potential conflicts of interest. Public-private partnerships can be a useful means of coordinating research among public and private research entities in a market-based economy. At the NIH, they are overseen by the NIH Public-Private Partnership Program (http://ppp.od.nih.gov/pppinfo/description.asp) which aims to facilitate partnerships that are "…science-driven, aim to improve the public health, and are structured to uphold the principles of transparency, fairness, inclusiveness, scientific rigor, and compliance with Federal laws and NIH policy."

## NOTES

1. E. Emanuel, D. Wendler, and C. Grady, "What Makes Clinical Research Ethical?" *Journal of the American Medical Association* 283, no. 20 (2000): 2701–2711.

2. C. Levine, "Has AIDS Changed the Ethics of Human Subjects Research?" *Law, Medicine, and Health Care* 16, no. 3–4 (1988): 167–173.

3. G. C. Persad, R. F. Little, and C. Grady, "Including Persons with HIV Infection in Cancer Clinical Trials," *Journal of Clinical Oncology* 26, no. 7 (2008): 1027–1032.

4. S. Rose and C. Pietri, "Workers as Research Subjects: A Vulnerable Population?" *Journal of Occupational and Environmental Medicine* 44 (2002): 801–805.

5. G. Kolata, "Lack of Study Volunteers Hobbles Cancer Fight," available at: http://www.nytimes.com/2009/08/03/health/research/03trials.html, accessed on May 4, 2010.

6. L. Wolf, "IRB Policies Regarding Finders Fees and Role Conflicts in Recruiting Research Participants," *IRB: Ethics and Human Research* 31, no. 1 (2009): 14–19.

7. L. Beskow, C. Grady, A. Iltis, J. Sadler, and B. Wilfond, "Points to Consider: The Research Ethics Consultation Service and the IRB," *IRB: Ethics & Research* 31, no. 6 (2009): 1–9.

8. C. Tishler and S. Bartholomae, "Repeat Participation among Normal Healthy Volunteers: Professional Guinea Pigs in Clinical Trials?" *Perspectives in Biology and Medicine* 46, no. 4 (2003): 508–520.

9. National Bioethics Advisory Commission (NBAC), *Ethical and Policy Issues in Research Involving Human Participants* (Bethesda: NBAC, 2001), chap. 5: Ensuring Voluntary Consent. available at: http://bioethics.georgetown.edu/nbac/human/oversumm.html, accessed on October 10, 2011.

10. US Code of Federal Regulations. Protection of Human Subjects. 45 Part 46. 117.

11. Department of Health and Human Services, *Institutional Review Board Guidebook*, chap. 3: Basic IRB Review, available at: http://www.hhs.gov/ohrp/irb/irb_guidebook.htm.

12. J. Hawkins and E. Emanuel, "Clarifying Confusions about Coercion," *Hastings Center Report* 35, no. 5 (2005): 16–19.

13. E. Emanuel, "Ending Concerns about Undue Inducement," *Journal of Law, Medicine, and Ethics* 32 (2004): 100–105.

14. N. Dickert, E. Emanuel, and C. Grady, "Decisions about Paying Research Subjects: Analysis of Current Policies," *Annals of Internal Medicine* 136, no. 5 (2002): 368–373.

15. 45.CFR.46.111 (7)(b)).

16. National Institutes of Health, "Guidelines for the Inclusion of Women and Minorities as Subjects in Clinical Research," in *NIH Guide for Grants and Contracts* (Bethesda, MD: National Institutes of Health, 1994); National Institutes of Health, "NIH Policy and Guidelines on the Inclusion of Children as Participants in Research Involving Human Subjects," in *NIH Guide for Grants and Contracts* (Bethesda, MD: National Institutes of Health, 1998).

17. C. Weijer and A. Fuks, "The Duty to Exclude: Excluding People at Undue Risk from Research," *Clinical and Investigative Medicine* 17, no 2 (1994): 115–122.

18. C. Weijer, "Evolving Ethical Issues in Selection of Subjects for Clinical Research," *Cambridge Quarterly Healthcare Ethics* 5 (1996): 334–345.

19. A. Wertheimer, "Exploitation in Clinical Research," in *The Oxford Textbook of Clinical Research Ethics*, eds. E. Emanuel, C. Grady, R. Crouch, R. Lie, F. Miller, and D. Wendler (New York: Oxford University Press, 2008), 201–210.

20. R. J. Sample, *Exploitation: What It Is and Why It's Wrong* (Lanham, MD: Rowan and Littlefield, 2003).

21. C. Pace, F. Miller, and M. Danis, "Enrolling the Uninsured in Clinical Trials: An Ethical Perspective," *Critical Care Medicine* 31, no. 3 (2003, Suppl.): S121–S125.

22. N. Dickert and C. Grady, "Incentives for Research Participants," in *The Oxford Textbook of Clinical Research Ethics*, eds. E. Emanuel, C. Grady, R. Crouch, R. Lie, F. Miller, and D. Wendler (New York: Oxford University Press, 2008), 386–396.

23. R. W. Grant and J. Sugarman, "Ethics in Human Subjects Research: Do Incentives Matter?" *Journal of Medicine and Philosophy* 29 (2004): 717–738.

24. E. J. Emanuel, "Ending Concerns about Undue Inducement," *Journal of Law Medicine and Ethics* 32 (2004):100–105.

25. N. Dickert, "Re-examining Respect for Human Research Participants," *Kennedy Institute of Ethics Journal* 19 (2009): 311–338.

26. S. D. Halpern, J. H. Karlawish, D. Casarett, J. A. Berlin, and D. A. Asch, "Empirical Assessment of Whether Moderate Payments Are Undue Inducements for Participation in Clinical Trials," *Archives of Internal Medicine* 164 (2004): 801–803.

27. E. Emanuel, R. Crouch, J. Arras, J. Moreno, and C. Grady (eds.), *Ethical and Regulatory Aspects of Clinical Research* (Baltimore: Johns Hopkins University Press, 2003).

28. We thank Barbara Karp, chair of the CNS IRB, who requested this consultation and worked in a very collaborative and effective fashion in developing the analysis as the consultation unfolded.

29. D. Begg, R. Brookland, J. Hope, J. Langley, and J. Broughton, "New Zealand Driver Is Study: Developing a Methodology for Conducting a Follow-up Study of Newly Licensed Drivers," *Journal of Safety Research* 34 (2003): 329–336.

30. *Guinea Pig Zero: A Journal for Human Research Subjects*, available at: http://www.guineapigzero.com/, accessed on June 30, 2010.

31. M. Valdman, "On the Morality of Guinea-Pig Recruitment," *Bioethics* 24, no. 6 (2010): 287–294.

# 3 Protecting Research Participants

Protecting research participants is perhaps the most widely endorsed and important requirement for ethical research. This requirement does not imply that clinical research must be risk free. Instead, it recognizes that clinical research necessarily involves uncertainty and risk, and it directs investigators, institutional review boards (IRBs), and ethics consultants to identify potential harms and implement appropriate safeguards to reduce their incidence and severity. Clinical research is justified only when the potential risks to participants are minimized, and any remaining risks are not excessive.[1] This chapter presents a collection of cases highlighting the ethical challenges that arise when assessing and minimizing research risks.

Independent and prospective review of proposed research studies provides an important way to discharge the obligation not to expose research participants to excessive risks. IRBs can require the elimination of unnecessary and duplicative interventions to the exclusion of groups that face significantly greater risks from participating in the research under review. While IRB review offers an important way to protect research subjects, it is limited by the fact that IRBs evaluate research studies prospectively, at which time it is unknown precisely which individuals will enroll. Because the level of risks posed by research interventions often depends on which individuals undergo them, this is an important limitation. Informed consent offers a mechanism to address partially this limitation. Explaining the nature of the study allows potential subjects to evaluate whether participation would pose excessive risks to them personally. IRBs also have the option of mandating assessment of the risk level for specific individuals at the time of enrollment. Investigators have an obligation to monitor subjects over the course of the research and ensure that the risk level remains appropriate, taking into account any changes to the circumstances or the subjects' health since the time of initial consent.

No matter how low the risks, clinical research is justified only when it offers individual and/or societal benefits sufficient to justify the risks and burdens to which the participating individuals are exposed. Most regulations specify only that research must have social value or offer the potential for clinical benefit. Left unspecified is whether it matters for this purpose what types of benefits might result from a given study. *Consult 3.1* focuses on whether certain types of benefits are inappropriate or insufficient to justify clinical research and the practice of exposing participants to research risks. This case involved a surgical study of transplanted tissues designed to produce purely cosmetic benefits. An investigator wondered whether potential clinical advances in reconstructive surgical procedures could justify the use of potentially life-threatening immunosuppressive therapy. This case also underscores the extent to which the Consultation Service must rely on others for their understanding of the relevant facts, raising questions regarding how far consultants should go to independently confirm the facts they are given before rendering an opinion.

Investigators and IRBs devote significant time and effort to designing research interventions to minimize risks, often putting in place mechanisms to continuously monitor and protect participants. In *Consult 3.2*, a pediatric research participant with an autoimmune disorder had an abnormal electrocardiogram after showing clinical improvement while on a study medication. Continued participation put him at additional risk and raised questions about whether the potential benefits of the study could justify his ongoing participation. New information regarding study interventions and subjects' circumstances can raise questions about the appropriateness of continuing a study and continuing the participation of specific research participants.

Determining the risk-benefit ratio of clinical trials is a difficult and, to some extent, subjective exercise. Risks can be difficult to estimate and evaluate, and reasonable people can reach different conclusions regarding the acceptability of research risks. Such variation can be especially problematic when research participants and investigators disagree. *Consult 3.3* raises questions about the proper balance between protecting participants from risk and respecting their autonomous choices. This case involved a young woman who expressed a desire to get pregnant while participating in a study that included pregnancy among its exclusion criteria. Complicating the analysis was the fact that she had not been able to ovulate before entering the trial, but the study drug had sufficiently normalized her hormonal cycles to make pregnancy possible. This consult required the research ethics consultants to consider the circumstances under which an investigator, IRB, or ethics consult service might overrule a participant's willingness to accept a given level of risk.

*Consult 3.4* raises questions about how investigators should proceed in response to a medical error that involved the potential failure to protect a research participant. The consult concerned an individual who, by accident, received an excessive dose of the study drug. Like the consults in Chapter 5: Balancing Clinical Research with Clinical Care, this case makes the point that clinical research often includes a good deal of clinical care. How should an investigator proceed when a serious clinical mistake has occurred? The case also raises concerns about the challenges of the consultation process, focusing on the competing roles, interests, and schedules that the research team, IRB, and Consultation Service bring to the case.

Protecting research participants, while important, is not the only ethical consideration that must be addressed when conducting clinical research. Some of the most difficult challenges in clinical research involve cases in which protecting research participants comes into conflict with other important values.

In *Consult 3.5*, the investigators presented a case in which protecting some individuals from risks seemed to require violation of a research participant's confidentiality. The case involved a man who had screened positive for a breast cancer gene but refused to share this information with his family, including his mother and two teenage daughters. The research team was worried that by disguising the truth, his daughters would go without important information that suggested they should seek screening and follow-up. The case highlights a tension between the research team's duty to protect a participant's confidentiality and the team's perceived duty to share clinically relevant information with people it could help. It also raises challenging issues about the interplay between ethics consultation and the law; legal concerns can complicate or conflict with the ethically appropriate course of action, raising questions about whether ethics consultants should ever provide advice that knowingly conflicts with what the law requires.

The theme of risks to individuals other than the research participants continues in *Consult 3.6*. This case raised questions about the scope of the requirement to minimize the risks of clinical research, both in terms of the types of risks that should be considered and in terms of who counts as a relevant at-risk party. The case involved a prospective research participant who would have to complete a 20-hour drive with a medically unstable relative in order to get to the National Institutes of Health (NIH) and enroll in a potentially beneficial treatment trial. Typically, minimizing the risks of research means focusing on harms faced by research participants that result from the interventions included in the study. But participating in clinical research can expose individuals to many risks beyond those posed by the specific interventions. They may face risks as the result of foregoing some activities while participating in research: for example, they risk losing wages due to absence from work. They also may face added risks in order to participate. This case underscores the fact that simply getting to the research site can pose significant risks to some people, including people who are not prospective participants.

Should IRBs take into account the risks individuals face in getting to the research site? If so, does it follow that individuals who live in locations remote from the research site should be excluded from research more often? Should IRBs evaluate risks to family members or other individuals who are part of research participants' lives when deciding the inclusion and exclusion criteria? Is this a matter of appropriately minimizing the risks of research, or potentially discriminating against those with large families? Is it ever appropriate to exclude an individual from research participation on the grounds that it would pose risks to a family member? Because there is no clear guidance in this area, the role of the Consultation Service was to help the investigator resolve some of these difficult questions.

## ■ CONSULT 3.1: JUSTIFICATION OF RESEARCH RISKS

### Reason for Consult

Dr. Paul Roberts, an NIH physician, requested an ethics consultation to evaluate whether it is acceptable to expose research participants to a risk of death in research designed to improve their appearance and functioning through reconstructive surgery.

### Narrative

Dr. Roberts is involved in a multicenter research protocol that involves transplantation of tissues of various types for important but nonessential cosmetic and functional benefit (e.g., surgery to correct disfiguring facial scars or limb transplantation). He explained that although the protocol has been approved by the IRB at each participating site, he and surgeons within the reconstructive surgery community are worried that the protocol is unethical because it involves the use of potentially life-threatening immunosuppressive therapy for the sake of improved appearance and functioning. These surgeons believe the risks are too great to be justified by either (1) benefits to the enrolled participants or (2) the clinical knowledge to be gained.

### Analysis and Recommendations

The consultants' understanding of the protocol is limited to the information presented by the requestor. As described, the protocol may be judged by some physicians as offering an unwise tradeoff of risks and benefits. Multiple IRBs have, however, approved the protocol. In addition, we assume that potential research participants will be informed of the risks and potential benefits, and the fact that the protocol involves research rather than standard medical care. Under these conditions, the consultants recommend that it is ethically acceptable to allow potential participants to decide whether to assume the risks of participating in the protocol.

### Authors' Commentary

This consult raises an important question about the extent to which protection of research participants is ensured by obtaining the voluntary, informed consent of competent individuals. In the present case, although the consultants did not see the study protocol, it appears that the potential participants—and not the ethics consultants—are in the best position to judge how much benefit they might derive from the surgery being conducted in the study. The risks of surgery can be appropriate to address serious limitations in functioning and at least some cosmetic concerns. For example, surgery to address disfiguring facial scars or limb functioning can provide enormous benefit. What constitutes a disfiguring scar or dysfunctional limb certainly is not clear, however, and individual judgment may vary widely. While this might suggest that investigators and IRBs should simply leave the decision of whether the risks are worth the potential benefits to potential participants, it also seems clear that people can make mistakes in this regard. Someone might, for example, choose to accept serious risks in order to have surgery to correct what in fact is a very minor concern.

In clinical practice patients are generally allowed to decide when the potential benefits of cosmetic surgery justify the risks, but even here there are limits. Surgeons should not agree to perform very risky surgery to correct something that even the individual agrees is a minor concern. Clinical research introduces the added concern of exposing individuals to inappropriate risks for the benefit of society. The details of clinical research studies typically are determined by what makes sense in the context of clinical care. For example, research studies do not evaluate the efficacy of bone marrow transplantation for minor concerns because bone marrow transplantation would not be offered for minor concerns in the clinical setting.

In contrast, cosmetic surgery is sometimes offered in the clinical setting for minor concerns. This raises the question of whether clinical studies should be designed to evaluate practices that are available in the clinical setting, or should be limited to practices in the clinical setting that are deemed appropriate. If there should be greater scrutiny of research, what standards should investigators and ethics consultants use to judge whether the benefits are sufficient to justify the risks involved? The U.S. regulations, like the regulations in many countries around the world, stipulate that the risks of clinical research must be justified by the potential benefits of the study to participants and others. Yet these regulations do not specify the types of benefits that should be considered to be sufficiently important, or those that might not be able to justify the conduct of a clinical trial and the associated risks to research participants.

When evaluating individual cases, ethics consultants often must decide when to defer to the judgments of others. There are numerous bodies that have responsibility for evaluating the appropriateness of clinical research. These include funders, research institutions, scientific review committees, IRBs, and the individual clinicians who conduct the research. A good deal of clinical research must be approved by an IRB before it can be conducted, and IRBs are charged with evaluating whether proposed studies are ethically acceptable. One might argue that if a duly constituted IRB approves a study, then that study should be treated, at least by ethics consultants, as appropriate. This view is supported by the fact that IRBs are in a position to evaluate the ethical acceptability of research studies based on all the relevant information. Ethics consultants, in contrast, are often limited, as in this case, to the information provided by requestors. At the same time, ethics consultants would seem to have a responsibility to evaluate cases based on their own judgment. This seems especially the case when a study offers what appears to be a clearly inappropriate balance of risks and benefits. Determining whether that condition is satisfied, however, requires an answer to the previous question of who is in a position to determine how much benefit a given study offers.

## ■ CONSULT 3.2: EVALUATION OF EVOLVING RISKS

### Reason for Consult

Dr. Franco Parnelli, an investigator, called the Consultation Service to discuss a pediatric research participant, Toby Roy, after new findings raised questions about whether Toby should be withdrawn from the study.

### Narrative

Toby, an 8-year-old boy, was diagnosed in infancy with a rare autoimmune disorder. Earlier this year, he came to the NIH and enrolled in a multicenter, double-blind, cross-over, placebo-controlled trial using an off-label medication (a medication being used for an indication other than the one for which it has Food and Drug Administration [FDA] approval). The purpose of the trial is to assess the safety and efficacy of the drug in the population of patients with his disorder.

Six months into the study, Toby had an abnormal electrocardiogram (EKG), which revealed ventricular hypertrophy (enlargement of the heart muscle) and premature ventricular contractions (extra heartbeats, an arrhythmia). According to Dr. Parnelli, consultations with a cardiologist revealed myocarditis (inflammation of the heart muscle). The cardiologist prescribed carvedilol and lisinopril, two cardiac medications.

Following Toby's abnormal EKG, Dr. Parnelli consulted with his IRB chair and the principal investigator at the coordinating center (not the NIH). The IRB chair advised Dr. Parnelli and his team to speak with the Consultation Service. In his initial meeting with the ethics team, Dr. Parnelli expressed his concern that continued participation in the study might entail a substantial risk for Toby. He and other members of his team also wished to determine whether Toby now met the exclusion criteria for the study. In the drug manufacturer's database, there were reports of infusion-related arrhythmias and decreases in ejection fraction (a measurement of the percentage of blood that leaves the heart each time it contracts). Therefore, the study protocol specifically excludes persons with "cardiomyopathy/congestive heart failure/arrhythmia (or New York Heart Classification III or IV disease) that would prevent adequate patient assessment or pose an added risk for study participants."

Dr. Parnelli also apprised the safety officer of the concerned data safety monitoring board (DSMB) about the developing situation. In his response to the investigators, the DSMB safety officer observed that the study drug was associated with arrhythmias but not myocardial toxicity. She noted that even if Toby did not meet the exclusion criteria, he may nevertheless be removed from the study if this was in his best interests; if, after further workup, Toby's cardiac status remained the same or improved, there would be less concern about continuing administration of the study medication.

The Consultation Service recommended that after these additional tests, the informed consent should be reviewed with the mother, including a discussion of alternative treatment options. Dr. Parnelli and his team agreed with this plan and prepared for Toby's scheduled return in 2 months.

\* \* \*

As scheduled, Toby and his mother returned to the Clinical Center 2 months later. Toby displayed improvement in his autoimmune disorder as manifested by an increased ability to perform activities of daily living and moderate exercise. Toby was scheduled for detailed cardiac testing to decide whether another infusion was appropriate. The DSMB and the principal investigator at the coordinating center advised Dr. Parnelli that if Toby's cardiac status remained unchanged or had improved, he should receive the next two infusions as outlined in the protocol. If Toby was allowed to continue, his cardiac status would have to be closely monitored.

Toby's mother was informed about the possible increased risk that the study drug posed to her son, given the relevant cardiac findings. In addition, she was told that although there appeared to be some improvement in Toby's physical functioning, it might be due to the treatment for his heart condition (initiated during his last visit to the NIH), rather than the study drug. Toby's mother was assured that steps would be taken to minimize risks from the study by admitting Toby to the intensive care unit and monitoring his cardiac status throughout the infusions, should he receive them.

Later that day, Toby's mother requested additional time to think about what she had been told and to consult with her son, along with Toby's father and his pediatrician, before she consented to proceed with the infusion. The next day, Toby's mother said that she would like to proceed with the scheduled infusions, if the team found no reasons to stop. She expressed hope that the infusion would benefit Toby but recognized that there were now some additional risks that were not apparent when she first consented to the study. She was informed that the findings of the cardiac workup—which would be available in several days—would be reviewed and discussed with her before a final decision was made about Toby's research participation.

Unfortunately, Toby's detailed cardiac evaluation showed severe, persistently poor left ventricular function with an ejection fraction in the range of 30% (a normal ejection fraction is usually 75%). It was concluded that receiving additional infusions in the study might pose an additional risk for Toby, in light of his cardiac status. Since the study was double-blinded, it was unknown whether Toby had already received or would be receiving the study drug or a placebo. If Toby were to receive the study drug and experience a severe reaction (such as anaphylaxis), there was a possibility that he would be unable to compensate due to his underlying heart condition.

Before reviewing these results with Toby's mother, Dr. Parnelli and two members of his team met with the Consultation Service to discuss the implications for Toby's ongoing participation and how this information might be communicated.

## Analysis and Recommendations

A decision about continuing Toby in the study should primarily be based on the degree to which his clinical findings present risk or alter the risk-benefit balance for him. Given the double-blind, cross-over design of this trial, it is not possible to know without unblinding Toby whether he has received placebo or active drug during his participation in the study thus far.

In general, the risks and benefits of such a study design are unpredictable for any research participant. This case is rendered particularly difficult because Toby's severe cardiac dysfunction was discovered after inclusion in the study— possibly altering his risk-benefit ratio midcourse. The study drug has been shown to increase risk in individuals with cardiomyopathy and arrhythmias, but it may also be of possible direct benefit to Toby.

If, in the opinion of the research team, the DSMB, and the cardiologist consultants, Toby's cardiac condition is either stable or improved, and there are no other protocol-related reasons to cancel or postpone his next infusions, it is ethically permissible to allow him to continue in the study. His continued participation would be ethically permissible as long as his cardiac status is carefully monitored during the infusions and risks are minimized. In this case, he should only continue with his mother's permission, obtained after clear review of the risks and benefits for Toby.

On the other hand, if the research team believes that there is increased risk and the risk-benefit assessment for Toby has changed given what is known about his cardiac function and the extent of additional risk from the drug infusion, it is ethically advisable to discontinue his participation in this study. In this case, recommendations should be made to optimize his clinical condition. The research team can suggest treatment options available outside of the study.

Consistent with the research team's inclination to incorporate more extensive baseline cardiac evaluations for future participants in the study, we recommend clarifying the protocol's criteria for cardiac monitoring, the exclusion criteria, and the study consent form.

## Authors' Commentary

Subsequent to this consult report, the investigators continued to meet with the IRB, cardiac consultants, and the Consultation Service ethicists. The research team eventually concluded that Toby's cardiac condition was sufficiently impaired to exclude him from the study. The research team, therefore, advised Toby and his mother that he would not receive additional infusions.

This consultation raises important questions about how to assess and react to new information obtained during an ongoing study. Investigators must be willing to reevaluate the risks and potential benefits for a given individual as additional clinical information and safety data become available. They must also be willing to communicate this information to participants so that participants can reevaluate their decision to participate. As this consult indicates, a reevaluation should be undertaken with a broad view toward the participant's best interests. Even in the context of potentially beneficial studies, it can sometimes be in the individual's best interest to halt treatment as new information changes the risk-benefit ratio.

In this case, the analysis of the changing risk-benefit ratio could have been more precise. The consult report states that if the situation had changed such that "there is increased risk and the risk-benefit assessment for Toby has changed given what is known about his cardiac function and the extent of additional risk from the drug infusion, it is ethically advisable to discontinue his participation in this study." It would have been more accurate to focus on whether the risks are no longer justified by the benefits; only then should his participation be discontinued. It is possible that even if there is increased risk and the risk-benefit assessment has changed, the risk-benefit ratio may yet be favorable and the best option for Toby would be to continue on the protocol.

The consult analysis could have also explored in more detail the ramifications of the trial's double-blind, cross-over design. There was no way to know whether Toby had already been given the active drug or a placebo, but in either case, his treatment status would have changed when the cross-over point was reached. This detail could have materially affected the risk-benefit analysis. For example, if Toby's mother understood the probability that he would be receiving placebo in the next phase of his participation, perhaps the uncertainty would have reduced the expected benefit to the point that they no longer outweighed the newly discovered risks.

The consult team appropriately discussed the fact that it is necessary for investigators to be flexible when considering the relevance of new information.

As was discussed in Chapter 2: Enrolling Research Participants, exclusion criteria cannot anticipate all potential risks that might preclude participation. Adequate protection of research participants will sometimes require investigators to weigh factors beyond those specifically enumerated in the protocol. A study team should be flexible enough to modify the protocol as needed in response to evolving clinical and scientific knowledge. When prompted with an unanticipated study risk, investigators should think carefully about whether it is appropriate and necessary to *(1)* change inclusion or exclusion criteria; *(2)* incorporate additional preenrollment screening measures to monitor for potential risk; and/or *(3)* implement ongoing safety tests and procedures to ensure that those who are enrolled are adequately protected. This flexibility is, of course, not only the responsibility of investigators. As this case demonstrates, the independent review provided by DSMBs and IRBs is another important way to protect research participants from emerging or changing research risks.

This consult also highlights the claim that informed consent should be understood as an ongoing process that continues over the course of research participation, as opposed to a one-time event at research enrollment. In particular, research participants should be kept informed of any changes to the protocol or their circumstances. Significant changes may even necessitate, as this case illustrates, the need to reevaluate study participation. The team appropriately reengaged Toby's mother to help her think through whether the additional risk should preclude his continued study participation. Unfortunately, this process was complicated by the fact that Toby's condition seemed to be improving while on protocol, but it was unclear whether the improvement was due to the study drug or the newly initiated cardiac treatment.

## ■ CONSULT 3.3: RESPECTING PARTICIPANT PREFERENCES WHILE MINIMIZING RISK

### Reason for Consult

Pat Ripley, a study coordinator, requested advice on how to respond to Mrs. Camille Henry's desire to get pregnant while on a protocol that explicitly lists pregnancy as an exclusion criterion.

### Narrative

In her meeting with the Consultation Service attending and fellow, Ms. Ripley explained that Mrs. Henry has lipodystrophy. As a result of her condition, Mrs. Henry also has severe insulin resistance, has very high triglyceride levels, and did not ovulate before entering the trial. The study drug she has been receiving in the protocol has largely normalized her hormonal cycles and triglycerides.

A year ago, an effort was made to withdraw the study drug. As a result, Mrs. Henry developed severe pancreatitis, leading to reinstitution of the study drug.

Mrs. Henry, now 27 years old, has married and wishes to become pregnant. There are no data on the study drug's effects on pregnant women or fetuses, though mouse studies show that it does cross the placental barrier. The company that provides the study drug requires that the protocol exclude pregnant or nursing women, and it requires the use of "effective birth control." Additionally, it is likely that pregnancy could have serious effects on Mrs. Henry's health, such as diabetes and preeclampsia.

As the meeting ended, Ms. Ripley mentioned that the study protocol is long term, and two-thirds of the participants are women with an average age of 22 years.

## Analysis and Recommendations

Our two primary recommendations are as follows:

1) The research team should discuss with Mrs. Henry her desire to become pregnant, including the possibility that pregnancy may seriously damage her health. She should also be informed that the protocol would have to be amended and reapproved by the IRB in order to allow her to continue receiving the study drug should she become pregnant. It is possible that the pharmaceutical company would not accept such an amendment or that the IRB would not approve it, and the result could be that Mrs. Henry is no longer able to receive the study drug.

2) The issue of pregnancy is likely to reoccur, given that two-thirds of the study participants are young women. It is therefore important that the principal investigator and study coordinators proactively anticipate and prepare for the event that other participants either become pregnant or express their wish to do so. The researchers need to determine whether the pharmaceutical company will allow them to amend the protocol to allow for some exceptions to the pregnancy exclusion, whether they wish to seek IRB approval for such an amendment, and whether they would make participants aware of this amendment if it is allowed by the pharmaceutical company and approved by the IRB. The Consultation Service is available to assist in any of these decisions or conversations.

## Authors' Commentary

Protecting research participants from risk is made challenging by the fact that clinical research often involves interventions, procedures, and medications about which little is known, including the extent to which they pose risks to those who undergo them. Indeed, the point of clinical research often is to determine whether and to what extent experimental interventions pose risks. Yet to approve studies designed to answer these questions, IRBs, funders, and investigators must first determine whether they pose acceptable risks. In the present case, it needs to be determined whether this study can include a woman who wants to become pregnant, in the absence of any data on the impact of the study drug on pregnant women or fetuses. This question was particularly salient because it will likely come up again; given the nature of the study, it is probable that other participants will either become pregnant or express a wish to do so.

One way to resolve this conundrum is to adopt a default approach in the face of insufficient evidence. The default typically taken by pharmaceutical companies in these cases is to exclude pregnant women from participating in drug studies and to require steps to ensure that participating women do not become pregnant. The problem, of course, is that this general approach makes it difficult, if not impossible, to evaluate what constitutes appropriate medical care for pregnant women.[2]

The alternative default in the face of insufficient evidence regarding risks is to disclose this uncertainty to potential participants, allowing them to decide for themselves whether to accept those risks. This is the approach taken in studies of first in human interventions where steps are taken to minimize risks, but it is acknowledged that the true risks are unknown and might be significant. This case also raises a question that will be continued in *Consult 3.6* about the extent to which risk evaluation should go beyond risks to the research participants to include risks to others, in the present case, the fetus. Alternatively, if one designs the study to evaluate whether the study drug poses risks to fetuses, one might conclude that the fetuses would qualify as participants in the study.

In standard cases, research interventions pose risks to participants by threatening a capacity or ability that the individuals have independent of the research. For example, most subjects have the ability for wound healing as the result of the presence of platelets in their blood. Some drugs can pose a risk to this capacity. In such cases, individuals can avoid the risk and preserve their capacity for wound healing by avoiding the research intervention in question. In the present case, by contrast, the study drug is responsible for Mrs. Henry's ability to become pregnant and also poses an unknown risk to fetuses and pregnant women. In this way, the present case eliminates one of the most effective responses to ethics consultation, namely, finding a way to avoid the concern. The team could not simply instruct Mrs. Henry to withdraw from the study, have a child, and then reenroll. In the absence of that option, the investigators, consultants, and IRB had to evaluate the risk-benefit profile presented by the research and decide who should make the final determination of whether the profile was acceptable in the present case.

## CONSULT 3.4: ADDRESSING MEDICAL ERROR

### Reason for Consult

Dr. Valerie Yu, a principal investigator, called to discuss whether it would be appropriate to keep a research participant, Mr. Crouch, on protocol after he received an incorrect (excessive) dose of a study drug.

### Narrative

Before the consult meeting, members of the Consultation Service obtained and read the study protocol. The study in question has been designed to evaluate an experimental drug for its possible efficacy in treating a devastating and progressive disorder that ultimately leads to death. Because of their degenerative disorder, it is expected that participants will lose decisional capacity over the course of the protocol and are asked to name a surrogate decision maker upon enrollment.

Mr. Crouch and his daughter, whom he appointed as his surrogate decision maker, both participated in the informed consent process. A member of the Department of Bioethics witnessed the consent process; she was not available to participate in the Consultation Service meeting but reported that Mr. Crouch and his daughter understood the risks, benefits, and alternatives to participation in the study and were committed to participating.

Dr. Yu and several members of her research team met with the Consultation Service. Dr. Yu told the ethics consultants that the protocol is highly controversial because it has been classified as high risk, and there is minimal expectation of benefit. Mr. Crouch was the first research participant enrolled in the trial.

With the first research intervention, Mr. Crouch accidentally received several times the dose of the experimental drug specified in the protocol. According to Dr. Yu, the presumed cause of this error is a medication infusion pump programming error, but this remains under investigation. While the investigation of possible causes continues, all protocol-related activity has been halted by the IRB. Mr. Crouch remains an inpatient at the Clinical Center. To date, he has suffered no apparent sequelae from the medical error. Both he and his daughter have been made aware of all developments.

Members of Dr. Yu's team explained to the ethics consultants that some limited data suggest the time sequence of doses may have an impact on the effectiveness of the experimental drug. The protocol was designed to reflect the data on time sequence, and Mr. Crouch's next dose of the experimental drug is due at the end of this week. Dr. Yu has communicated this to the IRB in a memo, but the IRB meeting is scheduled at its regular time a few weeks from now.

Mr. Crouch's daughter has written a strongly worded and heartfelt plea to the investigators and to the IRB, which was shared with the Consultation Service, asking that her father be allowed to continue with the study.

## Analysis and Recommendations

1) It is clearly recognized that the IRB has the authority and the responsibility to approve or disapprove continuation of the protocol. Although the daughter's letter is ardent, the IRB must weigh all available evidence on potential risks and benefits to reach its decision.
2) Because Mr. Crouch chooses to remain an inpatient at the Clinical Center while waiting for a decision, we recommend review at the earliest possible occasion.
3) The decision about the future enrollment of others into the protocol can be viewed separately from the decision regarding Mr. Crouch's continued participation. Consideration of a single patient treatment use from the FDA might also be a way to address the concerns relevant to his situation.
4) With so many charged and sensitive issues surrounding this protocol, it is recommended that every effort be made to facilitate an open and continuing dialogue among all involved parties.

## Authors' Commentary

Medication administration errors occur frequently, and steps must be taken to minimize their occurrence and to mitigate their effects. Investigators, IRBs, and medical institutions each have distinct responsibilities for protecting research participants from potential medication errors during the conduct of clinical trials. Investigators and other members of the research team are in the best position to identify possible sources of medical errors, and they are responsible for actively adjusting their study procedures to eliminate accidental harms. IRBs have the responsibility to ensure that investigators are doing everything in their power to avoid potential mistakes and have the regulatory authority, when necessary, to revoke or reject a study's authority to involve human subjects, if they are concerned that foreseeable risks have not been minimized.

Of note, this consult did not seem to include discussion of institutional interests or responsibilities. This possibility raises a more general question. Ethics consultants, like other consultants, often face the question of the extent to which the issues raised by consultation requests should be limited to the requestor and when other interested parties should be contacted. In the present case, the NIH provides personnel, equipment, and medical resources for the conduct of clinical research studies. Hence, the institution shares the investigator's responsibility for anticipating and preventing medication administration errors. The NIH Clinical Center, like other hospitals, has policies and practices in place to ensure high-quality clinical care. The submission of an incident report would have brought the present case to the attention of quality review bodies. The consultants must decide when to allow those mechanisms to operate independently, and when it is worth interacting with them directly to discuss the case. Similarly, ethics consultants are sometimes presented with cases that raise questions about the IRB review of a particular protocol. Even very qualified and well-intentioned committees make occasional mistakes. Thus, there can be reason for ethics consultants to approach these committees when questions arise. At the same time, such actions may be perceived as meddlesome and undermine the ethics consultants' standing with committee members.

This consult also raises two interesting issues about potential difficulties of the ethics consult process. First, there can be challenges associated with competing clinical and IRB timelines. Had the research participant received the appropriate dose, the next dose was scheduled for a week later. The IRB's next regular meeting would have been too late for the dose to be administered on the original schedule. The investigators believed that the scientific evidence favored administration of the next dose within a week. Therefore, it might have been appropriate for the Consultation Service to suggest that the IRB schedule an ad hoc meeting to discuss this issue. Second, there are questions about how much weight to give participant preferences in the face of competing evidence. When, if ever, should an IRB rely solely on a research participant's or surrogate's expressed preference when considering a potential protocol safety issue? The answer to this question is probably never. Individuals can be appropriately excluded from research when there are reasonable medical concerns about their safety or scientific justifications for their exclusion. In this case, the Consultation Service appropriately recommended that the daughter's letter was only one piece of evidence and must be weighed with the totality of the data at hand.

## CONSULT 3.5: RECONCILING CONFIDENTIALITY AND THE DUTY TO WARN

### Reason for Consult

Wanda Bandura, a social worker, called because a participant in a genetic study that has now been completed openly lied to at least one family member about his positive test result for *BRCA1* (mutation of this gene has been linked to hereditary breast and ovarian cancer). The team wonders how it might regain contact with him and address the possible health implications for his family members.

## Narrative

Ms. Bandura and members of the research team related the story of Mark Goldsmith, a 62-year-old male research participant, to the Consultation Service. In the course of an NIH protocol, Mr. Goldsmith was screened for *BRCA1*. He is part of a family that has borne a heavy burden of breast and ovarian cancer. The team reports that in the pretesting genetic counseling, Mr. Goldsmith understood the implications of *BRCA1* testing, both for himself and for his two teenage daughters. His stated position at that time was that, should he test positive, he would not inform his mother so as not to worry her, and would try to convince other siblings with the mutation to follow suit. Additionally, he requested—and the team agreed—that no test results be placed in his medical record.

The test was positive. On hearing the result, Mr. Goldsmith announced that he would lie to his mother. He did lie to his mother in front of members of the team. Regarding his daughters, he said he would "take care of" them but did not say that he would inform them of his results. The team notes that he seems to be a person who holds secrets. Since then, other family members have mentioned his "negative" test result to the team. Members of the research team expressed their suspicions that Mr. Goldsmith may have lied to his daughters in a way that might endanger their health.

The researchers worry that if the daughters falsely believe their father's test was negative, they will have no incentive to pursue screening and follow-up measures that are in fact warranted. Thus, if Mr. Goldsmith encourages this false belief, he will potentially endanger his daughters' health. If Mr. Goldsmith has actively deceived family members, this is a more serious problem than mere nondisclosure. The team has no certain knowledge of whether he has actively deceived his daughters, but they worry about this because they witnessed him actively deceiving his mother. The team has called Mr. Goldsmith twice to follow up. He has not returned either call.

Ms. Bandura articulated numerous concerns on behalf of the research team throughout the ethics consultation: How should they approach Mr. Goldsmith so as to regain constructive contact, and what should they do if he refuses all further contact? Do they have any responsibility to warn his daughters? Under what conditions would such a responsibility override their confidentiality agreement with this gentleman, and are those conditions satisfied in this case?

During the consultation process, the Consultation Service team identified two additional questions: If the participant rebuffs the research team's attempts to regain contact, how should they document their good-faith efforts? Should the research team adopt a general policy of documenting test results in participants' medical records?

## Analysis and Recommendations

### Problem 1: How to Approach the Participant So as to Regain Constructive Contact, and What to Do If the Participant Refuses All Further Contact

Mr. Goldsmith may be unaware of the research team's dilemma and moral anguish. We recommend that the team reach out to him in a spirit of candor about the problem his conduct has created for them. Being candid with him about their feelings might help them to feel that they have done their part in coping with the moral burden unfairly thrust upon them.

For instance, working on a default assumption that the participant will do what he said he would do—that is, "take care of" his daughters by encouraging them to go for the screening indicated—the team might consider telling him that they still feel caught in a bind. They have uncertain and conflicting evidence about whether he has encouraged his daughters to hold a false belief about his genetic status. They are troubled by the possibility of being party to a potentially harmful deception, especially since team members were present when the participant lied to his mother and did not correct his report.

### Problem 2: Has the Team Any Responsibility to Warn the Participant's Daughters? Under What Conditions Would Such a Responsibility Override Their Confidentiality Agreement, and Are Those Conditions Satisfied in This Case?

An exceptional breach of the confidentiality agreement might be entertained from the moral point of view, but only under conditions in which the unwarned person faces imminent, severe harm and is in a position to use the protected information to prevent that harm. Because Mr. Goldsmith's daughters are in their teens, they do not face any imminent, severe harm that could be prevented now. Special screening would not be indicated before age 25.

A further consideration is that the research team does not know for certain whether this individual has in fact lied to his daughters. Moreover, according to the Federal Privacy Act, it is legally impermissible to inform the daughters of their father's test result without his consent. Because the daughters are not NIH research participants, any independent contact with them could be construed as an implicit violation of the Privacy Act. Thus, in this case, protection of the participant's privacy is legally overriding.

## Problem 3: If the Participant Rebuffs the Team's Attempts to Regain Contact, How Should They Document Their Good-Faith Efforts to Do So?

Ideally, the research team's efforts to reestablish contact should be documented in Mr. Goldsmith's medical record, as would be customary, but they cannot document their efforts without mentioning his positive *BRCA1* test. Because the team made an explicit promise to Mr. Goldsmith not to document test results in his medical record, this route is closed. We recommend that the team document their efforts in the participant's research record, which already contains his test results.

## Problem 4: Problem 3 Raises a General Question as to Whether the Team Should Adopt a General Policy of Documenting Test Results in Participants' Medical Records

Although it is never possible to guarantee protection of a person's medical record against all breaches of security, it is a reasonable and customary place to keep health information private. Medical records are legally protected at least as well as the research records in which participants' test results are already documented. We recommend that the team consider adopting a general policy of documenting test results in participants' medical records.

### Authors' Commentary

There are strong legal and ethical norms in place to protect the confidentiality of research participants, but new technologies can raise novel ethical questions that push the boundaries of accepted standards. This case divided the research team, with some strongly arguing for protection of Mr. Goldsmith's confidentiality and some advocating in favor of the team's duty to warn. After extensive discussion of the relevant issues, the team unanimously decided not to contact Mr. Goldsmith's daughters, although they did take measures intended to maintain an open line of communication with him (regular phone calls and annual follow-up visits). This sustained contact was used as an opportunity to continue the conversation about the importance of truthfully conveying the positive *BRCA1* test result to his potentially affected daughters.

This consultation centers on the conflict between a research team's duty to protect confidentiality (especially when explicit promises were made to the participant) and the team's perceived duty to share clinically relevant information with the research participant's family. The duty to warn is typically invoked under extraordinary circumstances: when an individual is at risk for serious, imminent harm. Only in such extreme cases may a clinical researcher have duty to warn that can override a research participant's confidentiality. In most cases, like the one at hand, where genetic information is mainly relevant to the relatives' long-term health and well-being, the duty to warn becomes less compelling. Given this reality, some ethicists and genetic counselors have taken the position that there is a duty to "encourage, but not coerce, the sharing of genetic information in families."[3] In the end, the research team adopted this view, deciding against directly revealing the test results to the family, while continuing to actively encourage Mr. Goldsmith to disclose them voluntarily.

The case was further complicated by the research team's suspicion that Mr. Goldsmith was actively deceiving his daughters about the genetic test results. When someone simply chooses not to disclose his or her results, family members are free to seek out their own genetic testing. Based on false reports of a negative finding, however, the children would have understandably assumed that they could not have inherited the genetic mutation from their father. Accordingly, they would have had no reason to seek out independent testing, to their potential detriment. While this was troubling in its own right, members of the research team were particularly concerned about their potential complicity in the participant's deception, heightening concerns about some team members' professional and moral obligations.

A similar case is presented in Chapter 6: Navigating Interpersonal Difficulties. *Consult 6.1* involved an individual with a set of infectious diseases who refused to disclose his health status to his girlfriend. In both cases, the decision was made not to share information with the potentially affected parties, but it is worth noting that this was done for different reasons given the kinds of risks presented by genetic information versus communicable disease status.

Mr. Goldsmith's case also highlights the tendency for legal issues to bleed into ethics consultations. For example, a question was raised about how to document efforts to contact research participants, presumably in response to a fear of legal liability. Questions were also raised about where and how to document genetic test results, with potential ramifications relating to the discriminatory use of this genetic information in employment and health insurance contexts. This consult occurred prior to the passage of the Genetic Information Non-Discrimination Act of 2008 (GINA), which specifically prohibited discrimination based on genetic information when it comes to employment and health insurance.

As discussed in the Introduction to this book, it is prudent to distinguish purely legal issues from ethical concerns. The Consultation Service does not provide legal or regulatory advice, referring investigators to the Office of General Counsel when necessary. Furthermore, legal obligations can sometimes be inconsistent with the ethically appropriate course of action. Should consultants give advice that contradicts the law? In the present case, one might wonder whether there could be circumstances under which the ethically appropriate advice would be for the investigators to warn the daughters, despite the fact that doing so might conflict with the Privacy Act. When legal and ethical norms conflict, it is important to point out this tension to the requestor while encouraging the investigators to also consult with appropriate legal counsel.

## CONSULT 3.6: RISKS TO THIRD PARTIES

### Reason for Consult

Dr. Steve Diego, an investigator, called an urgent consultation to determine whether to enroll a young woman in a potentially beneficial trial, given the burdens enrollment would place on a family member.

### Narrative

Dr. Diego told the Consultation Service that he is conducting research to evaluate an experimental treatment for reducing the recurrence of blood clots. To be effective, the treatment must be started within 14 days of diagnosis. The protocol has enrolled 32 participants to date. Thus far, the treatment has been very effective, and no side effects have been identified.

Virginia Timmerman is a 19-year-old female. She was diagnosed with a blood clot 11 days ago. Ms. Timmerman contacted Dr. Diego about enrolling in the protocol after reading about his research online. According to Dr. Diego—the Consultation Service was unable to reach her by telephone—Ms. Timmerman reports that she is unable to afford a flight from her home in South Dakota to the research site. Ms. Timmerman cannot drive, but her sister has volunteered to drive her for the 24 plus hours required to get to the NIH.

Ms. Timmerman's sister is the primary caregiver for their elderly father. He was recently released from the hospital. He currently requires oxygen and is somewhat unstable. Ms. Timmerman's sister is unwilling to leave him home alone and, since there is no alternate caregiver, plans to bring him on the trip. Dr. Diego believes that enrollment in his study would provide an important potential benefit to Ms. Timmerman, but he is concerned that the long drive may pose significant risks to the father.

Dr. Diego asked that the Consultation Service provide an urgent recommendation on the grounds that Ms. Timmerman and her family would need to leave their home as soon as possible to ensure that they arrived at the NIH within the prescribed 14-day window.

### Analysis and Recommendations

Dr. Diego should consider whether it might be possible to provide the treatment to Ms. Timmerman near her home in South Dakota. If not, it would typically be up to the family to determine whether it is reasonable to place the father at risk for the anticipated benefit to Ms. Timmerman; however, if Dr. Diego has strong reason to believe that the decision to drive to the NIH is unreasonable, he may refuse to cooperate with it by refusing to enroll Ms. Timmerman.

If there are no scientific reasons against the inclusion of Ms. Timmerman in the trial, she cannot get treatment at home, and the sister's decision to drive from South Dakota does not seem unreasonable, then we would recommend that Dr. Diego offer Ms. Timmerman the opportunity to enroll. If Dr. Diego does decide to offer her the opportunity to enroll, he should ensure that she, her sister, and their father understand the nature of the study before they begin their long drive: that it is an experimental study whose main purpose is to obtain generalizable knowledge, that participation requires two repeat visits, and that care would not be available at the NIH should the father's condition destabilize.

## Authors' Commentary

In a subsequent conversation, Dr. Diego reported that he was able to locate a physician in South Dakota willing to provide the treatment to Virginia. With her family's support, Virginia made the decision to receive her care closer to home and ultimately did not make the trip to the NIH campus in Bethesda, Maryland. Although this case had a favorable resolution, cases like it continue to pose challenging ethical questions.

For example, it is important to ensure that clinical research does not pose inappropriate risks. This consult raised the question of the temporal and personal scope of this requirement. Should review committees, ethics consultants, and investigators consider risks that occur prior to research participation, such as the risks of driving to the research site? If one considers the risks of research to involve only the risks that result from research interventions per se, then the risks of travel typically would not constitute a risk of research. Alternatively, one might regard the risks of research, or at least the risks that IRBs should evaluate and minimize, to include all the risks that individuals will face as a result of enrolling in the study that they would not face if they decided not to enroll. While we can assume that Virginia would face some risks of driving absent the research, she would not face the risks of a 24-hour car ride.

Virginia's father similarly would not face these risks if Virginia did not pursue enrollment in Dr. Diego's protocol. Should risks that participation in research poses to third parties, especially family members, be taken into account? For example, should Dr. Diego take into account the risks to Virginia's sister of driving her car for 24 hours? While this seems at least not unreasonable, one might worry that this approach could be unfair. Would it lead, for example, to more frequent exclusion of individuals with large families? Further, it is not clear how investigators might operationalize evaluation of risks to family members. Would investigators be expected to ask potential participants how they will get to the study site and to determine what risks they and their family members will encounter? This case thereby highlights the possibility for ethics consultations to raise issues that require in-depth analysis of the kind that typically is not possible in the time frame allowed by most consultations. Ideally, the consultants would have asked Dr. Diego to give them a few years to develop an analysis of precisely which risks should be taken into account in evaluating the ethics of clinical research and determine where risks to family members as the result of driving to the research site come out in that analysis. Because ethics consultants do not have time for such analysis, they need to find ways to provide advice based on limited analysis and also to call for additional research to provide more in-depth analysis. While an emergency recommendation was rendered for Dr. Diego, the ethics consultants continued to consider the ethical implications of this case and used it as the basis for an Ethics Grand Rounds discussion at the NIH.

This consult highlights one way in which the ethics of clinical research are not exhausted by the regulations that govern it. Most regulations, including regulations in the United States, focus on evaluating and minimizing risks to research participants. It follows that there are no regulatory reasons to evaluate the risks to family members or to exclude Virginia from participating in the study. In fact, considering third-party risks is currently not accepted. It does not follow that there are no ethical concerns raised by Virginia's enrollment. There might be ethical reasons to exclude her, despite the fact that she satisfies the inclusion criteria for the study.

## ■ NOTES

1. E. J. Emanuel, D. Wendler, and C. Grady, "What Makes Clinical Research Ethical?" *Journal of the American Medical Association* 283, no. 20 (2000): 2701–2711.

2. M. Little, A. Lyerly, and R. Faden, "Pregnant Women and Medical Research: A Moral Imperative," *Bioethica Forum* 2, no. 2: 60–65; A. Lyerly, M. Little, and R. Faden, "Pregnancy and Research," *Hastings Center Report* 38, no. 6 (Nov.–Dec. 2008), inside back cover; A. Lyerly, M. Little, and R. Faden, "The Second Wave: Toward Ethical Inclusion of Pregnant Women in Clinical Research," *International Journal of Feminist Approaches to Bioethics* 1, no. 2 (Fall 2008): 5–22.

3. K. Offit et al., "The 'Duty to Warn' a Patient's Family Members about Hereditary Disease Risks," *Journal of the American Medical Association* 292, no. 12 (Sept. 22/29 2004): 1469–1473.

# 4 Conducting Research with Vulnerable Populations

U.S. federal regulations and international research ethics guidelines mandate special protections for individuals who are members of "vulnerable populations."[1] While appeals to the concept of vulnerability are common, and most people have an intuitive idea of what it means, it has proven difficult to pin down exactly what makes someone vulnerable. Consequently, determining what special protections vulnerable populations deserve and who exactly deserves them has proven elusive.

Some guidelines simply provide lists of vulnerable groups and specify that these groups should be provided with additional protections as appropriate. According to 45 CFR 46, vulnerable groups include "children, prisoners, pregnant women, mentally disabled persons, or economically or educationally disadvantaged persons."[2] The regulations go on to specify that additional safeguards should be "included in the study to protect the rights and welfare of these subjects."[3] The problem with simply enumerating groups that can be vulnerable is that the list tends to become so long that almost everyone qualifies as vulnerable. It then becomes unclear which protections could possibly be appropriate for the many and disparate groups on the list.

One way to address this concern is to provide a definition of vulnerability, which then determines which groups are in need of additional protections. On one plausible definition, vulnerable individuals are those who are unable, or less able, to provide informed consent. For example, the Belmont Report raises concerns regarding the enrollment of individuals who need extra protection due to their "dependent status and their frequently compromised capacity for free consent."[4] Other conceptions include the increased susceptibility of certain groups to research-related risks,[5] to exploitation,[6] or to just being wronged.[7] A different approach is to avoid the attempt to develop a single definition of vulnerability and to specify instead the grounds on which different groups are vulnerable and then describe which safeguards are needed to address their different vulnerabilities.[8]

Given the wide range of ways in which vulnerability has been understood, it is not surprising that ethical issues concerning vulnerable groups arise at almost every step in the research process. This is reflected by the inclusion of consultations involving vulnerable groups throughout this book. Chapter 1 includes consultations on starting research with HIV-infected individuals (*Consults 1.1 and 1.5*), individuals in developing countries (*Consults 1.2 and 1.5*), adults with potential cognitive limitations (*Consult 1.6*), and children (*Consults 1.4, 1.5, and 1.7*). Chapter 2 addresses issues related to enrolling children (*Consult 2.1*), individuals with mental illness (*Consult 2.2*), employees (*Consult 2.3*), and non-English speakers (*Consult 2.6(a)*) in research. Chapter 3 presents consultations related to minimizing risk in research involving children (*Consult 3.2*). Chapter 5 includes consultations on international research (*Consults 5.1 and 5.3*) and individuals with Alzheimer's disease (*Consult 5.4*), sickle cell disease (*Consult 5.5*), and HIV (*Consult 5.7*). Chapter 6 considers challenges that arise in research with minors (*Consults 6.2 and 6.3*), individuals who are alcohol dependent (*Consult 6.4*), or who are at the end of life (*Consults 6.5, 6.6., and 6.7*). Chapter 7 includes cases in determining posttrial obligations to children (*Consults 7.2 and 7.5*).

The present chapter presents consultations involving some key vulnerable populations: children, the cognitively impaired, patients in urgent need of treatment, the terminally ill, and the economically disadvantaged. One prominent group of vulnerable individuals not included in the present chapter is prisoners. In part, this reflects the nature of research at the National Institutes of Health (NIH) Clinical Center, which typically requires individuals to physically come to the Clinical Center. This often is not possible for prisoners. It also reflects the current state of research with prisoners. In the past, a good deal of research was conducted on prisoners since they were (literally) a captive population. Increased sensitivity to the ethical concerns raised by research with vulnerable groups led to greater protections for these individuals and attempts to protect them from exploitation by excluding them from clinical research.

Restricting the conditions under which members of vulnerable populations may be enrolled in research may have protected individuals from inappropriate enrollment. Yet this approach also raises concern that some vulnerable groups, especially prisoners, children, and pregnant women, have been excluded too often, resulting in a lack of systematic data on the conditions that affect them. Recognition of this concern has led to increased attention to the importance of finding an appropriate balance between protecting vulnerable populations and allowing research that is needed to promote their health and well-being.

Our first cases focus on children. Children can be vulnerable in several respects: they can be more susceptible to risk, they are dependent on adult caregivers, and they are incapable of giving their own consent (legally, if not always ethically). Because they are smaller and their development is not yet complete, children are often more susceptible to harm. For example, the effects of heavy metal contamination on the developing brains of fetuses and children are much worse than they are in adults. Thus, research procedures that are acceptable in adults may be excessively risky in small children. Concerns about risks for children are exacerbated by a paucity of data regarding these risks. New drugs and devices are frequently only tested in adults, even when they will be prescribed to children. For example, it is estimated that only 25% of drugs prescribed to children have been adequately tested in pediatric populations.[9] Of course, this problem cuts both ways: less research into the efficacy and safety of medicines that will be prescribed to children is both a reason to conduct more research and a reason to be cautious about the level of risk involved in research that is conducted. *Consult 4.1* concerns a study of transcranial magnetic stimulation (TMS), a technique that was proposed for studying neural development in healthy children and children with attention-deficit/hyperactivity disorder (ADHD). Safety data on TMS existed for adults, but not for children. The investigators proposed a study to evaluate the safety of TMS in children and called for ethics consultation when concerns were raised regarding the ethical appropriateness of enrolling children, especially healthy children, in the study.

The dependence of children played a key role in *Consult 4.2*. This consult involved a teenager—whom one would normally expect to have the ability to take part in decisions about his clinical care and research participation. However, the individual had an illness associated with cognitive decline, one which had recently resulted in the death of his older sister. The parents had not told the teen of his diagnosis nor his prognosis. The fact that he knew very little about his condition worried the team.

Many people who come to the Clinical Center are vulnerable because they are thought to have diminished capacity to consent. We would not want to accept the consent of someone who is incapable of understanding what is involved in research. Equally, however, we should not override the decisions of someone who actually has capacity, despite initial appearances. Along with other specialties, including psychiatry, members of the Department of Bioethics have been conducting capacity assessments since the inception of the Consultation Service. In the second part of this chapter, we explain our procedures for assessing potential participants' capacity to consent to research, their capacity to assign a surrogate decision maker to make decisions for them, and the appropriateness of surrogate decision makers. *Consult 4.3* describes an actual case in which we were part of the team assessing a potential participant and his possible surrogates.

Even when someone lacks the capacity to give consent, he or she may still be enrolled in some research by a surrogate decision maker. *Consult 4.4* illustrates some of the complications that can arise when obtaining surrogate consent. In this case, research participation looked like it might be in the interests of a critically ill individual, but her encephalitis rendered her unable to make decisions for herself. Following the process approved by the institutional review board (IRB), her husband was designated as the surrogate decision maker; however, he had not accompanied the prospective participant to the NIH, and he could not speak English. The analysis and recommendations for this consultation detail some of the procedures developed at the Clinical Center for dealing with cases like these.

*Consult 4.5* features a different type of vulnerability. An investigator studying brain tumors proposed harvesting tissue from recently deceased individuals. This would require bringing the individuals into the Clinical Center to die, and then taking brain tissue before releasing their bodies to their families. The vulnerability at issue in this case did not relate to capacity—only competent participants would be enrolled—and it was not a matter of increased susceptibility to harm, since the procedures would take place after death. But people who are dying, and their families, are already dealing with very difficult circumstances. It might seem unfair to burden them further, and inappropriate or disrespectful to make research-related requests at such a time.

The final consultation in this chapter demonstrates how the questions that arise with respect to vulnerable populations in practice can be quite different from those that are anticipated in guidelines. In *Consult 4.6* the Consultation Service was invited to help caregivers at NIH think through their obligations to an economically disadvantaged research participant. The participant was an Armenian citizen with familial Mediterranean fever (an inherited condition characterized by recurrent, painful episodes of inflammation) who did not have access to health care outside of NIH. Here, the participant's economic disadvantage did not give rise to concern that he might be exploitatively enrolled into research, the standard concern raised by this vulnerable group. Rather, the concern was that there did not seem to be any options for discharging him from the study in a way that would continue to address his health care needs. Consults 7.2 and 7.4 raise similar issues.

## Capacity Assessment Procedures

Some potential participants require additional protections because they are unable to give informed consent to research participation. Though the most obvious safeguard would seem to be to exclude such individuals, some research offers the potential for clinical benefit to participants, and other socially important research can be conducted only with individuals who are unable to give valid consent. As noted earlier, the U.S. federal regulations provide additional safeguards for research with children, prisoners, and pregnant women and fetuses. In contrast, there are no specific regulations for research with adults who cannot provide informed consent, beyond the possibility of obtaining consent from the subject's legally authorized representative. In the absence of more specific guidelines, some institutions have developed their own guidance.

The NIH Clinical Center developed a policy for research with cognitively impaired adults in 1987. These were likely some of the first guidelines of their kind. This policy was revised in 2003 and 2008, and *Consult 4.3* was conducted under the 2008 version of the policy. Following these latest revisions, the NIH Clinical Center developed instruments to assist consultants with implementing the protections called for by the policy. The policy stipulates that individuals should be evaluated when questions arise regarding their ability to provide initial or ongoing consent. This evaluation can be conducted by members of the research team or by the Ability to Consent Assessment Team (ACAT), an NIH Clinical Center group constituted to be independent of the research team that has been trained to evaluate individuals' ability to consent.

The ACAT's evaluation of an individual's ability to consent focuses on whether the person is able to consent to a specific protocol. The question is therefore not whether the individual has some general level of cognitive ability, but whether the person is able to understand and make an autonomous decision about participation in that study. It is thought that people who cannot give their own valid consent may still retain the ability to assign a surrogate decision maker. Very little has been written, however, on what is required to assign a surrogate for research purposes, and many research institutions simply accept surrogates who have been assigned to make clinical decisions. The NIH process stipulates that in order to assign a surrogate for research, individuals must be able to understand at least that *(1)* the surrogate will make decisions for him or her, *(2)* the decisions will be about undergoing procedures that may involve discomfort and risk, and *(3)* some of the procedures may have no chance of helping the individual but will be done to gather information that might benefit others.

One might argue that whomever an individual appoints should be allowed to make decisions according to his or her own lights. If I consent to be treated according to the decisions made by my surrogate, then the decisions my surrogate makes should be regarded as legitimate. Empirical studies find a wide range of views on the extent to which people would allow their surrogates leeway in making decisions for them. Many adults endorse significant leeway for their surrogates. These individuals appear willing to accept almost whatever decision their surrogate makes. However, many others are not willing to grant their surrogates significant leeway, and some do not want their surrogates to have any leeway beyond implementing their known treatment preferences.[10] In this context, NIH policy mandates an assessment of the appropriateness of surrogates. A determination that a surrogate is appropriate requires finding at least that the surrogate *(1)* understands the study involves research; *(2)* understands the risks, potential benefits, and alternatives to the study; and *(3)* has sufficient reason to believe participation in the study is consistent with the individual's preferences and values. Finally, the NIH policy requires that assent (i.e., affirmative agreement) should be obtained from research participants who are capable of providing it (regardless of the inability to give fully informed consent), and such participants' objections (dissent) should be respected. Evaluations of dissent can be especially difficult in individuals who are not able to provide informed consent. Often these individuals have difficulty communicating, and evaluation may have to be based on body language or other signs.

## CONSULT 4.1: EXPOSING CHILDREN TO RISK WHEN THERE IS NO PROSPECT OF DIRECT BENEFIT

### Reason for Consult

Dr. Michael Garnett, an NIH investigator, asked the Consultation Service to participate in a multidisciplinary meeting to discuss the appropriateness of exposing healthy children to research risks.

### Narrative

A meeting was called involving the investigators, members of the IRB, hearing consultants, and the Consultation Service to discuss Dr. Garnett's current research. At the start of the meeting, Dr. Garnett explained that he is studying ADHD in children using TMS, which is a procedure that uses magnetic fields to stimulate nerve cells in the brain. The study is attempting to identify brain changes associated with ADHD by comparing the results of TMS in healthy children to the results in children with ADHD.

The TMS procedure produces an acoustic artifact of approximately 120 decibels (dB) that has been shown to result in hearing damage in rabbits when performed without ear protection. It appears that no damage occurs in rabbits when earplugs are used. Previous studies have found no damage from TMS to the hearing of adults when earplugs are used. No studies looking specifically at the effects on hearing have been conducted in children. NIH investigators recently proposed an in-depth safety study to evaluate TMS in children, including healthy children. The proposed study would include hearing protection for all research participants, which would reduce the acoustic artifact to approximately 100 dB.

During the meeting, concern was expressed about the appropriateness of enrolling healthy children in the study. The U.S. federal regulations allow children, including healthy children, to be enrolled in research that does not offer them the potential for direct benefit when the risks are "minimal." The regulations define research risks as minimal when they do not exceed the risks "ordinarily encountered in daily life or during the performance of routine physical or psychological examinations or tests." In particular, questions were raised regarding whether the study was minimal risk, and whether it is appropriate to include children in research when there is no chance of benefit for them, even in the future.

### Analysis and Recommendations

There was agreement during the meeting that it is difficult to be confident of the risks associated with the safety study given the lack of data on TMS in children.

The safety study has specifically been proposed to provide such data, but the absence of data raises ethical concern over whether the study is acceptable.

While the precise risks of the study are unclear, it was agreed that participation in the study poses risks to hearing that are similar to and not greater than the risks posed to children's hearing by numerous sources in daily life. The fact that the risks of the TMS are no greater than the risks children ordinarily face implies that the study poses minimal risk and can be approved under the U.S. regulations for healthy children.

Even when studies pose minimal risk, it is important to reduce the risks to the extent possible. Thus, the Consultation Service recommended that the investigators consider whether it would be possible to further protect the children's hearing during the TMS in a way that could be replicated by studies using TMS. In addition, although there are no systematic data on TMS in children, it may be that other investigators have in fact conducted TMS in children. Hence, before conducting the study the investigators should attempt to determine whether other investigators have experience using TMS in children.

Some participants in the meeting expressed the view that a safety study would be more problematic in healthy children than in affected children. In particular, children with ADHD have at least some chance of benefitting in the future from the results of the safety study. At the same time, involving children with ADHD or some other condition in the study may increase the potential for therapeutic misconception, which is the mistaken belief that research procedures are in fact simply clinical care. The Consultation Service did not see a compelling argument for including or excluding healthy children. There are valid ethical arguments for enrolling both healthy and sick children, and there is no consensus in the field. In such cases, investigators' preferences are morally relevant and can be considered in the decision-making process.

## Authors' Commentary

The question raised by this consult, whether it is acceptable to expose children to research risks without the potential for clinical benefit, is one of the most enduring in research ethics. The U.S. research regulations, like the regulations in a number of other countries worldwide, allow children to be enrolled in research that does not offer the potential for clinical benefit when the risks are no greater than the risks ordinarily encountered in daily life.

It was noted in this consult that children are often exposed to sounds of 100 dB. This level is frequently present and even exceeded when individuals listen to music through headphones or at concerts, and when mowing the lawn. It follows that the risks of this study can be approved in children, including healthy children. As was also recognized in the consult report, however, the fact the study legally may be approved does not imply that it should be approved. The U.S. regulations define when IRBs may approve research. Not all research that satisfies the regulations is ethically appropriate. With respect to the present consult, there are some risks which are ordinarily encountered in daily life which seem unacceptable in the research context. For example, some children are raised close to environmental health hazards. This fact does not imply that it would be acceptable to conduct research that exposes children to the same level of risks. Instead, we would say that such risks are unacceptable and should be avoided in both contexts. This line of reasoning has led to substantial debate in the literature over which risks in daily life offer appropriate comparators for evaluating the risks of pediatric research.[11] In the present case, there was disagreement over whether the fact children ordinarily listen to music at 100 dB implies that research which involves noise at the same level is appropriate.

The present consult also addressed whether it is better to conduct research that does not offer the potential for clinical benefit with children who have the condition or illness under study, as opposed to conducting the research with healthy children. The U.S. federal regulations allow all children to be enrolled in research that poses minimal risks. In addition, the regulations allow research that poses a "minor increase" over minimal risk when it has the potential to yield generalizable knowledge about the participating children's disorder or condition. The justification for including the latter category might be based on a belief that it is more problematic to expose healthy children to research risks. Yet one might also argue that the fact some children have a disorder or condition provides a reason to provide them with extra protection, not a reason to subject them to additional risks. Subsequent research by members of the Department of Bioethics has explored this issue.[12]

## CONSULT 4.2: INFORMING A MINOR OF HIS DIAGNOSIS

### Reason for Consult

A research team requested an ethics consultation to assist them in thinking through the ethical issues involved in the case of a 17-year-old research participant who is not aware of his diagnosis or prognosis.

### Narrative

The Consultation Service met with several members of the research team to discuss the case of Jaime Gonzalez, a teenager with a diagnosis of LaFora's disease. LaFora's disease is a disorder in which polysaccharides deposit throughout the body. Deposition in the central nervous system (CNS) results in seizures, muscle spasms, and cognitive decline. The disease generally becomes evident in children at a relatively young age and most affected individuals die from complications in their late teens or early twenties.

Jaime began manifesting symptoms of LaFora's disease 1 year ago. Since then, he has started to experience seizures, difficulties with motor coordination, and decreasing strength in his upper and lower extremities. Jaime is participating in a research protocol testing the effects of a low-glucose diet on the progression of LaFora's disease. During the course of Jaime's research participation, it became evident to the clinical and research staff that Jaime has limited knowledge about his condition.

Jaime's sister died 2 months ago—at the age of 23—from complications of LaFora's disease. Her final years of life were quite difficult for the family, which caused Jaime's parents to decide against informing him that he has the same disease as his sister. According to the team and family, Jaime has not asked any questions about his disease, nor any questions about his prognosis. Nonetheless, members of the research team describe themselves as extremely uncomfortable with the situation.

## Analysis and Recommendations

While it is generally desirable that information not be withheld from 17 year olds, it is acceptable that this individual has been given limited information and has not been informed that he has the same illness that led to his sister's recent death. However, the Consultation Service recommends that if he asks questions about his own illness, his questions should be answered truthfully. In general, what Jaime ought to be told and how it should be disclosed is a decision that should be discussed with the family. The level of cognitive capacity he has at the time he asks will be an important factor in deciding what and how to tell him.

## Authors' Commentary

The ethics consultants recommended that the team need not inform Jaime of his diagnosis. However, if he asked directly, the consultants stated that the team should not lie to him. As we discuss later, this recommendation may have been due in part to the recognition that there can be more reason to provide a piece of information when a research participant requests it. In addition, the consultants' recommendations highlight a common view that there is an important ethical difference between withholding relevant information from someone and intentionally providing him with inaccurate information (see also Consult 3.5).

This case shows the importance of evaluating the circumstances and details of individual cases when providing ethics consultation. The consultants recognized that there is wide agreement on the importance of giving individuals accurate information. This is reflected in the view that minors typically should provide assent or positive agreement to their research enrollment and that this agreement should be based on an understanding of the relevant details, to the extent that the individual is able to understand them. In the present case, that principle would imply that Jaime should be informed that the study is designed to evaluate the impact of a particular diet on LaFora's disease and that he is being considered for the study because he has the disease himself. However, the typical teenager is one who is maturing and will develop increasing maturity and cognitive abilities over the coming years. In that case, there is a greater need to prepare him for adulthood when he will make his own decisions and consequently a greater need to inform him accurately. Jaime, in contrast, was almost certain to experience declining cognitive abilities. Hence, it may be that the principles regarding accurate information which apply to most 17 year olds do not apply in his case. In addition, the moral reasons in favor of informing this young man needed to be considered in the context of his having a sister who had recently died of the disease and the impact that such information might have on him. One way to understand this issue is in terms of the possible conflict between respecting individuals' ability to make their own decisions and protecting their interests.

In deciding whether to withhold information, one strategy is to try to discern whether the research participant wants to be informed. Typically, individuals should be provided with the information they want about the study in question, both as a way of respecting their preferences and because the information may be relevant to their decision about whether to participate in the study. Of course, the team could not directly ask Jaime whether he wanted to know that he had LaFora's disease without alerting him to his diagnosis. An alternative is to base one's approach on the behavior of the individual. In this case, Jaime had not asked any questions. One might regard that as a sign he did not want to know his diagnosis or prognosis. But this is not the only possible explanation of his silence. For example, it is possible that he assumed that since he had not been told his diagnosis that he had a treatable disease. Alternatively, he may suspect or have realized his condition. This possibility is given greater credence by the fact that he was experiencing symptoms and receiving treatment. Thus, failing to engage the issue might have left him isolated and unable to discuss his concerns with his family and care team.

An additional reason to provide teenagers, especially older ones, with accurate information is the assumption that once they become autonomous adults, there will be an obligation to inform them truthfully so that they can take control of their own medical care. Individuals who are provided with inaccurate information throughout their teen years and then suddenly given the truth are likely to respond negatively. This possibility provides an additional reason not to deceive, albeit one that may not have been applicable to the present case.

## CONSULT 4.3: ASSIGNMENT OF A SURROGATE DECISION MAKER BY A COGNITIVELY IMPAIRED RESEARCH PARTICIPANT

### Reason for Consult

Amir Zahid is being considered for a study which includes an IRB mandated requirement that all prospective participants be evaluated to determine whether they are capable of giving informed consent, and, if found unable to consent, evaluated to determine whether they are capable of designating a surrogate decision maker.

### The Narrative

The Consultation Service attending and fellow met with Mr. Zahid in his hospital room. He is a 20-year-old male with Fragile X (a disease associated with cognitive impairments). He lives with his two biological parents who brought him to the NIH for participation in a study that evaluates and is designed to better characterize Fragile X. The study has the potential to gather important information about the disease, but it does not offer participants the potential for clinical benefit. The IRB has mandated that potential research participants be evaluated by an independent team prior to being enrolled in the study. Individuals may be enrolled only if they can consent for themselves or if they have an appropriate surrogate who gives permission for them.

Mr. Zahid has an unremarkable medical history. He does not have a legal guardian or a previously appointed surrogate. In speaking with Mr. Zahid, the consultants find that he is willing to be at the NIH and supportive of the idea of doing things to help others. Mr. Zahid understands some aspects of the study but he does not understand enough to give valid consent. In particular, while Mr. Zahid understands the procedures involved, he does not understand the risks posed by the procedures (such as radiation risks). Based on what he can understand, Mr. Zahid assents to be in the study. Mr. Zahid's parents report that the procedures will not bother him and that he will emphatically let the staff know if he wants to stop being in the study or does not want to do something.

Because Mr. Zahid cannot give his own consent, the consultants considered next whether he could appoint a surrogate decision maker. Individuals who cannot give their own valid consent may in some cases retain the ability to assign a surrogate. Their discussion with Mr. Zahid proceeded as follows:

> Bioethics Consultant (BC): "Is there anyone you trust to help decide whether you should participate in research here?"

Amir Zahid (AZ): "Yes, my girlfriend. I really love her. She lives in Mendoza."

BC: "Could your girlfriend come here and help you decide whether to be in the research study?"

AZ: "No, she is far away, but that is okay. I can make my own decisions."

BC: "Who helps you make other important decisions?"

AZ: "I do."

BC: "Anyone else?"

AZ: "No, I can make my own decisions."

BC: "Is there anyone here that you trust who could help you decide whether to be in the research study?"

AZ: "No, ask me. I can make my own decisions."

BC: "Do your parents help you make important decisions, like going to the doctor and taking medicines?"

AZ: "Yes."

BC: "Do you think your parents help you make good decisions?"

AZ: "Yes."

BC: "Would your parents be good people to help you decide whether to be in the research study here?"

AZ: "Yes."

BC: "Do you trust your parents to make good decisions about whether you are in research?"

AZ: "Yes."

BC: "Here is a form you can sign to name your parents to help you make decisions about being in research here." (Provides form).

AZ: "Okay." (Signs form).

The consultants proceed to evaluate the appropriateness of Mr. Zahid's parents to serve as his surrogate decision makers. According to NIH policy, the determination that a surrogate is appropriate requires a finding that at least the following conditions are met: *(1)* the surrogate understands the study involves research; *(2)* the surrogate understands the risks, potential benefits, and alternatives to the study; and *(3)* the surrogate has sufficient reason to believe participation in the study is consistent with the individual's preferences and values. Discussion with the parents makes it clear that they meet all three conditions.

## Analysis and Recommendations

Based on these findings, the bioethics consultant determined that Mr. Zahid could designate his parents to be his surrogate decision makers with regard to his research participation. In addition, Mr. Zahid's parents are appropriate surrogates and can enroll him in this research study at the NIH. Finally, his assent also should be obtained prior to enrolment, and during his participation in the study.

## Authors' Commentary

Because the federal regulations do not provide specific guidance for research with adults who cannot give their own informed consent, there are no regulatory standards for who can serve as a surrogate for research purposes. NIH policy allows next of kin surrogates to make decisions in some cases but requires evaluation of their appropriateness. In addition, for research that poses more than minimal risk and does not offer a compensating potential for clinical benefit, NIH policy allows only surrogates who have been assigned by the individual to make decisions.

The present consultation highlights the importance of process, in addition to having the necessary regulations and guidelines. One might be concerned that, in the present case, the consultant inappropriately directed the choice of surrogate, effectively vetoing the choice of the girlfriend on practical grounds and recommending the parents instead. The young man who prompted this consult seemed clearly to endorse his parents as surrogates, but it was not his idea, at least initially. Even if one is not concerned in Mr. Zahid's case, there is clearly the possibility that how the options are presented and framed can influence the outcome of ethics consultations.

Another issue that arises in cases like these is the extent to which an impaired individual should have a say in his research participation. Most commentators agree that individuals who cannot consent should be informed to the extent they can understand and should be able to make decisions based on that level of understanding. This view is reflected in the NIH requirement that assent be obtained from those who retain the ability to provide it. This requirement highlights the fact that the appeal to a surrogate does not imply that the participant is to be excluded from the decision-making process. The surrogate does not always make decisions instead of the participant. Rather, the surrogate and participant, when possible, make decisions in tandem. This approach is important for respecting the individual and allowing him to continue to have some control over his life. In some cases, however, this approach raises the challenge of determining how to proceed in the face of a disagreement between a surrogate and participant. Typically, the default is that opposition from either party results in exclusion from research, although one might worry that this approach could preclude noncomprehending adults from being enrolled in research that offers an important potential for clinical benefit which they are not able to understand and which is unavailable outside of the research context.

## CONSULT 4.4: CONSENT FOR RESEARCH IN AN EMERGENCY

### Reason for Consult

Dr. Anna Rodriguez, a principal investigator, contacted the Consultation Service to discuss methods for obtaining informed consent from a cognitively impaired individual.

### Narrative

Ose Bannister is a 32-year-old female with cognitive impairment, presumed due to encephalitis (inflammation of the brain). Her family wishes to enroll her in a placebo-controlled trial of intravenous immunoglobulin G (IVIG). IVIG has shown some efficacy in animals and in a few individuals who received it on a compassionate basis (a special mechanism through which patients may obtain a drug that is not yet licensed), but it has not been approved for use in the United States. Data suggest that IVIG is relatively nontoxic, although these data are mostly from different patient populations.

Dr. Rodriguez reminded the Consultation Service team that the IRB classified the trial as posing a minor increase over minimal risk with a prospect of direct benefit. Following a previous research bioethics consultation, the IRB had waived (NIH Clinical Center policy) MAS 87-4 which, at the time, stipulated that only subject assigned surrogates could enroll individuals in research that posed greater than minimal risk, even when the research offered the prospect of clinical benefit to the subjects. The IRB stipulated that the closest first-degree relative could make enrollment decisions, even if not assigned by the prospective participant.

Upon her arrival at the clinical center, Mrs. Bannister was accompanied by three family members, including a sister. Her husband, who qualified as the surrogate based on the IRB-mandated hierarchy, remained at home with their children. He speaks Swahili but not English. Dr. Rodriguez contacted the Consultation Service to determine the best method for obtaining consent for Mrs. Bannister's admission to the Clinical Center as well as her enrollment in the IVIG protocol, if Mrs. Bannister is eligible.

### Analysis and Recommendations

The Consultation Service makes the following recommendations:

1) Fax the admission consent and the consent for research to the patient's husband.
2) By telephone, Dr. Rodriguez should take the husband through the two consent forms using a family member to translate.

3) Dr. Rodriguez should answer any questions, solicit the husband's permission, and have a witness who is with the husband sign the consent forms (this is per federal regulations on obtaining oral consent) and fax them back to the NIH.
4) Dr. Rodriguez should then call the husband directly using an independent translator, again explain the essential elements of informed consent, answer any questions, and again solicit the husband's consent.
5) The translator should have the husband write down in Swahili that the essential elements of consent were explained and that he consents, sign this statement, and fax it back to the NIH (this "short form" is also per federal regulations).
6) Per NIH policy for consent over the telephone, Dr. Rodriguez will write up this plan and solicit the agreement of her Institute Director and the IRB.
7) We suggest that the Dr. Rodriguez ask the husband to assign a family member who is with Mrs. Bannister at the NIH as the surrogate to make day-to-day decisions, although "major" decisions should still be made by the husband.

## Authors' Commentary

The NIH Clinical Center has policies detailing the conditions for obtaining oral (instead of written) consent, for unexpectedly having to obtain consent from someone who does not speak English, and for obtaining consent from a proxy decision maker. This consult was complicated principally because it was necessary to implement all three of these policies simultaneously.

The oral consent process (based on the U.S. federal regulations) requires that a written summary of the information that the person obtaining consent will provide to the potential research participant (or surrogate decision maker, as in this case) be approved by the IRB and then signed both by the person obtaining consent and by a witness to the oral presentation. It then requires that the person giving consent sign a short written consent form that states the following:

> Before you decide whether to participate, the researcher will tell you about *(1)* the purposes of the research; *(2)* how much of your time the research will take; *(3)* what research procedures you will undergo; *(4)* the risks to you of taking part in the research; *(5)* any benefits of the research to you or to other people; *(6)* how your confidentiality will be protected; and *(7)* what other options you may have instead of taking part in this research.

This form is available at NIH in a variety of languages, and it should be signed by the person giving consent in his or her native language.

Finally, the consult report mentions Medical Administrative Series Policy 87.4, which governs "Research Involving Adults Who Are or May Be Unable to Consent" (see Appendix). Some details of this policy were already explained in the introduction to this chapter. A previous consultation called by the investigators for this protocol had considered what to do for potential participants who could not consent, had no surrogate, and were not able to assign one. According to the policy at the time that consult was requested, enrollment of impaired participants in "more than minimal risk" research with a prospect of benefit (like the current case) required a bioethics consultation and a court appointed surrogate decision maker. The Consultation Service concluded that court appointment of a surrogate was not necessary for the present protocol and proposed the following:

> Rather, in certain circumstances, it may be acceptable for first-degree relatives (spouses, children, parents) or domestic partners to act as surrogate decision makers for impaired patients without involving the court.
>
> When relying upon a surrogate who has not been formally appointed by the patient or the court, we recommend an independent assessment of the surrogate's capacity as a research decision maker and his or her comprehension of the study. In this case, the assessment of the surrogate should include the following: *(1)* why the surrogate is interested in enrolling the subject in research; *(2)* what decision the surrogate thinks the subject would make about enrollment in research, if he or she were able; and *(3)* whether the surrogate understands that at the NIH he or she may have the option to enroll in a study of an experimental drug or in a study in which the subject will receive clinical management.

The present consultation, as well as several others, raised the question of whether the requirement of a court appointed guardian was an appropriate protection for individuals who could not provide informed consent, did not have a surrogate, and could not appoint one. This requirement was developed when institutions first began to rely on surrogates to make research decisions for cognitively impaired adults. The view was that an independent body should appoint the surrogate when research enrollment posed greater than minimal risk, even when it offered the potential for important clinical benefit. However, experience with this requirement led individuals at the NIH, including the members of the Consultation Service, to the view that this requirement constituted more of a burden on the family than a protection for the research participant. It forced families, who often lived at a distance, to remain in the area for weeks to months, hire a lawyer, and go to court. In the end, the burdens and costs did not seem justified, especially given that the courts typically appointed the next of kin as decision maker. This led to a change in NIH policy to allow decision making in some cases by close next of kin without a court appointment. This change lessened the burden on families, but it also decreased the independence of those who were evaluating the appropriateness of the next-of-kin surrogate. Under the revised policy, this determination is made by ethicists from the Consultation Service who are independent of the research study in question and often independent of the institute where the investigators work. However, they are still employees of the NIH. Precisely what level of independence is sufficient in this case remains an open question.

## CONSULT 4.5: RESEARCH WITH THE TERMINALLY ILL

### Reason for Consult

Dr. Fred Richmond, the principal investigator, called the Consultation Service to discuss issues relating to a protocol he is designing which involves the recently deceased.

### Narrative

In his conversation with the Consultation Service attending and fellow, Dr. Richmond explained that recent analysis of cells from gliomas (a type of brain tumor) suggests that the cancerous cells are neural stem cells that have accrued successive genetic mutations over time. It may therefore be useful to compare the genetic profiles of cancerous cells to "normal" neural stem cells from cancer patients. For glioma patients, the cause of death is not the bulk of the tumor—this is usually reduced adequately by neurosurgery—but cancerous cellular infiltrates of otherwise healthy regions of the brain. It would therefore also be useful to analyze these infiltrating cells in order to identify molecular targets for potential therapeutic agents.

Unfortunately, it is impossible to gather samples of normal neural stem cells or infiltrating cells from living patients without damaging normal areas of the brain. Furthermore, isolation of these cell populations from frozen samples is impossible. Therefore, Dr. Richmond argued that the only method of answering important questions related to glioma development and pathology is to harvest brain tissue from recently (within 1 hour) deceased individuals with glioma.

Tissue harvesting would involve bringing terminally ill individuals into the Clinical Center to die. Dr. Richmond recognizes that this raises important issues concerning the proper treatment of the dying and the recently deceased as well as their families. Nevertheless, Dr. Richmond noted that he would likely need only 5–10 brains to address the relevant scientific questions. This, coupled with the desire of a large number of individuals to donate tissue for research, should make recruitment relatively easy.

## Analysis and Recommendations

Given the significant symbolic value of the brain and the often delicate issues related to caring for the dying and their families, it will be important to implement the protocol in a manner that is sensitive and responsive to the concerns of all persons involved. Most of the potential concerns with this protocol involve the sensibilities of medical staff, research participants, and their families. Therefore, the greater the involvement of these parties in the protocol's development and during the course of its implementation, the better.

1) Recommendations for protocol development:
   The consult team suggests that prospective tissue donors and their families be consulted about the research plan, including their preferences for removal of the individual's body from the hospital room and its potential return. Dr. Richmond could also discuss the protocol with the nursing staff as well as the pain and palliative care team to solicit input on appropriate methods for dealing with the family and the body. Overnight stays should be made available for the family of anyone admitted under this protocol.
2) Recommendations for recruitment:
   The consult team and Dr. Richmond also resolved that (*a*) in order to facilitate family visiting, prospective participants would be recruited who are local to the Clinical Center, (*b*) only competent adults would be recruited, in order to preempt concerns over enrolling pediatric and incompetent participants, and (*c*) the research team would ensure that potential enrollees have access to expert end-of-life care outside the protocol in order to preempt potential concerns over undue inducement to enrollment. Participants should also be provided high-quality end-of-life care in the protocol to preempt concerns over exploitation of these individuals.
3) Recommendations for protocol implementation:
   The consult team and Dr. Richmond agreed that cardiac arrest should be used as the primary criterion for determination of death, as it avoids making judgments related to the brain activity of an already neurologically compromised individual. At the time of informed consent, families will be asked about their preferences for removal of their family member's body from the hospital room after death as well as for the return of the body after harvesting. These preferences would be reviewed, and amended if necessary, when the participant is admitted to the Clinical Center. Families would not be required to sign an additional consent document at the time of death, but they would be able to opt out of the harvesting procedure if they so chose.

## Authors' Commentary

There is nothing ethically problematic *in principle* about asking people to donate tissue for research after their deaths; however, in practice, a request to harvest parts of someone's brain so soon after death might constitute a further burden for an individual already dealing with a terrible illness and the impending end of life, and for family members who are experiencing the death of someone they love. This explains the focus in the analysis and recommendations on making sure that the research procedures were sensitive to the preferences of everyone involved, both in the development of the protocol and its implementation.

One possible objection to the analysis and recommendations is that families may opt out of the harvesting procedure after their loved one's death. Thus, some families might choose not to donate despite the fact that the decedent had clearly expressed a desire to do so.

## ■ CONSULT 4.6: CARING FOR THE ECONOMICALLY DISADVANTAGED

### Reason for Consult

Fiona Klein, a nurse, called on behalf of the primary care team to invite the Consultation Service to participate in a multidisciplinary meeting being held to develop a plan of care for a financially disadvantaged research participant.

### Narrative

The multidisciplinary meeting was held to discuss the case of Ara Petrosian, a 22-year-old Armenian citizen diagnosed with familial Mediterranean fever when he was in his mid-teens. Mr. Petrosian has widespread amyloidosis (abnormal protein deposits) in his heart, lungs, liver, and gastrointestinal system. He has a diagnosis of cardiomyopathy, which is currently stable. He receives dialysis three times a week and is fed through a gastric feeding tube.

The primary care team has increasing concerns about what resources should be provided to Mr. Petrosian. He currently needs two dental root canals, and the Clinical Center does not provide this service. Mr. Petrosian does not have insurance, and because he is not a U.S. citizen, he does not qualify for most public programs. If the primary care team is unable to find resources to pay for the root canals shortly, the teeth will have to be extracted at the Clinical Center. Mr. Petrosian and his father are apparently opposed to this option. Additionally, the primary care team expressed concern about how to continue paying for Mr. Petrosian's dialysis and other treatments.

Mr. Petrosian and his parents are staying at the Children's Inn (an inn on the NIH campus reserved for research participants and their families), and Mr. Petrosian's parents have been receiving food vouchers from the social workers. Next Friday marks the 120th night that Mr. Petrosian and his family have been at the Inn, and 120 nights is the maximum stay according to the Inn's policy. Mr. Petrosian has an uncle back home in Armenia who is willing and able to devote thousands—but not tens of thousands—of dollars to his medical care, if necessary. According to social workers present at the meeting, the parents state that they are unable to afford food and lodging off campus. The primary care team reports that the parents have been manipulative and appear to be suspicious that they and Mr. Petrosian are getting less because they are not Americans.

Five clinical options were presented and discussed by the team:

1) Mr. Petrosian could be transferred from NIH and potentially be sent back to Armenia to die at home.
2) Mr. Petrosian could remain as he is now, receiving hemodialysis, tube feedings, and experimental treatment to manage his serum amyloid (SAA) level.
3) Mr. Petrosian could receive a kidney transplant.
4) Mr. Petrosian could receive a kidney and heart transplant.
5) Mr. Petrosian could receive a kidney, heart, and bone marrow transplant.

The ethics consultants were asked for their input on the main ethical issues raised by Mr. Petrosian's case.

## Analysis and Recommendations

For now, the Consultation Service judges option 2 preferable. Long-term treatment to manage his SAA level could lead to some improvement of cardiac function, and this could eventually facilitate a kidney transplant. Continued treatment at NIH is warranted not only for beneficent reasons but also in order to answer scientific questions about treatment of amyloidosis and about the potential for organ damage from amyloidosis to be reversed with sustained normalization of SAA levels.

Kidney transplantation would be an appropriate goal. This would allow treatment with colchicine, the standard of care for familial Mediterranean fever, and unlike the experimental treatment, Mr. Petrosian could potentially obtain and afford colchicine should he return home to Armenia.

The family's preference would be for Mr. Petrosian to remain as in inpatient at NIH for the 6–12 months that would be necessary to determine whether there is a continued response to the experimental treatment. However, demand for inpatient beds and rooms at the Children's Inn exceeds supply. The clinical team appears to be willing and able to provide for Mr. Petrosian's clinical needs, including the experimental treatment and dialysis (although there are some concerns about personnel limitations for prolonged dialysis). The team is not, however, prepared to provide open-ended living expenses. The group discussed setting a transition timetable for Mr. Petrosian's family to learn to provide for daily care as an outpatient and to find alternative living arrangements.

The principal investigator will meet with the family and set a firm date after which they will no longer be able to stay at the Children's Inn or receive food vouchers. Kitchen facilities at the Inn will remain available for food preparation. The social worker will explore ways in which the family can reach out to and potentially be assisted by local community groups. The NIH patient representative, a designated liaison between research participants and the Clinical Center, is prepared to discuss concerns with the family and to emphasize that Mr. Petrosian is receiving care comparable to or better than most American citizens can access.

## Authors' Commentary

Though in this case the Consultation Service was used more as a sounding board for the care teams as they made their decisions than as a source of independent recommendations, it illustrates a relatively common dilemma that arises at the NIH Clinical Center. Ill research participants may not have access to health care elsewhere. Some of these participants are uninsured residents of the United States. Others, like Mr. Petrosian, are from abroad and would not get the level of care that they need back in their own countries. Naturally, the researchers and medical staff who look after these individuals feel an obligation to ensure that they continue to receive the best medical attention possible. This issue is considered at length in Chapter 5: Balancing Clinical Research and Clinical Care (see *Consult 5.3*) and in Chapter 7: Ending Research.

Research participants who lack access to health care outside of research are often considered more vulnerable to exploitation as a consequence: if they desperately need health care, they may agree to unfair or inappropriate research burdens and risks. But, perhaps even more than for other vulnerable groups, there is a counterbalancing danger in excluding them from research. If excluded, they are still unable to get the care they need; at least in research they could get that. The challenge that bioethics consultants face involves helping investigators design and execute studies in ways that benefit those people who need help the most without taking unfair advantage of their needs.

## NOTES

1. U.S. Code of Federal Regulations, Title 45 Part 46, "Protection of Human Subjects," 2005; World Medical Association, Declaration of Helsinki, 2008, Article 9; Council for International Organizations of Medical Sciences (CIOMS), "International Ethical Guidelines for Biomedical Research Involving Human Subjects," 2002, Guideline 13.
2. 45 CFR 46.111(a)(3).
3. 45 CFR 46.111(b).
4. The National Commission for the Protection of Human Subjects of Biomedical and Behavioral Research, *The Belmont Report: Ethical Principles and Guidelines for the Protection of Human Subjects of Research* (Washington, D.C.: Department of Health, Education, and Welfare, 1979).
5. Levine et al., "The Limitations of 'Vulnerability' as a Protection for Human Research Participants," *The American Journal of Bioethics* 4, no. 3 (2004): 44–49.
6. R. Macklin, "Bioethics, Vulnerability, and Protection," *Bioethics* 17, no. 5–6 (2003): 472–486.
7. S. Hurst, "Vulnerability in Research and Health Care; Describing the Elephant in the Room?" *Bioethics* 22, no. 4 (2008): 191–202.
8. C. C. Denny and C. Grady, "Clinical Research with Economically Disadvantaged Populations," *Journal of Medical Ethics* 33 (2007): 382–385.
9. R. Roberts, W. Rodriquez, D. Murphy, and T. Crescenzi, "Pediatric Drug Labeling: Improving the Safety and Efficacy of Pediatric Therapies," *Journal of the American Medical Association* 290 (2003): 905–911.
10. L. Ayalon, "Willingness to Participate in Alzheimer Disease Research and Attitudes Towards Proxy-Informed Consent: Results from the Health and Retirement Study," *American Journal of Geriatric Psychiatry* 17 (2009): 65–74; J. Karlawish, J. Rubright, D. Casarett, M. Cary, T. Ten Have, and P. Sankar, "Older Adults' Attitudes Toward Enrollment of Non-competent Subjects Participating in Alzheimer's Research," *American Journal of Psychiatry* 166 (2009): 182–188; S. Y. H. Kim, H. M. Kim, K. M. Langa, J. H. T. Karlawish, D. S. Knopman, and P. S. Appelbaum, "Surrogate Consent for Dementia Research: A National Survey of Older Americans," *Neurology* 72 (2009): 149–155.
11. D. B. Resnik, "Eliminating the Daily Risks Standard from the Definition of Minimal Risk," *Journal of Medical Ethics* 31 (2005): 35–38; D. Wendler and L. Glantz, "A New Standard for Assessing the Risks of Pediatric Research: Pro and Con," *Journal of Pediatrics* 150 (2007): 579–582.
12. S. Shah and D. Wendler, "Interpretation of the Subjects' Condition Requirement: A Legal Perspective," *Journal of Law, Medicine, & Ethics* 38, no. 2 (2010): 365–373; D. Wendler, S. Shah, A. Whittle, and B. Wilfond, "Non-Beneficial Research with Individuals Who Cannot Consent: Is It Ethically Better to Enroll Healthy or Affected Individuals?" *IRB: Ethics and Human Research* 25 (2003): 1–4.

# 5 Balancing Clinical Research and Clinical Care

In the course of clinical research, healthy volunteers and patient participants alike may present with preexisting health problems or develop new health problems that require medical attention and treatment. A requirement of ethical research is respect for the rights and welfare of participants; this requirement can involve monitoring participants throughout their research participation, notifying them of changes in their clinical status, and providing them with appropriate treatment, if necessary.[1] There are, however, numerous ways to interpret and fulfill this obligation—one of several obligations that research teams must thoughtfully balance. The consultation reports collected in this chapter reveal some of the ethical challenges that can arise when participants' clinical needs are in tension with clinical research. In particular, this chapter will focus on ancillary care obligations, management of incidental findings, enrollment of the uninsured in clinical trials, the therapeutic misconception, off-study access to experimental treatments, and noncompliance with clinically indicated care.

Appreciating the differences between clinical care and clinical research can be difficult for participants as well as for clinical researchers who may struggle to reconcile their roles as health care providers and researchers. Although there is no ironclad distinction between clinical care and clinical research, there are significant ways in which they differ.[2] First, the goal of clinical care is to benefit the current patient. By contrast, the goal of clinical research is to benefit future patients by advancing knowledge of disease, palliative treatments, or curative interventions. Second, many research methods, including randomization, use of placebo controls, and blinding, are unique to research and have no corollary in clinical care. Third, whereas the risks entailed by interventions in clinical care are justified by the potential benefits to the patient, clinical research protocols often include research procedures that carry risk or burden without compensating benefits to the study participant. Risks and burdens that may be borne by the research participants are justified by the potential value of the knowledge gained. Finally, the physician's obligation to promote the patient's interests and to advocate, within bounds, on the patient's behalf is quite powerful. By contrast, clinical investigators have a strong responsibility to promote the integrity of their data and cannot have the same kind of relationship with study participants.[3] These substantive differences give rise to unique ethical tensions in the context of clinical research.

Before a study begins, researchers may have reason to believe they will encounter unmet medical needs in their study population. This is often the case when research is conducted in the developing world, where resources are scarce and access to medical care is limited. In *Consult 5.1*, researchers heading to Africa to conduct health screenings of approximately 8,000 families anticipated encountering numerous health problems in their participants, including symptoms of sexually transmitted infections (STIs). The research team came to the Consultation Service to determine whether they had an obligation to provide ancillary care and to determine how a need for ancillary care would best be met. Ancillary care is care that is not necessitated by requirements of scientific validity or safe trial conduct, and not required to fulfill promises of care to participants or redress injuries incurred in the course of participation in research.[4] In the literature, there is a general consensus that clinical researchers and their sponsors have some ancillary care obligations.[5] Yet existing guidance on the extent of these obligations and how one might fulfill them is unsatisfactory, as regulations and guidelines rarely address ancillary care issues specifically and sometimes appear contradictory. Like the NIH research team that brought *Consult 5.1* to the Consultation Service, many researchers and sponsors strongly feel a need for clearer guidance about ancillary care. Additional populations that would benefit from clear guidance include members of study populations, those normally responsible for a study population's health care, and institutional review boards (IRBs). Questions about ancillary care obligations are expected to become increasingly prevalent and pressing in the future as more research is conducted in the developing world, and this topic continues to be an area of great interest in the research ethics community.

In *Consult 5.2* a researcher came to the Consultation Service questioning the appropriateness of conducting clinical magnetic resonance imaging (MRI) scans and reporting incidental findings to research participants. An incidental finding "is a finding concerning an individual research participant that has potential health or reproductive importance and is discovered in the course of conducting research but is beyond the aims of the study."[6] As some scholars have noted, despite the fact that these incidental findings should not be "unexpected" since investigators can predictably expect to find things that they aren't actively seeking, the research community has not reached a consensus on how to handle this kind of information. This consult report explores the controversy surrounding the ethical appropriateness of returning individual research results.

Even with a well-conceived plan for addressing incidental findings, researchers can still be faced with unforeseen complications, as occurred in *Consult 5.3*. A participant was enrolled in a study involving a peripheral blood stem cell transplant; the transplant was both clinically indicated and a part of the research protocol. His brother was flown to the National Institutes of Health (NIH) from abroad to serve as a stem cell donor. When the brother arrived, however, he was found to have an assortment of serious medical conditions that made donating stem cells considerably riskier for him than for the "average" person. Using the brother as a donor significantly increased the chances of a good outcome for the participant; however, using the brother as a donor also raised the question of the research team's obligation to provide the brother with medical care.

Though many ethical questions concern how much clinical care should be provided to research participants, there are also times when it is necessary to determine how much clinically indicated care can be ethically *withheld* for research purposes. This was the question in *Consult 5.4*. While screening a potential participant for enrollment in a depression protocol, researchers noted early signs and symptoms of Alzheimer's disease. For reasons of scientific validity, the research study was designed such that the participant could not enroll and also take donepezil hydrochloride, a medication that can slow the decline in activities of daily living and improve neuropsychiatric symptoms in patients with Alzheimer's disease. It is not unusual for researchers to identify tension between different requirements of ethical research—here, scientific validity and respect for participants—and to need to balance or specify the requirements so as to satisfy both.[7] In this case, however, ethical analysis was complicated because the potential participant was uninsured and lacked access to health care. Therefore, she could not afford to obtain a prescription for donepezil hydrochloride if she did *not* enroll in the trial. Within the bioethics literature, ambiguity persists regarding whether, and to what extent, the economically disadvantaged might be vulnerable in a research setting.[8] Enrolling participants in research who could not otherwise afford or access health care leads to numerous ethical concerns. Exploitation, which occurs when one party takes unfair advantage of another, is prominent among these concerns and was the primary concern of the requestors who brought this case to the Consultation Service.[9]

In the course of research, a research team may gain a new appreciation of the clinical significance of a participant's condition. As a result, the team may perceive a need for clinical care where no care or more-limited care was previously indicated. This was the case in *Consult 5.5*, where some participants enrolled in a natural history study of pulmonary hypertension in sickle-cell disease were found to have a higher than expected mortality rate. The researchers sought advice from the Consultation Service to discuss the moral implications of their findings and how to address the participants' newly recognized clinical needs without compromising the scientific validity of their work. One factor contributing to the ethical concerns in this case was the lack of a standard of care for treating pulmonary hypertension in sickle-cell disease patients. The lack of a standard, which was the crux of this consultation request, underscores how difficult it can be to distinguish between research and care in practice. One ethical concern raised by the research team was that in seeking evidence to support the development of a standard of care for patients with the dual-diagnoses of sickle cell anemia and pulmonary hypertension, they might reinforce a therapeutic misconception. A therapeutic misconception "exists when individuals do not understand that the defining purpose of clinical research is to produce generalizable knowledge, regardless of whether the participants enrolled in the trial may potentially benefit from the intervention under study or from other aspects of the clinical trial" and arises in many interventional studies.[10]

Although some participants struggle with the therapeutic misconception, others understand clearly research methods including blinding, randomization, and placebo controls and can become frustrated with the implications for their own personal care. A research participant anonymously contacted the Consultation Service in *Consult 5.6* to discuss her participation in a double-blinded, randomized controlled trial. After several years of participating in research, she believed that the experimental drug under study was a "miracle drug" and that her declining medical condition was the result of receiving a placebo. This consult explores whether a research participant has an ethical claim to investigational drugs, an issue that was contemporaneously explored by the courts in the *Abigail Alliance* case.[11] This consult also ties to the discussion of the ethics of placebos offered in Chapter 1: Starting Research and issues related to posttrial access that are discussed in Chapter 7: Ending Research.

Poor compliance and noncompliance—when individuals do not adhere to their prescribed treatment—are concerns familiar to clinicians and researchers alike. Individuals demonstrating poor compliance may not take medications as indicated (e.g., incorrect frequency or dosage), not avoid other incompatible or contraindicated medicines, or not adopt recommended lifestyle modifications.[12] For clinical researchers, participant noncompliance typically raises concerns about the scientific validity of findings, as discussed in Chapter 6: Navigating Interpersonal Difficulties. Interestingly, in *Consult 5.7*, a research team came to the Consultation Service with ethical concerns about a participant who was largely compliant in her research participation but consistently demonstrated poor compliance with her clinical care obtained outside the NIH. The team wondered whether allowing her to continue participating in research was tantamount to condoning noncompliance or made them complicit in her noncompliance. This consultation was very revealing: even when a trial does not explicitly include any clinical care components, it may be necessary to balance clinical care and clinical research.

## CONSULT 5.1: FULFILLING ANCILLARY CARE OBLIGATIONS

### Reason for Consultation

Maryellen Timmons, a research coordinator for a behavioral study in an under-resourced third world country, asked the Consultation Service whether researchers were obligated to treat STI symptoms screened for during the course of a study recruitment strategy. She also wished to discuss broader guidance regarding ancillary care obligations that her institute might provide to researchers when they encounter research participants who do not have easy access to medical treatment outside research participation.

## Narrative

The study Ms. Timmons described proposes to investigate a nonpharmaceutical intervention for adolescents who have HIV-infected parents. A large number of families will be screened to yield a study sample of families where at least one adult is HIV-positive and at least one child stays at home. The potential target families will undergo a health screening conducted by health professionals from the national university. The health screening will include testing for HIV infection and an STI symptom assessment, among other items.

Individuals diagnosed with conditions such as hypertension or HIV infection will be referred to local public health clinics. In addition, the principal investigator proposes that the health professionals conducting the screening will treat individuals who have STI symptoms according to a syndromic management protocol developed by the national Ministry of Health (MoH). It is believed that the health professionals who are part of the research team have previously undertaken syndromic management of STIs within the target community according to the MoH guidelines; however, on this occasion they are being compensated as research personnel through the university, rather than being paid as public health workers.

The principal investigator is skeptical that referring symptomatic individuals for treatment of STIs to local health facilities will be effective, as she believes it unlikely that they will seek treatment at the local clinics. Furthermore, she suspects that if cash vouchers are provided to these persons, they may be used to make other purchases (e.g., food).

## Analysis and Recommendations

There is currently no standard NIH policy on ancillary care obligations, no widely established standard practice in current research protocols, and no generally accepted consensus position on ancillary care obligations. A position paper from a recent international conference on ancillary care responsibilities concludes that researchers are responsible for anticipating which ancillary conditions they are likely to encounter during the course of their study and for planning how they might deal with these ancillary care obligations in partnership with collaborators.[13] The scope of these obligations, however, might vary considerably and should be evaluated on a case-by-case basis. Sometimes research participants should be offered treatment when it can be provided without imposing onerous burdens on the research team, while referrals to existing health care facilities may suffice in other cases.

The Consultation Service recommends that following considerations may be useful in determining the nature and scope of ancillary care obligations that accrue to researchers during the course of a particular study:

1) What ancillary care needs are likely to be encountered?
2) To what extent can the identified ancillary care needs identified in question (1) be met by the existing local health system?
3) How strong is the researchers' responsibility to address ancillary care needs, taking into account the severity and acuity of the predictable care needs, the extent of the relationship between researchers and participants, and the foreseeable financial and personnel costs of providing ancillary care?

In this particular case, the researchers expect to find STIs during the course of recruiting for the study. Therefore, developing a plan for how to deal with this predictable ancillary care need is indicated. The extent of this ancillary care obligation should be agreed upon by the principal investigator, the sponsoring agency, and collaborating institutions. Either providing STI treatment to symptomatic individuals encountered in screening or referring the participants to existing health care facilities is ethically acceptable.

Since the principal investigator is doubtful that the participants will choose to get treatment outside the study on their own, a case can be made for treating symptomatic individuals during the initial screening for the study, especially if the health professionals conducting the health screening already use the MoH protocol for syndromic management of STIs within the target community and are known within the community for performing this service, and the cost of treating these STI symptoms does not jeopardize the study.

As far as general guidance, the institute could recommend that researchers anticipate ancillary care needs which will arise predictably during the course of their research and include a plan for how they will deal with them. The exact scope of the response would be determined on a case-by-case basis. It may be possible, however, to construct a set of institution-specific broad guiding principles based on the kind of considerations we have outlined earlier.

## Authors' Commentary

Within the literature there is little formal guidance on ancillary care and significant disagreement on the extent and source of ancillary care obligations. One extreme view is that clinical researchers should provide participants all ancillary care that a physician would provide a similarly situated patient. The Declaration of Helsinki states that "the health of my patient will be my first consideration," suggesting that researchers are akin to physicians.[14] By contrast, others hold that because researchers are chiefly scientists and participants are volunteers, there are no fundamental reasons for providing ancillary care.[15] One of the most explicit statements regarding ancillary care can be found in the CIOMS/WHO International Ethical Guidelines for Biomedical Research Involving Human Subjects, which state that "although sponsors are, in general, not obligated to provide health care services beyond what is necessary for the conduct of research, it is morally praiseworthy to do so."[16] This guidance can be interpreted to mean that no requirement to provide ancillary care exists.

As can be seen in this consult report, the lack of established guidance on ancillary care obligations can leave researchers confused about the extent of their obligations and how they might fulfill them. Participants at a workshop on ancillary care obligations wrote: "Leaving the moral burden of assessing ancillary-care claims and the logistical burden of planning for them in the hands of individual principal investigators is unfair, unduly exposing them to controversy and charges of unethical behavior. It is also inefficient and unlikely to ensure that ancillary care is always provided when it should be."[17]

As a result of this case and similar cases brought to the Consultation Service, members of the Department of Bioethics have published on ancillary care obligations and contributed to ongoing discussions about the extent to which investigators are responsible for providing medical care for incidental conditions identified among research participants.[18] Generally, they have taken a moderate viewpoint, arguing that researchers do not have the obligation to treat participants as though the researchers were their personal physicians but that substantive fiduciary obligations require provision of some ancillary care (see also the discussion in Chapter 6: Navigating Interpersonal Difficulties). The three considerations outlined in the consultation report echo the framework offered by Richardson and Belsky to determine the stringency of obligations.[19] This case, as with others, highlights the difficulty of making ancillary care decisions when research is conducted in developing countries.

Significantly, an ethical obligation to provide ancillary care may be modulated by tension between the goal of advancing science and the importance of caring for research participants. Provision of ancillary care can conflict with the defining goal of clinical research in two main ways: *(1)* provision of ancillary care can divert resources—financial and human—from the research enterprise; and *(2)* provision of ancillary care can interfere with a research protocol if providing individualized care requires protocol deviations, for example, by confounding analysis or requiring participants to be dropped or excluded.

## CONSULT 5.2: DISCLOSURE OF INCIDENTAL FINDINGS

### Reason for Consultation

Dr. Kasimir, a principal investigator, contacted the Consultation Service to request assistance in answering the following questions: Should a clinical-grade MRI scan be required for all participants who undergo a research-grade MRI scan? If clinical scans are required, what measures should be taken to best implement this requirement?

### Narrative

Dr. Kasimir asked the Consultation Service for input on a Clinical Center policy that requires clinical MRIs for all research participants who receive research-grade MRI scans. The Clinical Center policy states, "Clinical screening scans must be obtained at least once a year on all participants or as specified in the IRB protocol." Dr. Kasimir had questions about the clause "or as specified in the IRB protocol," which seems to permit an IRB to approve less frequent scans and, perhaps, to waive the requirement for a clinical scan entirely. However, in practice, all Clinical Center participants in NIH protocols that involve research MRI scans are required to undergo clinical MRI at least once a year.

Prompted by Dr. Kasimir's concerns, the consult team conducted close analysis of the ethical issues raised by this requirement, including four questions in particular:

1. Should clinical scans be required for all participants who undergo a research MRI?
2. Should individuals be required to provide informed consent specifically for the clinical MRI?
3. Should individuals be allowed to opt out of the clinical MRI but still participate in research when a clinical MRI is not required for research purposes?
4. How should staff respond to individuals who decline to receive MRI results?

### Analysis and Recommendations

1. Requiring a clinical MRI: This requirement is well intentioned and likely benefits at least some research participants. In addition, there are no decisive ethical objections to the requirement. Thus, in our judgment, the requirement is ethically permissible, and those who do not think it is the best approach should, nonetheless, have no serious ethical qualms about following it. Later we consider whether this requirement is preferable, all things considered.

2. Informing participants: Research participants are not informed prospectively of many routine screening tests (e.g., sodium, CBC). However, brain MRI is not a routine screening test, and the literature suggests that experts are divided on whether clinical MRI is in the interests of asymptomatic individuals. This debate focuses on the potential negative psychological and social implications of false positives and findings of unknown clinical significance, as well as the risks of follow-up diagnostic procedures. Given these concerns, we believe participants should be informed of the risks and potential benefits of the clinical MRI and of the conditions under which they will be informed of any findings. This information would allow individuals to decline to participate in the study if they prefer to avoid the clinical MRI.
3. Opt-out option: We believe consideration should be given to allowing individuals to opt out, or to allowing the IRB to decide whether participants may opt out. If an informed participant does not want to undergo clinical MRI, and there are no strong reasons to believe she is making a clinically significant error, it seems the participant should be able to participate in research without undergoing the scan, assuming it is not needed for research purposes.
4. Individuals who do not want MRI results: Individuals should be able to decline to receive information of no or of unknown clinical significance. In contrast, individuals should be informed of findings that indicate a clinically significant and treatable abnormality and should be informed prospectively that they will be so informed. This approach allows individuals to decline to participate in the research if they want to avoid such information.

The Consultation Service has two additional recommendations:

1. Threshold for informing: Further analysis should be conducted to determine the threshold for disclosure of MRI findings to participants and whether this threshold should be consistent across the NIH. Should disclosure include all findings, only findings that may be clinically significant, or only findings that are of known clinical significance?
2. Need for data: The NIH requirement gains support from the assumption that having a clinical scan is in research participants' interests. However, it appears there are insufficient empirical data to evaluate this assumption. Thus, assuming the requirement remains unchanged, we strongly recommend that the NIH develop a protocol to systematically evaluate individuals who undergo a clinical scan to determine whether the benefits of clinically significant findings outweigh the burdens of undergoing a clinical scan (particularly when meeting the requirement entails an

additional scan) and the risks of false positives and findings of unknown clinical significance.

These six recommendations leave the question of whether it is preferable to require a clinical MRI, all things considered. The Consultation Service believes that several considerations are central to this determination:

1. Research participants' expectations: Some participants may mistakenly assume that if they undergo a research brain MRI, and no abnormality is detected, then there is no possibility of a brain abnormality. This is a valid concern, which provides some support for the requirement of a clinical brain MRI. However, this concern exists for other research procedures as well. For example, participants who undergo a cardiac scan for research purposes may mistakenly assume that if no abnormality is detected, there is no possibility of cardiac disease. Assuming the NIH does not, and probably should not, require a complete clinical workup of all research participants, this potential misapprehension will have to be addressed generally, independent of whether clinical MRIs are required. In addition, while a policy requiring clinical MRIs—and informing individuals that they will be performed—is responsive to this "therapeutic misconception" as it pertains to MRIs in particular, it has the potential to foster misapprehension in other individuals. That is, individuals who are informed that the investigators will conduct a clinical MRI may mistakenly conclude that NIH investigators perform a complete clinical workup. To address this concern, it may make sense to explain the possibility of incidental findings generally to research participants and describe the individual procedures, including research MRI, solely in research terms. Using this approach, investigators would treat MRIs as research procedures and have them read as needed for research purposes, with a plan in place for how to handle incidental findings. This approach is consistent with the report of an NIH workshop, in which the majority felt that requiring a clinical scan "for each participant would be overly costly and impractical considering the unknown incidence of true-positive, clinically significant incidental findings in asymptomatic individuals."[20]

2. What is appropriate care in the research context? The fact that research scans amount to substandard clinical care provides reason to require a clinical MRI. At the same time, it is not the role of the NIH to provide clinical care that is independent of research and doing so, especially when it is resource intensive, may conflict with the NIH's mandate to conduct research. Moreover, current debate suggests that clinical scans are not standard of care for asymptomatic individuals and raises concern about the potential for false positives.

3. Enhancing research benefits: While clinical investigators are not obliged to provide clinical care, they should enhance the benefits of research participation when doing so requires little effort or resources and provides important benefit. Having a trained radiologist read the research MRI or a clinical MRI involves relatively little effort for potentially very important benefit. In particular, it allows investigators and the NIH to avoid the tragic and potentially legally culpable possibility of missing a significant finding. Unfortunately, the NIH cannot immunize itself nor research participants against the possibility of missing a treatable condition in a research participant. And the NIH cannot require a complete clinical workup to look for all possible findings. For example, we do not require a dermatologist or oncologist to check every research participant for melanoma. Full evaluation of this issue would require a comprehensive comparison of the benefits and negative effects of clinical brain MRI, compared to other clinical procedures. The fact that there is debate regarding the wisdom of clinical brain MRI in asymptomatic individuals suggests that clinical MRI may not provide a reliable or cost-effective way to enhance the benefits of research participation.

In summary, there are valid reasons for requiring a clinical MRI and valid arguments against requiring it. On this issue, reasonable persons can disagree. Our analysis suggests that there are at least some reasons to question whether the requirement of a clinical MRI represents the best approach. Given this possibility and the complexity of the issue, and the fact that it involves existing NIH policy, the bioethics consultants will recommend to the Clinical Center Ethics Committee, which has responsibility for evaluating Clinical Center policies, that it take up this question. We will recommend that the Ethics Committee evaluate, and consider the best way to implement, the recommendations described here and consider in more depth whether requiring clinical scans is preferable, all things considered.

## Authors' Commentary

An incidental, or secondary, finding is a potentially clinically significant piece of information learned in the course of research, but not related to the condition(s) directly under study. There has been an active debate in the research ethics literature about the return of these findings to individual research participants, but a consensus has not yet emerged.[21]

It was in the context of this unsettled debate that the NIH policy under question emerged. A paper published several years before this consultation occurred found that abnormal results were discovered in 18% of healthy volunteers at the NIH who underwent computed tomography (CT) scan, with 2.9%

requiring routine or urgent follow-up.[22] This study led to a concern that when screening healthy volunteers, the NIH might miss clinically significant findings. As a result of this study, the policy requiring clinical-grade MRI scans was implemented. Some investigators in the intramural research community saw this policy as a barrier to research, arguing that it unduly hindered the performance of studies, imposed an unnecessary burden on research participants, and was difficult to put into practice.

This internal NIH debate about the appropriate level of clinical care that must be provided in a research context echoes some of the issues raised by scholarly conversation around the broader questions relating to return of individual research results. At one extreme, some have taken a research-focused approach, arguing that the goal of research is to produce generalizable knowledge for societal benefit; the return of individual results is inappropriate because it is inconsistent with this broad goal and could foster a therapeutic misconception.[23] In contrast, others have taken a patient-focused approach, arguing that the principles of respect for persons, beneficence, and reciprocity imply an individual right to learn clinically relevant information about oneself.[24] Of course, there are a number of moderate positions between these two extremes, most of which assert that incidental findings should be returned under a limited set of circumstances.[25] These moderate positions focus on a number of factors when determining whether to return a given finding, including the clinical validity, significance, and utility of the information in question.

The controversy surrounding return of incidental research findings seems unlikely to dissipate, particularly as new diagnostic and imaging technologies are introduced. For example, the development of next-generation genomic sequencing capacity has exponentially increased the amount of data that can be analyzed for a given individual, increasing the likelihood that genetic research will produce secondary findings that may be more or less clinically relevant. As investigators, ethicists, and IRBs continue to struggle with whether and how to return individual results, particularly in genetic research, they will have to face a difficult series of emerging issues: respecting participant preferences, managing participant expectations, and ensuring adequate informed consent; defining the scope of an investigator's obligation; and ensuring that investigators have the appropriate resources and capacity to return results.[26]

In the year after this consultation, NIH began grappling with the question of whether to revisit this policy. A number of internal NIH advocates, including representatives from the Consultation Service, began to argue that the policy should be revised or rescinded. This reversal raises a number of process-related issues. First, the recommendations in a given consult can have implications beyond the limited set of facts in the case at hand, potentially influencing institutional policies and practices. Sometimes, it can be appropriate to incorporate policy questions into the consult analysis. Second, ethics consultants must be willing to revisit even the most carefully reasoned conclusions as more information becomes available and the thinking on an issue develops. Interestingly, in a previous consultation, the Consultation Service team stated that the "ethics consultation team endorses the policy of performing clinical MRI scans on healthy volunteers who participate in functional MRI protocols." On subsequent analysis, as seen in this consultation report, the Consultation Service team came to a more tentative conclusion and raised a number of concerns about the risk-benefit ratio of requiring MRI scans.

## CONSULT 5.3: OBLIGATIONS TO INDIVIDUALS TANGENTIALLY RELATED TO RESEARCH

### Reason for Request

Bill Sanders, a nurse practitioner, contacted the Consultation Service attending to request her participation in a multidisciplinary meeting. A potential stem cell donor flown in from Lebanon has presented with a host of serious and unexpected medical conditions, but he reportedly still wants to donate to his brother who is enrolled in a transplant protocol. There are ethical questions about the risks of donation and whether, given this risk, the donation should go forward. Regardless of whether donation is appropriate, there is also a question of NIH's obligations to provide medical care to the donor.

### Narrative

Mr. Sanders described the case of Rafiq Haddad, a 27-year-old male research participant who requires a stem cell transplant (an infusion of healthy stem cells, the immature cells from which all blood cells develop). Due to a rare autoimmune disorder, his prognosis without a stem cell transplant is unclear; it is estimated to be anywhere from 0 to 20 years with supportive care. A human leukocyte antigen (HLA) matched transplant—one where the donor is immunologically compatible with Rafiq—is associated with approximately a 10% risk of death and a 90% chance of curing the disease in the recipient. Rafiq lives near NIH and has access to medical care outside of NIH.

Rafiq's 36-year-old brother, Hakim Haddad, is thought to be the only HLA identical matched donor for Rafiq. There remains, however, a slim chance that as-yet-untested relatives would match. Hakim lives in Lebanon with his wife and children, and he has been flown to NIH to donate stem cells to Rafiq. In general, an estimated 30% of participants otherwise eligible for a stem cell transplant find a matching donor.

The research team was aware that Hakim had diabetes prior to his arrival at NIH. However, after Hakim arrived at NIH, it was found that he has numerous serious medical conditions, including hypertension, coronary artery disease, severe renal insufficiency, and a lung mass. Given his multiple comorbidities, the possibility that he will eventually develop renal failure requiring dialysis is high. It is the medical team's understanding that Hakim has limited access to medical care in Lebanon and may not be able to get dialysis there.

Hakim's medical conditions make donating stem cells considerably more risky for him. Standard donation involves aphaeresis (the donor blood is passed through a machine that removes the stem cells). Aphaeresis is preceded by granulocyte colony-stimulating factor (G-CSF)-induced mobilization; G-CSF causes more stem cells to be available in the blood. Hakim might not be able to tolerate G-CSF without first having cardiac stents or bypass surgery, because of the risk of myocardial infarction associated with G-CSF-induced mobilization. If Hakim were to have stents placed or bypass surgery, there is a substantial (estimated to be 10%–30%) risk of inducing renal failure, though members of Hakim's family have reportedly expressed willingness to donate a kidney should it be needed.

Had the research team been aware of the extent of Hakim's medical problems, he would not have been brought to the NIH to be a donor. All other donors to date have been otherwise healthy and there have been no deaths or serious complications at the NIH from the donation of peripheral blood stem cells. However, provided that Hakim's lung mass is not cancer, he reportedly does not meet any explicit exclusion criteria for stem cell donation.

The research team noted that bone marrow donation under general anesthesia is a possible alternative strategy for Hakim. This procedure would reportedly reduce the risk of renal failure, but it presents Hakim with an estimated 5% risk of a cardiac event. Hakim is reportedly adamant in his desire to donate stem cells to his brother.

Finally, Hakim's renal insufficiency has worsened since arrival at the NIH, which could possibly be secondary to treating his hypertension, an iatrogenic effect of the dye load from cardiac angiography, or an indication of rapidly progressive kidney disease.

## Analysis and Recommendations

According to clinical team members at the interdisciplinary meeting, stem cell donation by aphaeresis does not appear to be an option for Hakim. The risk is too high without cardiac surgery, and cardiac surgery would be difficult for Hakim to obtain due to his limited resources and the fact that there is not a cardiac surgery protocol at the NIH. The only potentially acceptable method for donation appears to be a bone marrow harvest under general anesthesia, which reportedly involves a much greater risk of serious morbidity than is typically incurred.

Nonetheless, there are ethical considerations in favor of permitting Hakim to donate bone marrow:

1. Hakim may have a well-informed, autonomous desire to donate stem cells in order to help his brother. The decision to accept even extraordinary risks for the benefit of others can be reasonable in some cases—perhaps especially for close family members, or when one's natural prognosis is poor regardless of the risks of donation.
2. Despite the high risk of donation, it may be that the total expected medical benefit of donation outweighs the risks. That is to say, reportedly, it is likely that donation would significantly extend Rafiq's life without shortening Hakim's life, and without donation it is likely that neither Rafiq nor Hakim will live long.

The Consultation Service does not, however, recommend donation at this time. In addition to concerns about potential harm to Hakim, there are prudential concerns about the reported level of risk:

1. The level of risk involved in Hakim's donation would reportedly be an unprecedented break from standard practice at the NIH and possibly in clinical practice generally. To accept a level of risk to a donor higher than normally considered acceptable could be precedent setting and should receive a more thorough and broad discussion at the NIH than the Consultation Service can provide. This discussion might include other NIH transplant programs, IRB members, NIH administrators, and the Clinical Center Ethics Committee, among others.
2. If Hakim were to die or suffer serious injury in the course of a donation that would normally be regarded as too risky, there is significant potential for the appearance of exploitation because Hakim has been brought here from a developing country to be involved in research.

This recommendation assumes that the reported 5% risk of a serious cardiac event is accurate, and that such a risk is truly unprecedented for donation. It would also be relevant if there were any feasible options remaining for a less risky donation, for instance, if a bone marrow harvest could be performed without general anesthesia. It might also be worth exploring whether any of Hakim's children are suitable donors.

One component of the broader discussion about acceptable risks to donors should address the possibility of having independent evaluators for donors and recipients. In the present case, concerns about conflict of interest are mitigated because Rafiq's clinical team appropriately sought outside clinical evaluations and an ethics consult to discuss Hakim's interests.

In the course of the interdisciplinary meeting, one of Rafiq's physicians suggested that the ethics consult team members meet with Rafiq and Hakim before making any recommendations. The consult team decided against this, because regardless of the sincerity or reasonableness of the brothers' wishes, allowing Hakim to donate seems inadvisable at this time. However, if in the final judgment of the clinical team, it is appropriate for Hakim to donate, the Consultation Service would be willing to meet with Rafiq and Hakim to help ensure valid informed consent.

The question of what the NIH owes to Hakim was also discussed at the interdisciplinary meeting. Because NIH is a research institution, it cannot offer Hakim long-term medical care. However, because Hakim has formed a relationship with the NIH clinical team and because his condition may have worsened since coming to NIH, in addition to a flight home, Hakim should be offered a reasonable level of clinical support while he is here. This may include recommendations for medical management of his problems and a summary of diagnostic and treatment recommendations for him to provide to his local physician, a supply of medications that he is currently receiving, referrals to community resources for the remainder of his stay in the United States, and if potentially beneficial, a lung mass biopsy. Hakim should also be offered the chance to participate in medically beneficial research if there is any for which he is eligible, including research that might treat conditions revealed by the biopsy if he receives one.

In summary:

1. Hakim should not be accepted as a stem cell donor because broader dialogue should precede any decision to deviate significantly from a commonly accepted level of risk.
2. There should be further broad discussion of acceptable levels of risk for donors at the NIH.
3. Discharge planning for Hakim should include providing a supply of medications to last at least until Hakim returns home, referrals for further medical care while he is in the United States, and a summary of his treatments for his home physicians.

## Authors' Commentary

As explored in Chapter 3: Protecting Research Participants, deciding who counts as a research participant can be difficult. Investigators and IRBs are used to balancing the risks and benefits of research for a single participant. It becomes decidedly more complicated when one has to balance the risks to a potential donor against the benefits for a primary research participant. In this case, based on available evidence, the Consultation Service team determined that the risks to the donor were too high to justify the potential benefit to the primary participant. Of course, this discounts the possibility that a reasonable donor would be willing to rationally accept a high level of risk because of a sincere desire to help a loved one. As a point of process, it is interesting to note that the participant and his brother were not included in this consultation although the Consultation Service normally promotes the involvement of all stakeholders. Although the consult report mentions Hakim's possible altruistic interests, the decision to exclude Hakim and Rafiq precluded further exploration of this position.

The case also raised a second, less typical issue related to donor motivation and autonomy. Normally, a case of directed donation to loved ones can raise concern about the potential for implicit (or explicit) pressure from family.[27] In this case, there is an added concern about the donor feeling pressure to donate in order to receive ancillary care. It is possible that prior to arriving at the NIH, the donor did not have complete information about his health status. The process of coming to the NIH and learning that he needed urgent medical care could have, at least in part, motivated him to continue participating in order to receive ancillary care for his now apparent conditions that would have been unavailable to him at home. Of course, this assumes that the research team had an obligation to provide ancillary care. Does an investigator's obligation to provide ancillary care extend to nonparticipants brought to the NIH to help enrolled research participants? In this case, the research team arranged for the donor's long-distance travel, which could have exacerbated his condition. As such, at the very least they had an obligation to stabilize him before sending him home.

Finally, this consultation raises questions about institutional obligations to provide care to someone who has limited access to care elsewhere. This theme is reflected in other cases we have had that raised questions about taking care of uninsured participants and participants whose immigration status is unclear. The Clinical Center is a hospital that provides clinical care, but it does so under the umbrella of its research mandate. These roles can come into tension because, while individual participants can benefit from participation in research protocols, the NIH's mission is to devote federal resources toward the development of medical advances that will benefit society as a whole.

## ■ CONSULT 5.4: WITHHOLDING CARE FOR REASONS OF SCIENTIFIC VALIDITY

### Reason for Consultation

A research team wants to know whether it is ethical to enroll a potential participant with early signs of Alzheimer's disease in their trial given that they would need to require that she not take a clinically indicated medication for the duration of the trail.

### Narrative

While screening Juana Hernandez, a 63-year-old Hispanic female, as a prospective participant in a depression protocol, the research team noted early signs of Alzheimer's disease, which were confirmed by a consulting NIH geriatrician.

In addition to depression, Ms. Hernandez has history of alcohol abuse, panic attacks, and social anxiety. Normally, she doesn't leave her neighborhood.

While both standard care for depression and the drug used in the protocol are compatible with donepezil hydrochloride (the relevant treatment for Alzheimer's disease), and while Alzheimer's disease is not strictly speaking an exclusion criterion for the depression protocol, the depression protocol disallows participants to take donepezil hydrochloride for reasons of scientific validity. Hence, for Alzheimer patients with the financial means to procure donepezil hydrochloride, the standard clinical recommendation would be not to enroll in the depression protocol.

Ms. Hernandez, however, is uninsured, and could not procure donepezil hydrochloride without filing for disability. She would find it difficult to file for disability on her own since she is depressed, estranged from family and friends needed as signatories, and barely literate. Because Ms. Hernandez works from time to time, if she files for disability from outside the protocol, her application might be rejected. Even if ultimately successful in obtaining disability status, the process might take up to 5 months, according to NIH social workers.

On the other hand, participants in the depression protocol benefit from generous access to social workers, who could potentially help Ms. Hernandez file for disability. Moreover, that protocol involves access to many types of medical care, including Alzheimer's treatment, for 3–4 months after the trial. In other words, as soon as the trial ends (in 2 months), Ms. Hernandez could start taking donepezil hydrochloride, initially provided by the research team and later, in virtue of her new disability status, by the state. Ms. Hernandez is interested in enrolling in the trial, both in order to avail herself of these benefits and out of altruism. She said that even if the protocol did not involve access to social work and drugs, she would want to participate. The medical team wanted to ensure that it is ethical to allow Ms. Hernandez to enroll in the trial.

After meeting with the research team, the Consultation Service attending and fellow met with Ms. Hernandez. She reports feeling happier since starting to come to the Clinical Center for checkups. She is impressively conscientious and responsible. Ms. Hernandez explained that 3 years ago, when she was still insured, she received antidepressants and only stopped taking them because she was laid off and became uninsured. She seems to understand her Alzheimer's diagnosis well.

Over the course of their meetings, the Consultation Service team identified as an additional concern that Ms. Hernandez lacks a Durable Power of Attorney ("DPA").

## Analysis and Recommendations

The researchers all seemed to agree that enrollment would be in Ms. Hernandez's best interests. There was, however, a certain concern about exploitation: NIH, an arm of the government, is taking advantage of the failure of the government to provide access to basic medical treatment. The participant said that she would enroll even absent the benefits in terms of social work services and free drugs; moreover, exploitation is mitigated by the fact that, to provide these benefits, the NIH will expend considerable effort.

The Consultation Service recommends that the team invite Ms. Hernandez to enroll in the depression trial and that social workers assist her in applying for disability and in finding a legal guardian. The attending ethicist also suggested that the research team inform the clinical director and, toward the next annual review, the IRB, of this experience.

## Authors' Commentary

This consultation report identifies exploitation as a particular concern when enrolling the uninsured in clinical research trials. Exploitation is usually understood as using people as a mere means for the ends of others and/or as taking unfair advantage of people.[28] Either or both senses can be applicable in the clinical research context. For example, individuals may be used for the good of others without being treated respectfully, or they may accept considerable risks in research for less than fair benefits because of their limited bargaining power.

Treating people as a mere means can be minimized in clinical research by assuring that participants understand the purpose of the research and voluntarily agree to participate because they believe it to be a valuable activity. Ms. Hernandez's reported altruistic motivation to participate suggests that she is not being used merely as a means to others' ends. It can be more difficult to determine whether participants are being treated unfairly—that is, if they are receiving an unfair level of benefit, and this seems clearly to be the definition of exploitation that was the source of ethical concern for the research team. Can it be exploitative to enroll individuals lacking access to health care in clinical trials?

Certainly, unfairness exists in the background circumstances of the participant at the center of this consultation. In her daily life, she lacks access to health care that would improve her health and well-being. By recruiting this participant—or any uninsured person who is motivated to participate in research because of lack of access to health care—investigators *do* take advantage of unfairness. Yet taking advantage of a person's unfair background conditions does not entail that one is taking unfair advantage of that person, and there need not be anything inherently exploitative about enrolling the uninsured in clinical research.[29] IRB review and approval, when done correctly, should ensure that the risks and benefits a trial offers to participants are reasonable regardless of whether a participant is insured.[30] If a study offers benefits or reasons to participate that justify the risks of participation and that participants accept, it does not exploit participants, even if lack of health care strongly influences their decision to enroll.[31] From the perspective of the ethics consultants and the research team, this participant would receive a number of benefits in exchange for her participation in the IRB-approved depression protocol; these included availability of social work, free drugs, assistance accessing health care resources in the community, and psychological gains.

Arguably, the ethics consultants could have taken their analysis further and asserted that it would be unfair *not* to enroll this participant simply because she lacks access to health care. Excluding an uninsured person seeking to participate in research could mean eliminating an option for possible therapeutic benefit for an individual who has few such options (for further discussion, see Chapter 2: Enrolling Research Participants). Although participation in research "cannot and should not serve to remedy inequities in health care delivery," it should not be denied to the uninsured.[32] Much attention has been focused on the ethical concerns created by international disparities in access to health care and to the attendant ethical concerns of exploitation and fair subject selection. Nevertheless, the ethical questions attendant to domestic disparities in access also demand our attention and will persist even as more Americans obtain health insurance.

## CONSULT 5.5: MEETING CLINICAL NEEDS WITHOUT COMPROMISING SCIENTIFIC VALIDITY

### Reason for Request

Dr. Walter Greene, a physician, called on behalf of his research team to discuss the ethics of an ongoing protocol in which participants have an unexpectedly high mortality rate. The team's first concern is that their natural history study could become morally problematic. Their second concern, in view of a higher-than-expected mortality in a subgroup of participants, is how to offer treatment without compromising the scientific validity of the research.

### Narrative

This research team is studying pulmonary hypertension (elevated blood pressure in the arteries of the lungs) in individuals with sickle-cell disease (SCD). SCD, also known as sickle-cell anemia, is a chronic anemia characterized by destruction of red blood cells and by episodic blocking of blood vessels. Blocked vessels can cause pain, infections, and organ damage.

Dr. Greene explained that in order to obtain reliable data on the prevalence, severity, and impact of pulmonary hypertension in this population, the research team recruited individuals with SCD broadly and tested them for the presence of pulmonary hypertension. The results of this screening were shared with participants, and, with their consent, with their physicians. The purpose of this disclosure was that participants be able to benefit from clinical treatment, where indicated, following the screening. When the study began, it was thought that individuals with mild pulmonary hypertension were not at high risk of complications. Participants diagnosed with mild pulmonary hypertension were therefore told that they had pulmonary hypertension; however, they were also told that it was not clear that this finding had clinical significance for them.

An intermediate analysis now shows that the mortality of individuals with mild pulmonary hypertension is higher than expected. The data safety monitoring board (DSMB) has requested that treatment be offered to participants with pulmonary hypertension, even if it is mild, and Dr. Greene agrees that this needs to be done. However, he and the members of his team told the Consultation Service that they are concerned about to how best to do this without compromising the scientific validity of the natural history study, and how to deal with the fact that some of their participants now seem to have been falsely reassured about their prognosis.

In this case, circumstances are complicated by the fact that several treatments have been approved for pulmonary hypertension, but none have been scientifically tested in individuals whose pulmonary hypertension is a result of SCD. Their efficacy for this population is not clearly established. Treatments considered by the team include the medication sildenafil and oxygen, both of which have been used in pulmonary hypertension but not tested in SCD patients, and hydroxyurea or exchange transfusions, which are known to be beneficial in SCD, but have not been tested for efficacy in SCD-related pulmonary hypertension. Currently, there is therefore no established standard of care for SCD-related pulmonary hypertension.

## Analysis and Recommendations

The research team's first concern regarded the ethics of conducting a natural history protocol. The mortality rate of the total sample of participants on the protocol was not higher than expected in a population of patients with SCD, but the mortality among participants with mild pulmonary hypertension was higher than expected. In light of this, and given the prevalence of SCD in the African-American population, the investigators were concerned that their study could lead to concerns about race and exploitation, echoing the Tuskegee study of untreated syphilis.

We suggest that, since test results and their implications are shared with the participants, and treatment recommendations are made, this is not a concern as long as treatment is available to participants and they receive all relevant information that could affect their care. Because there is no established standard of care for SCD-related pulmonary hypertension, the treatment offered to these research participants should be based on the best available knowledge and reflect what a clinician would be expected to offer them were they not participating in research. As the standard of care evolves, the information and treatment made available to the participants should be adapted accordingly.

The research team's second concern was that offering care on the protocol should not compromise the scientific validity of the natural history study. According to Dr. Greene, however, making these treatments available on protocol would have scientific merit independent of the possible benefit to participants. Since no scientifically proven treatments exist for pulmonary hypertension associated with SCD, even limited data on a small sample would yield information that would be scientifically valuable in planning larger studies.

Several additional issues were identified by the Consultation Service:

- Providing treatment on the protocol is complicated by the fact that community resources are lacking to manage SCD and pulmonary hypertension.
- It was not clear to the research team how best to inform participants in the mild pulmonary hypertension subgroup, who had been previously reassured, that their risk may have been underestimated.
- The team was in the process of expediting a treatment protocol for which the individuals in the mild pulmonary hypertension subgroup would have been good candidates. There was therefore a concern that informing them that their risk was higher than expected might create undue influence to enroll in a treatment protocol.

Since community resources are lacking for the treatment of SCD, and some SCD patients lack health insurance, it is not clear that adequate treatment is indeed available off protocol for some of these individuals. It is important to note here that this is a case where the ethical conduct of research is rendered more difficult by the existence of a separate problem of distributive justice regarding access to medical care. The team should address this by helping participants gain access to appropriate care whenever possible. An automatic referral to a social worker for prospective participants who do not have adequate management of their SCD outside the NIH would be one way to address this.

Offering scientifically unproven but possibly effective therapeutic interventions on the protocol could reinforce the "therapeutic misconception," that is, the perception by participants that the research is being conducted primarily to benefit them personally. For this reason, alternatives to enrolling in research should be made explicit to them. Treatments that have been approved for pulmonary hypertension should be mentioned and recommended realistically. Where uncertainty persists as to their efficacy in SCD, this should be stated also.

Participants should be informed of the higher-than-expected death rate, especially those participants who have been previously reassured that their condition did not greatly increase their risk. Realistic information about treatment options, including the fact that these therapies have not been tested in SCD patients, should also be provided.

Though disclosure is important, information should be communicated with sensitivity to its frightening nature. One issue is that this information contradicts previous, reassuring information given to these individuals. Wording should, however, be clear and precise. Vague wording can be misinterpreted in two ways: (1) allowing underestimation of the risk it conveys or (2) allowing presumption of the worst-case scenario. Difficulty is increased by the fact that one has to be cautious about the inferences that can be made from the current mortality data. Not all causes of SCD-related death seem to be known, and a link to pulmonary hypertension is therefore not definite. If more information can be obtained to help clarify this, it should be done. The limitations of this new knowledge should be conveyed to the participants as well.

## Authors' Commentary

Like *Consult 5.4*, this consultation raises questions about enrolling the uninsured and those with a lack of access to health care in clinical research. This consultation, however, highlights a different ethical concern: that clinical research may offer services or other goods sufficiently attractive to potential participants to impair decision making.[33] This concern is often termed "undue inducement." The core worry is that individuals are offered some good that is so large as to be irresistible in the context; this leads the individual to exercise poor judgment and assume a substantial risk of harm or forsake deeply held values.[34] Undue inducement is a common charge in biomedical research and an ethical concern that is raised in guidelines and regulations.[35] Although money is the paradigmatic source of concerns about undue influence, offers of medical care might also affect judgment, and this has been cited in the literature on enrolling the economically disadvantaged in research.[36] The possibility that treatment would be an undue influence is mentioned in passing in this consultation but possibly deserves more attention.

Because there are limited resources in the community to treat SCD and some individuals with a diagnosis of SCD lack insurance, there are reasons to think that participants may be motivated to participate in research when they otherwise might not. Accepting free health care in exchange for participation in research does not necessarily indicate an impaired consideration of risks. Certainly, in this consultation, an offer of health care would be an inducement—a good offered to encourage participant enrollment. But is it undue? According to Emanuel, offers of goods or services, no matter how large, do not constitute undue inducement if the activities are legal, ethical, and prudent, even if they entail some risk, as long as the risk is reasonable.[37] If the study receives

IRB approval, we can assume that the risk-benefit ratio is favorable and that a reasonable person could choose to participate. Furthermore, the lack of a standard of care for treating pulmonary hypertension in SCD suggests that participation in research may be in the participants' best interests, preferable even to receiving care in the community. This is, perhaps, a counterintuitive but illuminating conclusion.

This consultation also raised questions about therapeutic misconception. A number of definitions for therapeutic misconception have been proposed in the literature; confusion about what the purpose of research means to a participant is integral to most.[38] A definition proposed by a collaborative group of bioethics scholars states that a therapeutic misconception "exists when individuals do not understand that the defining purpose of clinical research is to produce generalizable knowledge, regardless of whether the participants enrolled in the trial may potentially benefit from the intervention under study or from other aspects of the clinical trial."[39] Research participants often mistakenly believe that they will receive direct medical benefit from procedures that are solely intended for research purposes.

The therapeutic misconception is ethically significant because informed consent is essential to most ethical research.[40] There is reason to be concerned about the adequacy of informed consent when participants fail to comprehend how trial participation differs from medical care; one cannot give fully informed consent to participation in research without understanding that clinical management decisions, unlike those in the context of medical care, are not entirely guided by individualized medical judgment.[41] Consistent with the Consultation Service recommendations, efforts by researchers to dispel the therapeutic misconception are considered imperative. Five dimensions of research that should be understand by trial participants include scientific purpose; study procedures—those intended primarily or solely to generate scientific knowledge rather than patient care; uncertainty; adherence to protocol; and the role of the clinician as investigator.[42] Informed consent was discussed in Chapter 2: Enrolling Research Participants, but it is worth considering how tensions between research and care can raise the need for additional participant protections and refinement of the consent process.

## CONSULT 5.6: ACCESS TO EXPERIMENTAL DRUGS OUTSIDE A STUDY PROTOCOL

### Reason for Consult

A female research participant who wished to remain anonymous called to ask about the possibility of receiving a drug being offered in the treatment arm of a double-blind, placebo-controlled trial.

## Narrative

In a telephone conversation with the Consultation Service attending, the anonymous caller gave the following information: She has been enrolled in a double-blind, placebo-controlled trial for 3 years. Her disease has taken a significant turn for the worse, and she has concluded that she is on the placebo arm. The protocol specifies that at the end of the trial (approximately 12–15 months from now) all participants will receive the study drug. Her personal physician advised her to ask the investigators to allow her to receive the study drug now. She called to ask whether the investigators could or would respond to this request, to be reassured that it is acceptable to make this request, and to express disgruntlement with the placebo-controlled study design.

The caller was clearly very frightened, and she said a number of times that the drug is a "miracle drug" (though once she qualified that it was "for some people"), and that she would do anything to get it ("stand on my head, be their guinea pig, pay for the drug").

## Analysis and Recommendations

The ethics consultant offered sympathy and told the caller that, due to her desire for complete anonymity, and a resultant lack of knowledge about the details of the protocol, it is impossible to clearly assess whether the investigators are obligated or able to provide her with the drug. The ethics consultant suggested that the investigators would know this information and asked how she felt about talking to them. She spoke very highly of them and said she was comfortable speaking with them about her situation. The ethics consultant offered to arrange a meeting with members of the Consultation Service and the investigators, or a meeting with just the Consultation Service, but she decided to first discuss her situation with her investigators and only call back if she needed more support.

The caller said that she didn't like the placebo-controlled trial design and was told that she was not alone in that feeling, but that all the protocols here go through extensive review and that the placebo control would only be allowed if there were good reasons for it. Unsurprisingly, she wasn't very satisfied by that but said she would talk to the investigators about it. She did not wish to leave her contact information, but she took the ethics consultant's phone number and said she would be in touch again later.

## Authors' Commentary

This consult was unusual in that it was unilaterally initiated by a research participant without the knowledge of the research team. It was difficult to provide her with a thoughtful analysis in the absence of key details about the protocol and her condition. In fact, it did not seem that she wanted to engage in an extended conversation about the ethical issues raised by her case; she seemed to be primarily seeking affirmation that it was appropriate for her to approach the research team. As a result, the consult focused on process, trying to help the participant develop an acceptable strategy for approaching the investigators with her questions and concerns. We do not know the ultimate outcome or whether the researchers allowed her early access to the study drug.

This consult arose just around the time that the courts were considering the Abigail Alliance case, which addressed whether terminally ill patients had a constitutional right to investigational drugs. Advocacy groups had criticized the FDA's compassionate use policy as being unduly restrictive and sought to change the regulations.[43] The case specifically involved the FDA's refusal to promulgate new regulations that would allow terminal patients to buy drugs that had not yet received FDA approval. An appellate court found that there was a constitutional right to obtain unapproved but potentially life-saving investigational drugs.[44] This controversial ruling was short lived; the full Circuit court reheard the case and overturned the decision, and the Supreme Court declined to hear the case.

This consult, and the Abigail Alliance case, highlight the frequent tension between the broad social goals of clinical research and the realities faced by severely or terminally ill individuals. While participants can sometimes obtain direct benefit from experimental interventions, certain kinds of research (e.g., double-blind, placebo-controlled studies and Phase I trials) justifiably involve enrolling participants with extremely little prospect of direct benefit. Clinical research is primarily aimed at producing knowledge to improve society, a goal that can be at odds with a specific participant's desire to access an intervention of last resort. Furthermore, allowing individual access to investigational drugs outside of a protocol could have practical consequences. Such a right might create a disincentive to enroll in placebo-controlled studies, reducing the ability to measure true safety and efficacy of a drug. It also places physicians in a difficult position with regard to helping patients evaluate the risks and benefits of an experimental treatment: desperate patients with no further approved therapeutic options will demand treatment with an unproved drug that often will provide little or no benefit, while potentially exposing themselves to serious harm.

## ■ CONSULT 5.7: NONCOMPLIANCE

### Reason for Consult

Dr. Alex Norton, a physician-researcher, contacted the Consultation Service to determine whether it is appropriate to keep a research participant who has poor compliance with her primary medical care on a protocol that offers no prospect of direct benefit.

## Narrative

Dr. Norton and diverse members of the research team, including the research nurse, and a nurse practitioner from the HIV/AIDS clinic came to the Department of Bioethics for the consultation. To begin the meeting, Dr. Norton described the research participant, Janelle Soffee. She is a 37-year-old female infected with HIV. Her medical history is significant for hypertension, diabetes type II (for which she requires medication), chronic renal insufficiency, and obesity. She has a history of poor compliance with her medical treatment.

In 2006, Ms. Soffee enrolled in a NIH protocol that involves once or twice yearly leukopheresis (a procedure by which the white blood cells are removed from her blood for use in research). The research involves minimal risk and offers no prospect of benefit to participants. Participants are only paid a small amount to reimburse them for travel expenses. The team reports that Ms. Soffee understands the research will not benefit her, and she is strongly motivated to participate in the study to help others with HIV infection.

In the past, Ms. Soffee received her primary medical care at the NIH as part of a different protocol. Some members of the research team in attendance at the consultation meeting were previously involved in her health care. They reported that, during that time, Ms. Soffee was periodically noncompliant. At the completion of the protocol, the NIH stopped providing primary care to Ms. Soffee, and the team helped her arrange alterative medical care outside the NIH.

During the week prior to the consultation meeting, Ms. Soffee came to the NIH for a scheduled leukopheresis appointment. At that time, she reported poor compliance with her hypertension and diabetes medications. Her blood pressure was slightly elevated, and her blood sugar was extremely elevated. Ms. Soffee's elevated blood pressure and blood glucose did not pose an increased risk with leukopheresis. However, in light of her clinical status and out of an abundance of caution, the decision was made not to do the research procedure.

Members of the research team spoke with Ms. Soffee about her poor compliance. They report that she understands that her noncompliance jeopardizes her health and research participation, and this is very upsetting to her. It is unclear to the research team what explains her continuing poor compliance. On several occasions she has met with social workers at the NIH to try to identify and address the causes of her noncompliance, with little apparent improvement.

The primary question for the Consultation Service team was how to handle Ms. Soffee in the future. Additionally, the research team felt it would be useful to develop a framework for how best to work with other noncompliant participants.

## Analysis and Recommendations

In general, poor compliance with primary medical care can raise a number of ethical concerns for researchers, depending on the specific circumstances.

1. *Poor compliance may undermine the data obtained from participants.* If poor compliance undermines the validity of the data, and this situation cannot be remedied, the participant should be excluded from the study.
2. *Poor compliance may increase the risks of research participation.* If poor compliance increases the risks of research beyond an acceptable level, the participant should be excluded. Poor compliance that increases risks, even when these risks remain within an acceptable level, raises concern that the study is violating the requirement to minimize the risks of research. To address this concern, the team should take reasonable measures to minimize the risks (e.g., counseling, acute interventions). If these measures are unsuccessful, the research will expose the participants to risks that, while acceptable in absolute terms, are higher than they need to be. This situation might be problematic if some of the increased risks involve the potential for serious harm, especially when there are participants available who could replace the participant and do not face a risk of serious harm. At a minimum, participants should be informed of the ways in which their noncompliance increases their risk and may affect their participation.
3. *Participation in research may encourage or increase poor compliance.* If study participation somehow encourages poor compliance, and there is good reason to think the participant would be significantly better off outside of research, the participant should be excluded from the study.
4. *Research might exploit participants by taking advantage of their problems and noncompliance to get them to participate.* To address this possibility, the team should evaluate whether the participant wants to participate independent of the poor compliance. The team also can address the concern of exploitation by taking steps to help the participant be compliant.
5. *Poor compliance may signal that the participant lacks capacity to understand.* If this is a concern, the participant's capacity should be assessed. The Clinical Center has a Capacity Assessment Team available to provide assistance in this regard. If a participant is found to lack capacity, he or she should be excluded from research or have an appropriate surrogate provide permission on his or her behalf.
6. *Poor compliance may reflect a desire to refuse medical care or participation in research.* To address this concern, participants' reasons for poor compliance and views of medical care and research participation should be evaluated. In some cases, it may be useful to have this evaluation conducted by a neutral third party.
7. *Over time, researchers may become complicit in, or seem to be condoning or enabling, the participant's poor compliance and consequent decline.* To address this concern, researchers should make clear that they view poor compliance as problematic and take steps to help the participant become compliant.
8. *Payment may represent an undue inducement to participants to participate in research.* Concerns of undue inducement arise when payment may entice

individuals to participate in research that is contrary to their long-term interests. To address this concern, the team should evaluate whether the payment level is excessive and consider whether participants clearly would be better off not participating in the research.

9. *Working with noncompliant participants can be emotionally burdensome.* Some of this burden may stem from concerns that participants' participation in research is unethical. This concern should be addressed by evaluating the prior considerations. Even when participation is ethical, and appropriate steps are being taken to help the individual be compliant, working with noncompliant individuals can be emotionally burdensome. The team should recognize this burden and consider measures to reduce it (e.g., rotating who interacts with the participant). In some cases, if the burden is substantial and the benefits to society and the participant of the participant's participation are minimal, the team might consider excluding the participant.

To what extent are these ethical concerns relevant to Ms. Soffee's research participation?

1. Her poor compliance does not appear to undermine the validity of the data obtained from her. According to the primary investigator, an elevated hemoglobin A1C, for example, does not affect the analysis of her white cells.

2. Her poor compliance may slightly increase the risks of leukopheresis. For example, her elevated blood sugars may increase her risk of phlebitis (inflammation of a vein). The team believes her poor compliance increases her risk *within* the minimal risk range but does not increase the risks beyond the minimal risk threshold.
Ms. Soffee should be made aware of the increased risks she faces due to her noncompliance. She should also be informed that poor compliance may result in her eventual exclusion from the study due to safety concerns. While the risks to her are minimal at this point, it is a requirement of ethical research that research-related risks are minimized to the extent possible. To address this concern, the team should continue to pursue efforts to increase Ms. Soffee's compliance. In addition, if the risks due to poor compliance seem substantially elevated, the team may elect to postpone the procedure, even when it remains within the range of minimal risk.

3. Her participation in research appears to be increasing rather than decreasing her compliance with her medications. At NIH clinic visits, the research team reviews Ms. Soffee's clinical history and encourages her to be compliant.

4. According to the research team, Ms. Soffee's poor compliance is not increasing her willingness to participate in research. Her participation

reflects an altruistic desire to aid others and contribute to the development of treatments for future patients.
5. It appears that Ms. Soffee understands the implications of her noncompliance and the fact that the research will not benefit her clinically.
6. She continually expresses a desire to receive treatment. She does not refuse care and accepted interventions during her last clinic visit, including insulin to bring down her blood sugar. The source of her poor compliance is unknown.
7. To keep from becoming complicit or seeming to condone or enable Ms. Soffee's poor compliance, the team should continue to express their concern regarding her poor compliance and take steps to help her become compliant.
8. Undue inducement is not a concern in this case. Payments are modest, and Ms. Soffee gains indirect psychological benefit from participating in the study.
9. The research team has a close and long-standing relationship with Ms. Soffee, and this may enhance the staff's emotional burden associated with her noncompliance. It is especially difficult and frustrating to witness an individual's decline when it is due to poor compliance, and the clinicians are unable to fix things. The benefits that society and Ms. Soffee gain from her participation clearly seem to outweigh the emotional burden. The team may want to consider ways to distribute the burden if it becomes more serious.

## Recommendations

1. Inform Ms. Soffee that she faces increased research-related risks due to her poor compliance and that at some point she will be excluded from the study if her status continues to deteriorate.
2. The research team should take concrete steps, consistent with their status as researchers, to encourage better compliance by Ms. Soffee and thus reduce the risks she faces. One possibility would be to set explicit thresholds for her test results, beyond which leukopheresis will be rescheduled. Another option would be to require her to see her primary care physician prior to leukopheresis. At the same time, the team should be careful not to present absolute limits that may be difficult to enforce permanently if Ms. Soffee fails to meet them. While it has been attempted in the past, it may make sense to periodically require Ms. Soffee to meet with a counselor to discuss her poor compliance.
3. The team should continue to assess over time the emotional burden that is posed by Ms. Soffee's participation in the study, including measures to reduce this burden.

## Authors' Commentary

Many types of care are delivered in clinical research. In randomized controlled trials, for example, control treatments are integral to study design. In some trials, clinical care is promised to participants as an inducement to participate in research or provided in recognition of an ancillary care obligation. In yet other trials, participants receive medical care to optimize them for participation in research or to redress study-related complications or injuries. Unlike the other cases presented in this chapter that focused on how participation in research should affect the delivery of clinical care, the ethical analysis for this consultation focused on how clinical care delivered outside of a trial might affect research participation. At times, a participant's clinical care may affect his or her research participation in straightforward ways. For example, noncompliance may unfavorably alter the risk-benefit ratio of research and result in the participant meeting exclusion criteria; or noncompliance might result in the collection of incomplete or incorrect data, which might also merit exclusion.[45] In this case, however, the researchers worried that allowing Ms. Soffee to participate in research made them party to her noncompliance and complicit in her unnecessary clinical decline.

Noncompliance can have many causes: individuals may be in denial that they have a medical problem; they may grow tired of unpleasant side effects; the cost of treatment may be too burdensome; or they may find it difficult to adhere to a complex treatment regimen.[46] In some cases, individuals lack trust in their care team or have diminished expectations of success in light of previous experiences. Ethics consultants often do not have the ability to diagnose the causes of noncompliance, but it is an appropriate role for research ethics consultants to make referrals to other services—for example, to social work or psychiatry—or for the consultant to participate in multidisciplinary meetings focused on noncompliance. As mentioned in the consult, the research team had already tried several times without success to understand and remedy the causes of Ms. Soffee's noncompliance; in parallel with continued efforts to understand her lack of adherence to medically indicated care, the research team called the Consultation Service to request assistance in understanding the ethical implications of ongoing noncompliance.

Readers may find the structure of this consult report somewhat unusual: first, numerous potential ethical concerns are raised; then, the extent to which each concern is applicable to the case at hand is analyzed. For the Consultation Service attending and the fellow who wrote this report, the structure fulfilled two needs. The first need was pedagogical. The research team had requested recommendations specific to Ms. Soffee's situation but also wanted guidance on how to think about noncompliant research participants in the future. This structure allowed the Consultation Service to outline ethical considerations relevant to poor compliance and to demonstrate how they could be applied to a particular case. The second need was practical but may be less apparent to the reader. The research team came to the Consultation Service without a clear ethical question but with strong misgivings about Ms. Soffee's continued research participation. The Consultation Service utilized the consultation meeting to pinpoint the ethical concerns prompting the research team's unease and drafted the consultation report to reflect this deductive process. Typically, the Consultation Service allows the requestor to define the scope of the consultation question; in this case, however, the ethics consultants needed to help define the question and ensure that no member of the research team's ethical concerns were overlooked.

## ■ NOTES

1. E. J. Emanuel, D. Wendler, and C. Grady, "What Makes Clinical Research Ethical?" *Journal of the American Medical Association* 283, no. 20 (2000): 2701–2711.

2. The National Commission for the Protection of Human Subjects of Biomedical and Behavioral Research, *The Belmont Report: Ethical Principles and Guidelines for the Protection of Human Subjects of Research* (Washington, DC: Department of Health, Education, and Welfare, 1979).

C. Fried, *Medical Experimentation: Personal Integrity and Social Policy* (New York: American Elsevier Publishing Co., 1974).

3. S. Sollitto, S. Hoffman, M. Mehlman, R. Lederman, S. Youngner, and M. Lederman, "Intrinsic Conflicts of Interest in Clinical Research: A Need for Disclosure," *Kennedy Institute of Ethics Journal* 13, no. 2 (2003): 83–91.

P. Appelbaum, L. Roth, C. Lidz, P. Benson, and W. Winslade, "False Hopes and Best Data: Consent to Research and the Therapeutic Misconception," *Hastings Center Report* 17, no. 2 (1987): 20–24.

4. H. Richardson and L. Belsky, "The Ancillary-Case Responsibilities of Medical Researchers: An Ethical Framework for Thinking about the Clinical Care That Researchers Owe Their Subjects," *Hastings Center Report* 34, no. 1 (2004): 25–33.

L. Belsky and H. Richardson, "Medical Researchers' Ancillary Clinical Care Responsibility," *British Medical Journal* 328 (2004): 1494–1496.

5. N. Dickert and D. Wendler, "Ancillary Care Obligations of Medical Researchers," *Journal of the American Medical Association* 302, no. 4 (2009): 424–428.

Participants in the 2006 Georgetown University Workshop on the Ancillary-Care Obligations of Medical Researchers Working in Developing Countries, "The Ancillary-Care Obligations of Medical Researchers Working in Developing Countries," *PLoS Medicine* 5, no. 5 (2008): 709–713.

6. S. Wolf, F. Lawrenz, C. Nelson, et al., "Managing Incidental Findings in Human Subjects Research: Analysis and Recommendations," *Journal of Law and Medical Ethics* 36, no. 2 (2008): 211–219.

7. E. J. Emanuel, D. Wendler, and C. Grady, "What Makes Clinical Research Ethical?" *Journal of the American Medical Association* 283, no. 20 (2000): 2701–2711.

8. C. Grady, "Vulnerability in Research: Individuals with Limited Financial and/or Social Resources," *Journal of Law and Medical Ethics* 37, no. 1 (2009): 19–27.

The Council for International Organizations of Medical Sciences (CIOMS) in collaboration with the World Health Organization (WHO), *The International Ethical Guidelines for Biomedical Research Involving Human Subjects*, 2002.

The National Commission for the Protection of Human Subjects of Biomedical and Behavioral Research, *The Belmont Report: Ethical Principles and Guidelines for the Protection of Human Subjects of Research* (Washington, DC: Department of Health, Education, and Welfare, 1979).

World Medical Association, *The Declaration of Helsinki: Ethical Principles for Medical Research Involving Human Subjects*, 2008.

9. A. Wertheimer. *Exploitation* (Princeton, NJ: Princeton University Press, 1996).

10. G. Henderson, L. Churchill, A. Davis, et al., "Clinical Trials and Medical Care: Defining the Therapeutic Misconception," *PLoS Medicine* 4, no. 11 (2007): 1735–1738.

P. Appelbaum, L. Roth, C. Lidz, P. Benson, and W. Winslade, "False Hopes and Best Data: Consent to Research and the Therapeutic Misconception," *Hastings Center Report* 17, no. 2 (1987): 20–24.

F. Miller and S. Joffe, "Evaluating the Therapeutic Misconception," *Kennedy Institute of Ethics Journal* 16, no. 4 (2006): 353–366.

11. E. J. Emanuel and C. Grady, "Four Paradigms of Clinical Research and Research Oversight," *Cambridge Quarterly of Healthcare Ethics* 16 (2006): 82–96.

12. B. Spilker, "Methods of Assessing and Improving Patient Compliance in Clinical Trials," *IRB* 14, no. 3 (1992): 1–6.

13. Participants in the 2006 Georgetown University Workshop on the Ancillary-Care Obligations of Medical Researchers Working in Developing Countries, "The Ancillary-Care Obligations of Medical Researchers Working in Developing Countries," *PLoS Medicine* 5, no. 5 (2008): 709–713.

14. World Medical Association, *The Declaration of Helsinki: Ethical Principles for Medical Research Involving Human Subjects*, 2008.

15. H. Richardson and L. Belsky, "The Ancillary-Case Responsibilities of Medical Researchers: An Ethical Framework for Thinking about the Clinical Care That Researchers Owe Their Subjects," *Hastings Center Report* 34, no. 1 (2004): 25–33.

16. The Council for International Organizations of Medical Sciences (CIOMS) in collaboration with the World Health Organization (WHO), *The International Ethical Guidelines for Biomedical Research Involving Human Subjects*, 2002.

17. Participants in the 2006 Georgetown University Workshop on the Ancillary-Care Obligations of Medical Researchers Working in Developing Countries, "The Ancillary-Care Obligations of Medical Researchers Working in Developing Countries," *PLoS Medicine* 5, no. 5 (2008): 709–713.

18. N. Dickert and D. Wendler, "Ancillary Care Obligations of Medical Researchers," *Journal of the American Medical Association* 302, no. 4 (2009): 424–428.

19. L. Belsky and H. Richardson, "Medical Researchers' Ancillary Clinical Care Responsibility," *British Medical Journal* 328 (2004): 1494–1496.

H. Richardson, "Gradations of Researcher's Obligation to Provide Ancillary Care for HIV/AIDS in Developing Countries," *Health Policy and Ethics* 97, no. 11 (2007): 12–17.

H. Richardson and L. Belsky, "The Ancillary-Case Responsibilities of Medical Researchers: An Ethical Framework for Thinking about the Clinical Care That Researchers Owe Their Subjects," *Hastings Center Report* 34, no. 1(2004): 25–33.

20. Illes et al., "Incidental Findings in Brain Imaging Research," *Science* 311 (2006): 783–784.

21. F. Lawrenz and S. Sobotka, "Empirical Analysis of Current Approaches to Incidental Findings," *Journal of Law, Medicine and Ethics* 36 (2008): 249–255.

S. M. Wolf, "The Challenge of Incidental Findings," *Journal of Law, Medicine and Ethics* 36 (2008): 216–218.

22. G. Katzman, A. Dagher, and N. Patronas, "Incidental Findings on Brain Magnetic Resonance Imaging from 1000 Asymptomatic Volunteers," *Journal of the American Medical Association* 281, no. 1 (1999): 36–39.

23. E. W. Clayton, "Incidental Findings in Genetics Research Using Archived DNA," *Journal of Law, Medicine, and Ethics* 36 (2008): 286–291.

F. A. Miller et al., "Duty to Disclose What? Querying the Putative Obligation to Return Research Results to Participants", *Journal of Medical Ethics* 34 (2008): 210–213.

24. F. G. Miller, M. M. Mello, and S. Joffe, "Incidental Findings in Human Subjects Research: What Do Investigators Owe Research Participants?" *Journal of Law, Medicine and Ethics* 36 (2008): 271–279.

D. I. Shalowitz and F. G. Miller, "Disclosing Individual Results of Clinical Research," *Journal of the American Medical Association* 294 (2005): 737–740.

25. V. Ravitsky and B. S. Wilfond, "Disclosing Individual Genetic Results to Research Participants," *The American Journal of Bioethics* 6 (2006): 8–17.

26. B. E. Berkman and S. C, Hull, "Ethical Issues in Genomic Databases," *Encyclopedia of Applied Ethics*. 2012.

27. R. D. Truog, "The Ethics of Organ Donation by Living Donors," *New England Journal of Medicine* 353, no. 5 (2005): 444–446.

28. C. Grady, "Vulnerability in Research: Individuals with Limited Financial and/or Social Resources," *Journal of Law and Medical Ethics* 37, no. 1 (2009): 19–27.

A. Wertheimer, *Exploitation* (Princeton, NJ: Princeton University Press, 1996).

29. C. Pace, F. Miller, and M. Danis, "Enrolling the Uninsured in Clinical Trials: An Ethical Perspective," *Critical Care Medicine* 31, no. 3 (2003): S121–S125.

30. C. Denny and C. Grady, "Clinical Research with Economically Disadvantaged Populations," *Journal of Medical Ethics* 33 (2007): 382–385.

31. C. Grady, "Vulnerability in Research: Individuals with Limited Financial and/or Social Resources," *Journal of Law and Medical Ethics* 37, no. 1 (2009): 19–27.

32. C. Pace, F. Miller, and M. Danis, "Enrolling the Uninsured in Clinical Trials: An Ethical Perspective," *Critical Care Medicine* 31, no. 3 (2003): S121–S125.

33. C. Denny and C. Grady, "Clinical Research with Economically Disadvantaged Populations," *Journal of Medical Ethics* 33 (2007): 382–385.

34. E. J. Emanuel, "Undue Inducement: Nonsense on Stilts?" *The American Journal of Bioethics* 5, no. 5 (2005): 9–13.

35. United States Department of Health and Human Services, National Institutes of Health, Office for Human Research Protections, The Common Rule, Title 45 (Public Welfare), Code of Federal Regulations, Part 46 (Protection of Human Subjects), Subparts A-D, 2001.

The Council for International Organizations of Medical Sciences (CIOMS) in collaboration with the World Health Organization (WHO), *The International Ethical Guidelines for Biomedical Research Involving Human Subjects*, 2002.

36. C. Grady, "Vulnerability in Research: Individuals with Limited Financial and/or Social Resources," *Journal of Law and Medical Ethics* 37, no. 1 (2009): 19–27.

C. Pace, F. Miller, and M. Danis, "Enrolling the Uninsured in Clinical Trials: An Ethical Perspective," *Critical Care Medicine* 31, no. 3 (2003): S121–S125.

37. E. J. Emanuel, "Undue Inducement: Nonsense on Stilts?" *The American Journal of Bioethics* 5, no. 5 (2005): 9–13.

E. J. Emanuel, "Ending Concerns about Undue Inducement," *Journal of Law, Medicine, and Ethics* 32 (2004): 100–105.

38. National Bioethics Advisory Commission, "Ethical and Policy Issues in International Research: Clinical Trials in Developing Countries," available at: http://bioethics.georgetown.edu/nbac/clinical/Chap1.html, accessed on February 11, 2010.

P. Appelbaum, L. Roth, C. Lidz, P. Benson, and W. Winslade, "False Hopes and Best Data: Consent to Research and the Therapeutic Misconception," *Hastings Center Report* 17, no. 2 (1987): 20–24.

39. G. Henderson, L. Churchill, A. Davis, et al., "Clinical Trials and Medical Care: Defining the Therapeutic Misconception," *PLoS Medicine* 4, no. 11 (2007): 1735–1738.

40. Nuremburg Military Tribunal, from U.S. v. Karl Brandt et al. "The Nuremburg Code," available at: http://ohsr.od.nih.gov/guidelines/nuremberg.html.

The Council for International Organizations of Medical Sciences (CIOMS) in collaboration with the World Health Organization (WHO), *The International Ethical Guidelines for Biomedical Research Involving Human Subjects*, 2002.

United States Department of Health and Human Services, National Institutes of Health, Office for Human Research Protections, The Common Rule, Title 45 (Public Welfare), Code of Federal Regulations, Part 46 (Protection of Human Subjects), Subparts A-D, 2001.

World Medical Association, *The Declaration of Helsinki: Ethical Principles for Medical Research Involving Human Subjects*, 2008.

41. F. Miller and S. Joffe, "Evaluating the Therapeutic Misconception," *Kennedy Institute of Ethics Journal* 16, no. 4 (2006): 353–366.

42. G. Henderson, L. Churchill, A. Davis, et al., "Clinical Trials and Medical Care: Defining the Therapeutic Misconception," *PLoS Medicine* 4, no. 11 (2007): 1735–1738.

43. P. D. Jacobson and W. E. Parmet, "A New Era of Unapproved Drugs: The Case of Abigail Alliance v Von Eschenbach," *Journal of the American Medical Association* 297, no. 2 (2007): 205–208.

44. *Abigail Alliance for Better Access to Developmental Drugs v Von Escenbach*, 495 F.3d 470 (DC Cir 2006).

45. B. Spilker, "Methods of Assessing and Improving Patient Compliance in Clinical Trials," *IRB* 14, no. 3 (1992): 1–6.

46. A. L. Gifford, J. E. Bormann, M. J. Shively, et al., "Predictors of Self-Reported Adherence and Plasma HIV Concentrations in Patients on Multidrug Antiretroviral Regimens," *Journal of Acquired Immune Deficiency Syndromes* 23, no. 5 (2000): 386–395.

# 6 Navigating Interpersonal Difficulties

Medical researchers, nurses and other clinical staff, research participants, and participants' family members are all individuals with varied histories, beliefs, experiences, values, and preferences who are quite likely to be dealing with complicated and difficult circumstances. As such, they will sometimes disagree. This is all too common in hospital-based research. Prospective participants and their loved ones may find themselves in alien and uncomfortable surroundings, may be frightened, and may be very ill. In medical care, uncertainty about a patient's diagnosis, prognosis, and appropriate treatment plan can increase the possibilities for disagreement and misunderstanding. Patients and their families may be asked to make decisions that they do not feel equipped to make, and members of the medical team may have their own views about what the correct choice is. In clinical research, this element of uncertainty is frequently exacerbated, since the purpose of research is to find the answers to unsolved problems of human health.

Although our ethics consultations almost invariably must take account of the human element, this chapter presents cases in which the relationships between people are central to the ethical questions raised. The first four cases can be described as involving people refusing to do what most reasonable people would generally agree they should do. The difficult question in these cases is not what should ideally be done, but what to do in the face of problematic behavior. The remaining four cases can reasonably be described as cases of disagreement, in which the people involved have well-intentioned but divergent views about the right course of action. In all cases involving interpersonal issues, the ethics consultant must give particular consideration to the elements of process described in the Introduction to this book. The consultation process usually benefits from including all the stakeholders in the case. When interpersonal difficulties are involved, it is all the more important that the process be and be seen as transparent, sensitive, and fair. One of the more useful tools at a bioethics consultant's disposal is the ability to facilitate clear communication among the parties involved.

Clinical research participants, like clinical care patients, entrust their personal and medical information to health professionals with the understanding that it will be kept confidential. Indeed, the standard template for intramural National Institutes of Health (NIH) consent forms includes an assurance of confidentiality that is often supplemented with a description of additional, study-specific protections. Sometimes, however, other considerations favor providing confidential medical information to a third party. For example, legal requirements to breach confidentiality exist if child abuse is suspected or if participants have certain reportable diseases. There may also be ethical reasons to breach confidentiality. This frequently occurs when a duty to provide information is not being fulfilled by a patient or research participant (as occurred in *Consult 3.5*). In *Consult 6.1*, a research participant with serious and contagious infections wanted to keep his disease status hidden from his live-in girlfriend. Given her risk of infection, the research participant had an ethical duty to inform her, a duty that he did not intend to fulfill. Members of the medical team caring for him felt they had conflicting duties to warn her and to maintain his confidentiality.

The context of clinical research also generates some distinctive ethical quandaries regarding people who have difficulty doing what is expected of them. *Consults 6.2* and *6.3* deal with prospective participants whom researchers thought were likely not to comply with research requirements. Noncompliance, otherwise referred to as nonadherence, can be ethically problematic for several reasons. First, a participant's noncompliance may be associated with heightened risks; there may therefore be an obligation on researchers to exclude participants who are more likely to be noncompliant in order to protect them. Second, data collected from noncompliant participants are more likely to be biased, inaccurate, or incomplete, thereby compromising the integrity of the study while wasting resources that could be used for participants who are more likely to help advance the study's aims. Yet if research subjects are not compliant for reasons that are beyond their control, excluding them from beneficial research may be unfair.

In *Consult 6.2*, a 14-year-old boy was referred to the NIH for participation in an allogenic stem cell transplant protocol (that is, a transplant using stem cells harvested from a matched donor's bone marrow). He would have been the first participant in this protocol but had behavioral problems such that the team doubted whether he would adhere to the complex drug regimen required. In *Consult 6.3*, a father wanted to enroll both himself and his young son as healthy volunteers but had problems with making and keeping his appointments. In both cases, the study team wanted to know if they could or should prospectively refuse enrollment on behavioral grounds for otherwise qualified potential participants. Other situations involve participants whose noncompliance emerges only when they are already enrolled into research at the NIH. This may add further complications; for example, if a participant who receives an intervention requiring long-term monitoring (e.g., an experimental transplant) is lost to follow-up, his safety may be at risk. In addition, researchers may have a more difficult time discharging research participants with whom they have developed a relationship, and they may be worried about compromising study data by removing someone.

Sometimes research participants make decisions that put others at risk. In the Clinical Center, as in other hospitals, the staff must consider the treatment of each individual against the backdrop of its care for others. *Consult 6.4* describes the case of a long-time participant in a natural history protocol for postoperative cancer survivors. This participant carried methicillin-resistant staphylococcus aureus (MRSA) and has alcoholism. Because MRSA is highly antibiotic resistant and can lead to life-threatening infections, carriers are normally isolated to avoid affecting others in hospital settings. When this research participant was found intoxicated on a ward that included immune-compromised participants, the medical team wanted to know whether and how she could be safely discharged, given the risks she posed to others and her reluctance to seek treatment for alcoholism. Cases like these are complex because of the multiple people whose safety is involved, the relationship of care that develops between long-time research participants and their care team, the resources (or lack thereof) that discharged research participants have to access care outside the NIH, and the personalities involved. Difficult ethical questions go hand in hand with delicate social interactions.

Although interpersonal issues arise when people are behaving problematically, they most often arise in the context of well-intentioned disagreements. There are many ethical issues about which reasonable people disagree, and research ethics consultants are often called upon to mediate these differences and help research teams and participants identify acceptable solutions. Many of our consults involve disagreements about how to treat very ill research participants who cannot make decisions for themselves. In these cases, the default option—to ask the individual what he or she prefers—is not available, yet urgent decisions must be made. As described in Chapter 4: Conducting Research with Vulnerable Populations, when a research participant lacks the capacity to consent for himself, a surrogate decision maker may make decisions about care and/or research participation on his behalf. The surrogate is expected to make the decisions that she believes the participant would have wanted, or, where she has no evidence about the participant's preferences, to make decisions in his best interests. However, surrogates, like participants, may make decisions that conflict with those recommended by professional caregivers.

In *Consult 6.5*, the mother of a man dying of leukemia insisted on treatment that the medical team regarded as futile. Not only did further treatment interventions, such as blood transfusions, hold no prospect of benefit, they would use up scarce and expensive resources that could help other research participants. This consult required careful consideration of how to respect the family's concerns while conveying the limits to the interventions the team were prepared to perform. *Consult 6.6* describes a case in which these roles were reversed. The research participant's wife had decided to withdraw life support on the basis of his previously stated wishes, his continued suffering, and his poor prognosis, but the team was reluctant to give up treatment that it saw as beneficial.

Cases like these two, painful as they are for all involved, involve relatively straightforward disagreements. Even more complicated issues may arise when there is also disagreement within the medical team or the family, or when there are doubts about the appropriateness of a surrogate decision maker. *Consult 6.7* describes one way this issue arose at the Clinical Center. Members of the clinical research team were worried about the surrogate their participant had chosen. Not only did he question their clinical judgments, but they were also concerned that he might make decisions that were not in the participant's best interests and which conflicted with her previously stated wishes. This case unfolded over the course of four separate consultations while the woman's health and cognitive capacity deteriorated, and it required consideration of whether and when surrogate decision makers may be overridden.

Our final case involves a conflict related to a participant's religious convictions. *Consult 6.8* describes a research participant who had signed a consent form to undergo medically indicated surgery but who also had religious beliefs that forbade the blood transfusions that he might need. The surgeons did not want to proceed if they could not give transfusions that might be medically necessary but that left the research participant with an apparent choice between his health and his faith. In both research and clinical care, it is generally accepted that autonomous individuals have the right to refuse potentially life-saving and beneficial interventions, such as blood transfusions, on the basis of their religious beliefs. Likewise, surrogate decision makers generally may refuse such care on behalf of others only where a previously competent individual's own wishes are clear. What remains unresolved is how the importance of respecting such deeply held beliefs should be balanced against the moral integrity of health care workers who do not want to be complicit in a harm they could avoid.

## CONSULT 6.1: OBLIGATIONS TO PREVENT HARM AND PROTECT CONFIDENTIALITY

### Reason for Consult

Jeanette King, a nurse, contacted the Consultation Service to discuss staff concerns about a research participant with a number of infectious diseases. Members of the research staff are concerned about how to balance their responsibility to protect the participant's confidentiality against his girlfriend's right to know that she is at risk of becoming infected. The Consultation Service was invited to participate in a multidisciplinary meeting including members of the research team and the hospital epidemiology service.

### Narrative

Jim Elon is a 26-year-old male research participant with human T-lymphatic virus type 1 (HTLV-1) and hepatitis B virus (HBV) infections. During his stay at the Clinical Center for an inpatient research protocol, Mr. Elon was on respiratory isolation to rule out tuberculosis (TB) infection. Mr. Elon's girlfriend, Michelle, visited him over the weekend. Against medical advice, she spent the night in Mr. Elon's room but did not wear a mask as would be indicated by the possibility of TB infection. When questioned, Michelle was unconcerned about the risk of TB and said that she would already be infected with anything that Mr. Elon has, having lived with him for 2 years.

Mr. Elon was released from the NIH and returned to Houston. Before he left, he made clear to the staff—including his nurses, his attending physician, and the research nurse—that he did not want any information about his medical condition to be shared with family or friends. During his girlfriend's visit, it became clear to the clinical staff that she likely does not know of Mr. Elon's HTLV-1 and HBV status or that she is at risk for transmission.

The research team related that, before Mr. Elon left, several members of the medical staff spoke with him about the importance of sharing information about HTLV-1 and HBV infection with Michelle. According to individuals present for that conversation, Mr. Elon adamantly insisted that he did not want the information shared, although he did indicate that he uses a condom during sexual intercourse. When pressed by the bioethics consultants to think about why Mr. Elon might not want to have this information shared with his girlfriend, the research team stated that he is generally secretive about aspects of his life, and it is not clear to them why he did not want to share his medical information.

A central point of discussion during the consult meeting was the Public Health Service (PHS) 5/3/90 sex partner notification policy, which pertains specifically to HIV infection. This policy requires NIH staff to inform partners (directly or through the public health department) if research participants refuse to do so themselves. If there are enough details available in cases of other infectious diseases—like HBV and HTLV-1—to determine that an individual is at risk of infection, and the consequences of that infection are serious, the policy supports a "discretionary disclosure" to partners of infected individuals by clinicians. HBV infection is a reportable disease to public health departments, although it is typically reported as a "case" without specific patient identifiers.

According to the members of the hospital epidemiology service, there is approximately a 30%–35% annual risk of transmission of HBV, which leads to a 1% chance of death and a 10% chance of chronic active HBV disease. Though HTLV-1 can be transmitted sexually or through needles (though much less frequently than HBV), its primary mode of infection is through breastfeeding (25%–30%). There is a 2%–4% risk of dying from HTLV-1 infection, primarily via adult T-cell lymphoma or a progressive neurological syndrome.

Over the course of the consultation, it became clear that members of the research team had several concerns about this case. There was disagreement about how reasonable it was to expect Michelle, the girlfriend, to take responsibility to protect herself from sexually transmitted diseases in general, and whether diseases related to HBV and HTLV-1 infection are beyond the general knowledge of the public. Research team members were also concerned about whether notifying Mr. Elon's girlfriend in this case meant that they would have to notify partners of individuals affected with HBV in every case.

## Analysis and Recommendations

The Consultation Service summarized the tensions between maintaining the research participant's confidentiality and breaching it. Reasons in favor of maintaining confidentiality included the fact that infectious disease status is private information over which a person is entitled to maintain control and the importance of preserving trust between individuals and their health care providers. The reasons in favor of breaching confidentiality included protecting the public's interests and preventing harm to an individual. Legal considerations were also discussed: NIH medical records are maintained under the Privacy Act system, which permits exceptions to requiring consent for disclosure of these records in order to protect the safety of others.

The Consultation Service recommended that partner notification is not appropriate in this situation, given that it is not clear that Mr. Elon is having unprotected sex, nor whether the girlfriend has been immunized for HBV. In addition, there had been no discussion of the couple's intentions to have children. The Consultation Service shares the research team's concern that by disclosing details of Mr. Elon's medical history to his girlfriend, they would be likely to sever the opportunity for an ongoing relationship with him. Maintaining an ongoing relationship to follow-up may provide a mechanism to reiterate persistently over time the importance of informing Michelle about her risks.

## Authors' Commentary

The decision for the research team not to inform Mr. Elon's girlfriend about her risk of various infections—in order to protect the research participant's confidentiality—was a defensible though controversial conclusion 10 years ago when this deliberation took place. It might be less defensible and more controversial today. Although the sexual partner notification policy that is followed by the NIH is specific to HIV infection, it may be the case that its requirements are also applicable to other infectious disease as well. Given that policies do not directly address disclosure requirements for non-HIV-infected individuals, but some (like the Privacy Act) leave open a narrow range of circumstances in which a duty to warn might override the obligation to protect confidentiality, a careful analysis of potential harms and the likelihood that they would materialize without a breach of confidentiality was warranted in this case. This was indeed the approach taken by the Consultation Service.

The Consultation Service team involved with this case acknowledged that there were facts about the risks of transmission that were unknown (e.g., whether the girlfriend had been immunized, was having unprotected sex, etc.) and felt that these uncertainties weakened the arguments in favor of notifying her against Mr. Elon's explicit wishes. The team also acknowledged the importance of maintaining a good relationship with the research participant over time, which would be important both to provide optimal care to him but also, at least theoretically, to encourage him to notify his sex partners about his status. This approach was similar to the one discussed in *Consult 3.5*, where the research team hoped to maintain contact with a research participant to encourage him to notify his daughters of the result of a genetic test that may have clinical implications for them.

A follow-up conversation with Jeanette, the consult requestor, revealed some important additional details that were not captured in the earlier narrative summary. First, Mr. Elon had ended the relationship with his girlfriend by the time of his 4-month postdischarge follow-up visit, and he never informed her about his infection status. The hope that the team would be able to counsel him over time to disclose that information himself did not materialize. We also learned that the research participant had human papilloma virus (HPV) infection in addition to the other infections enumerated in the consult report. Given that he had obviously visible genital warts as a result of the HPV infection, according to Jeanette, it is possible that Mr. Elon's girlfriend was already aware of her risk of sexually transmitted infections even without an explicit disclosure by the research participant. This is one additional factor that might have helped justify a decision not to inform the girlfriend.

The analysis described in the consultation report did not, however, address some additional considerations that would argue in favor of disclosure by the research team.[1] First, disclosure to the girlfriend could help reduce the risk of her transmitting potential infections (of which she was possibly unaware) to others. Transmission from people who are not aware of their infection status accounts for 54%–70% of new HIV infections,[2] for example. Second, disclosure could also enable her to receive treatment for infections that she might not be aware she had. Data suggest that contact tracing (the systematic identification of sexual partners) can be a cost-effective way to identify newly infected individuals in order to treat them, which can significantly reduce the morbidity or even mortality associated with infection.[3]

Although the NIH sexual partner notification policy remains unchanged since the time of this consult, the Centers for Disease Control (CDC) has revised its recommendations for "partner counseling and referral service programs"[4] for HIV and other infectious diseases within that timeframe. Specifically, the CDC has endorsed a shift in emphasis away from self-referral (as the least effective method for notifying partners) toward provider referral (as the most effective methods for notifying partners) to facilitate access to infectious disease counseling services. It also defines a broader role for public health resources for these counseling services.[5] This reasoning, and the most recent data about the infectious disease transmission risks, might well lead to a different conclusion than the one drawn by the Consultation Service team a decade ago.

## CONSULT 6.2: EXCLUDING A NONCOMPLIANT PARTICIPANT FROM A STUDY WITH THE PROSPECT OF DIRECT BENEFIT

### Reason for Consult

Dr. Jari Hyypiä, the principal investigator, called for advice concerning a pediatric research participant and his potential inability to comply with an allogenic stem cell transplant protocol.

### Narrative

Dr. Hyypiä came to the Consultation Service to discuss the case of Michael, a 14 year old diagnosed earlier in childhood with chronic granulomatous disease (CGD, a disease in which immune system cells called phagocytes do not function properly). Michael was referred to the NIH from an outside hospital for participation in an allogeneic stem cell transplant protocol (i.e., involving stem cells that are harvested from a matched donor's bone marrow). He was admitted to the protocol, with his 17-year-old sister as the planned human leukocyte antigen (HLA) matched donor.

According to the research team, Michael has been seen at the NIH for 18 months and is currently being treated for infection. Recently, concerns arose over increasing behavioral problems and noncompliance. In the previous month, for example, Michael was noncompliant with his regimen of antibiotics and care of his central line while home in New Jersey. A psychiatric consult was called, which indicated that he has mild mental retardation (IQ of 67) and a predisposition toward violent behavior.

In conversation, Dr. Hyypiä acknowledges that it might be in Michael's interest to receive the transplant; however, he voiced the research team's significant concerns about having a noncompliant individual be the first to enroll in a protocol that requires a rigorous regimen of procedures and drugs. Lack of compliance could jeopardize not only Michael's safety and well-being but also the integrity of the study.

### Analysis and Recommendations

There is no general requirement to accept individuals into research protocols. Nevertheless, given the relationship between Michael and the research team and his established interest in receiving a bone marrow transplant at the NIH, options for allowing him to continue on the protocol were explored.

As discussed during the ethics meeting, the Consultation Service recommended conducting a time-limited trial of three standard drugs to treat Michael's underlying condition, during which time his compliance with the medications, required visits, and some additional behaviors would be evaluated. To implement this plan, the team was advised to meet with Michael and his mother to convey their concerns about his behavior and compliance, and establish a behavioral contract that sets forth the conditions of enrollment at different stages, including the possibility of not receiving a transplant here if Michael is unsuccessful in meeting initial expectations.

## Authors' Commentary

In the analysis of this case, it was noted that there is no general right to enroll in research at the NIH, though people should not be unfairly excluded. The purpose of clinical research is the generation of scientific knowledge that may advance human health, not the benefit of individual research participants. Researchers therefore have a degree of discretion about whom to enroll into their studies, especially if the choice may unnecessarily interfere with scientific goals like maintaining the integrity of the data. Protocols that involve relatively rare diseases tend to be small and only enroll a few participants; therefore, one noncompliant participant represents a tremendous expenditure of resources and could skew the data substantially. In addition, the transplant procedure being used was relatively untested in this context. As the first potential participant in this study, the participant could therefore be exposed to unknown risks, and his noncompliance could make it difficult to separate research risks from risks that could have been avoided if he had taken his medications.

Nevertheless, research participants at the NIH may not have other good options for treatment for their conditions, and relationships of care may develop between participants and researchers. Although the purpose of this kind of research is ultimately to generate scientific knowledge, the research also takes on a therapeutic orientation in which researchers may feel they have strong duties not to abandon individuals that they can help. This was a primary motivation behind exploring options to keep this adolescent research participant on the transplant protocol.

An additional concern that was not raised in this consult is that the bone marrow harvesting procedure exposes the donor sibling to risks that might not be justified if the recipient is not going to be compliant with the treatment regimen. The need to establish a compliant pattern of behavior, with the mother's involvement, is an important way to protect the donor from being exposed to risk of harm in a futile attempt to help her brother.

## CONSULT 6.3: EXCLUDING A NONCOMPLIANT PARTICIPANT FROM A STUDY WITH NO PROSPECT OF BENEFIT

### Reason for Request

Dr. Olivia Schrader, an NIH investigator, contacted the Consultation Service to discuss whether concerns about compliance and various behaviors on the part of a prospective healthy volunteer were sufficient to justify not enrolling him or his son in a protocol.

### Narrative

A healthy adult male and his 6-year-old son wish to enroll as healthy volunteers in a protocol led by Dr. Schrader. This protocol evaluates body mechanics in order to develop better treatments for persons with cerebral palsy. For healthy volunteers, the protocol has negligible risk and no prospect of medical benefit.

The father and son made an appointment to enroll in the protocol but failed to appear for evaluation and did not call or contact the clinic. Approximately 1 week later, the father called to reschedule and reported that they had missed the previous appointment because of a family emergency. The research coordinator attempted to reschedule, informing the father that the lab could not guarantee a particular day in advance but would try to accommodate his requested date.

The father called the research coordinator several times over the next week and became increasingly impatient and upset about not being guaranteed the enrollment date he preferred. The research coordinator was troubled by the father's tone and suggested that it would be better to communicate only via e-mail. At this point, the father responded angrily by e-mail to the research coordinator and also contacted Dr. Schrader to express his displeasure. Dr. Schrader consulted with the lab director and determined that it would be best to exclude the father and son from the study due to concerns about the father's demands and the resource constraints in the laboratory. The lab director requested input from the Consultation Service on how to proceed.

### Analysis and Recommendations

Prospective research participants do not have a right to be included in research, but they do have a right to have their potential inclusion evaluated fairly. The participants' previous failure to appear on time for enrollment and subsequent difficulty finding a mutually acceptable rescheduling date constitute a sufficient reason to exclude the prospective participants. Excluding them on these grounds is not unfair or invidious. That the study is a one-time evaluation with no prospect of medical benefit and that the laboratory is currently understaffed both provide additional justifications for exclusion. While the Consultation Service did not believe that exclusion was obligatory in this case, it believed that it is permissible. The Consultation Service communicated this opinion to the research team, and they elected not to enroll the prospective research participants.

An additional issue came up during discussion. Some of the scheduling difficulties were related to the pediatric volunteer's simultaneous enrollment in another protocol, raising the possibility that the pediatric volunteer was enrolled in multiple other protocols. The NIH patient representative was contacted, and upon reviewing the father and son's records, she determined that the pediatric volunteer was only enrolled in one other protocol, although the adult volunteer was enrolled in several protocols.

## Authors' Commentary

As in *Consult 6.2*, this case acknowledged that although there may not be a right to enroll in research at the NIH, people should not be unfairly excluded. Since researchers have stronger reason to enroll research participants whom they can help, it seems reasonable to decide to exclude the father and son from participation in this study as healthy volunteers, while coming to a different conclusion in another study involving the prospect of direct benefit to an adolescent participant.

The possible enrollment of the pediatric volunteer in multiple other protocols ultimately did not factor into the Consultation Service's recommendations. Enrollment in multiple protocols as a pediatric healthy volunteer could be problematic, however, if, for instance, it required missing school, particularly since the pediatric volunteer had to travel to the NIH from out of state. Another potential concern would be that enrollment in multiple studies could interfere with the quality of the data. For example, if a trial was testing a drug for safety, then enrollees in that trial should not be in another safety trial; otherwise, the investigators would not know which drug was responsible for negative effects. Still another concern is that multiple blood draws and other study procedures across several studies could pose cumulative risks that are above the threshold of risk that children are usually permitted to be exposed to in research. Discovering that a pediatric research participant was enrolled in multiple studies in a burdensome manner might have provided additional support for excluding that research participant from further studies, especially given that they held no prospect of benefit for him. *Consult 2.5* contains further discussion of the ethical implications of participants enrolling in multiple protocols.

## CONSULT 6.4: DISCHARGING AN AT-RISK PARTICIPANT

### Reason for Consult

Sarah Rich, a member of the research team, contacted the Consultation Service to discuss how to responsibly care for and discharge a research participant suffering from alcoholism and potentially placing other hospitalized research participants at risk.

### Narrative

According to Ms. Rich, Francine Winters came to the NIH to participate in a protocol as a healthy volunteer. During screening, however, a tumor was discovered, and Ms. Winters was enrolled as a research participant in a relevant natural history study. The tumor was surgically removed as part of that protocol. Ms. Winters still comes to the NIH regularly for research follow-up visits. Although Ms. Winters has excellent doctors that she sees outside of the NIH, the research team here continues to follow her. Ms. Winters carries methicillin-resistant staphylococcus aureus (MRSA) and is an alcoholic.

Ms. Winters arrived for a research follow-up visit intoxicated. She was admitted to the Clinical Center as an inpatient for detoxification. She was supposed to be discharged however, two days before her planned discharge, Ms. Winters left the unit on which she was staying and procured three bottles of rum. A search for Ms. Winters found her on the bone marrow transplant unit, intoxicated and speaking with the nurses. Because she carries MRSA and will not remain on the appropriate unit, the Clinical Center staff feels that Ms. Winters poses a significant risk to the immunocompromised individuals on the bone marrow transplant unit and to other inpatients at the NIH for whom MRSA infection could be lethal.

Now that Ms. Winters completed the detoxification program, the research team agrees that it is time for her to be discharged from the NIH. Her boyfriend, however, will not allow her to return to the home they share, and she has no other family who can help care for her. In addition, Ms. Winters's insurance company will no longer cover treatment for her alcoholism. Although it was suspected that she has ample resources at her disposal, Ms. Winters continually refuses to pay for services at a private residential treatment facility.

Ms. Winters underwent a psychiatric consultation. The psychiatrist did not feel that Ms. Winters was suicidal at the time of the consultation but expressed concern that if Ms. Winters was discharged, she could check into a hotel, begin drinking again, and potentially become suicidal. The research team contacted the Consultation Service regarding how to proceed ethically in light of this information and Ms. Winters's complicated psychosocial situation.

## Analysis and Recommendations

Although the risks that Ms. Winters posed to other inpatient research participants at the NIH lent this case greater urgency, the Consultation Service first considered the ideal clinical course for Ms. Winters, and then considered whether her interests did indeed compete with the interests of other research participants at the NIH.

Without any clear indications of suicidal ideation, discharging Ms. Winters seemed to be clinically appropriate for the following reasons: discharge was consistent with the standard of care, given that Ms. Winters had completed the detoxification process and was not considered to be at medical risk from alcohol withdrawal. In addition, referring her to a rehabilitation hospital or extending her stay at the NIH to address her drinking did not seem appropriate given that she had not yet expressed any motivation to stop drinking. Her boyfriend's refusal to allow Ms. Winters to return home complicated this matter, making it more difficult to find a safe place to which Ms. Winters could be discharged. Nevertheless, given the psychiatrist's assessment of the behavior patterns of alcoholics, it seemed appropriate to discharge Ms. Winters and wait until she was ready to pursue rehabilitation.

If, prior to discharge, it became apparent that Ms. Winters was at risk of committing suicide, the research team would have had to reassess the appropriateness of keeping her at the NIH or transferring her to another facility. Unless the research team acquired evidence that Ms. Winters was suicidal, attempting to find a place where Ms. Winters could be safely discharged seemed to be the best clinical course.

Two additional ethical considerations further supported this course of action. First, given that Ms. Winters posed a risk to other research participants in the Clinical Center, and that the NIH has a responsibility to protect these individuals, discharging Ms. Winters allowed the NIH to meet this responsibility. Second, providing treatment for Ms. Winters's alcoholism would be considered ancillary care because it is unrelated to the natural history protocol in which she is enrolled. The NIH does not have a responsibility to provide alcohol treatment or sanctuary for Ms. Winters, and the concern that she might harm other research participants by exposing them to MRSA gives additional justification for this conclusion. Had Ms. Winters become suicidal, the NIH might have had a responsibility to provide this ancillary care. Under the prevailing circumstances, however, it was consistent with NIH's ethical responsibilities to discharge Ms. Winters.

Recommendations:

1) Plan to discharge Ms. Winters the afternoon of the consult.
2) Arrange a conversation between Ms. Winters, her boyfriend, and a social worker to discuss options.
3) Look into private treatment facilities and check whether Ms. Winters (or her boyfriend) would be willing and able to pay for one of these.
4) If this is not an option, be in contact with the local emergency housing services.

The Consultation Service acknowledged that the plan might need to be revised, depending on how further conversations progressed, and recommended that the research team discuss plans to deal with Ms. Winters in the future, assuming that she might return to the NIH for research follow-up visits.

## Authors' Commentary

This consult involved a research participant who presented with multiple issues that were unrelated to the reason she came to the NIH: to enroll as a healthy volunteer. The first unexpected finding, a tumor, was relatively easily addressed via treatment under a different research protocol. Other findings (e.g., MRSA infection, alcoholism) were not relevant to this treatment protocol but were nonetheless significant to the participant's health and/or to the safety of other participants at the NIH. This consult raises questions about the scope of the research teams' obligations to provide ancillary care to Ms. Winters for these unrelated conditions. In their discussion of ancillary care obligations, Belsky and Richardson acknowledge that the entrustment is partial because research participants entrust only specific aspects of their health to researchers, and that researchers are not obliged to assume responsibility for all aspects of participants' health care. Ancillary care obligations are limited by factors such as the intensity and duration of the researcher–participant relationship and the participant's vulnerability and dependence on the researcher.[6]

The NIH infrastructure was already equipped to handle ancillary care needs related to MRSA infection, which was more of a threat to other participants (particularly those with immune deficiencies), than to Ms. Winters herself. The NIH, like many hospital settings, can manage the risks of infection to others through the use of inpatient isolation units, for example. The NIH's ability to manage this risk was, however, complicated by other behavioral health issues such as Ms. Winters's alcoholism, which either directly (leading to the desire to leave the unit to acquire alcohol) or indirectly (impairing her judgment about risk taking) led to noncompliance with the isolation requirements. The NIH attempted to support the participant through detoxification for her alcohol dependence in parallel to her enrollment on the treatment protocol, but she was not compliant with that intervention.

These issues were still further complicated by the participant's lack of social support outside of the NIH and lack of health insurance coverage for alcohol treatment outside of the NIH. These factors made her more dependent on the free care and support available at the NIH. The research team struggled with the appropriateness of terminating their provision of ancillary care services, especially given her vulnerability and dependence on them. The Consultation Service's analysis took into account that this participant had completed her treatment protocol for the tumor, that efforts had been made to treat her alcohol dependence, and that she was relatively stable (i.e., not suicidal) to come to the conclusion that on balance, the researchers owed her no further duty of ancillary care. This was further corroborated by the fact that she posed an ongoing risk of infection to other participants at the NIH, a risk that she was not cooperative in helping to manage.

In follow-up, we learned from the consult requestor that after she was discharged from the NIH, Ms. Winters checked herself into a 30-day alcohol rehabilitation facility and thereafter patched up her relationship with her boyfriend and her life. She moved to Seattle with her boyfriend and has remained sober since.

## CONSULT 6.5: FUTILE CARE

### Reason for Consult

Dr. Ronald Samuels, an NIH fellow, asked the Consultation Service to assist his research team in arriving at end-of-life care decisions in the face of disagreement between the team and the research participant's surrogate decision maker.

### Narrative

In a phone call with members of the Consultation Service, Dr. Samuels related the medical history of Stephan Wooten, an adult male with leukemia. Mr. Wooten underwent a stem-cell transplant in March 2004 and has received several courses of chemotherapy, both standard and experimental, with no response. He has lost the capacity to make decisions for himself, is in critical condition in the intensive care unit (ICU), and the research team feels that his death is imminent. Stephan's mother—whom he appointed as his surrogate decision maker—does not perceive shifting to comfort care as an acceptable strategy.

At his mother's insistence, Mr. Wooten regularly undergoes blood draws to monitor his status and receives interventions to deal with infections and correct his chronically low blood cell counts. In light of the inability to address successfully his underlying illness, the research team perceives these interventions as futile care. In addition, at his mother's request, Mr. Wooten has not been receiving pain medication. She wishes to maintain his alertness, which the research team thinks is not in his best medical interest.

At the end of this initial phone conversation, the Consultation Service offered to meet with Dr. Samuels, the medical team, and Mr. Wooten's mother. The research team, requested, however, to talk with the Consultation Service independently. Before talking with the mother, they wanted to address their concerns about the ethics of using certain interventions, such as blood transfusions that are medically inappropriate at this point, considering that they are not prolonging Mr. Wooten's life significantly. Moreover, both blood and ICU beds are in limited supply, so that using them for Mr. Wooten requires taking away resources that could be used to help others.

## Analysis and Recommendations

There is no ethical obligation to provide futile care, even if patients, research participants, or family members demand it. The research team stands on solid ethical ground with regard to withholding certain treatments while providing appropriate palliative care. We note, however, that there is an ongoing debate in the literature regarding the definition of futile care and who decides when to withhold further interventions. In most cases, we tend to rely on the individual's wishes. We offer our analysis here while acknowledging that this issue can be contentious.

In this particular case, the attempts to treat Mr. Wooten's leukemia have gone beyond the standard of care and the demands of the family have been unrealistic. At this point, it is appropriate for the research team to take the position that further interventions would be futile because they have done all that they can to address the underlying illness, and it is now appropriate to focus on the goal of making the dying process as comfortable as possible.

The research team's concern about the allocation of resources is valid. An argument can be made regarding the ethics of using scarce resources, which would be particularly supported if the institution has a uniformly applied set of guidelines for forgoing interventions. In the absence of such an institutional policy, the researchers should base treatment decisions on an assessment of what is beneficial for the individual participant. The research team should consider what the standard of care is in such cases. It is fair to treat Mr. Wooten in the same way that other participants are treated under similar circumstances.

With regard to communicating with the family, it is important to make sure the team agrees on a unified approach so that the family is not exposed to conflicting messages, which may aggravate the situation. One possible approach at this point would be to avoid explicit discussion and not push the family anymore regarding decisions that are at the heart of the conflict, such as a transfer to hospice care or the institution of a do-not-resuscitate (DNR) order. Alternatively, it is possible to develop a plan of care that involves withholding treatments that are not medically indicated and to present this plan to the family. With this approach, it is advisable to minimize further conflict with family members by letting them know that every possible medically beneficial intervention has been performed to treat the underlying illness and that, at this point, comfort care is in the best interest of Mr. Wooten. It is also advisable to bring to their attention that Mr. Wooten is dying of his leukemia and not because he is being denied care.

Following discussion with the Office of Legal Counsel and in agreement with Clinical Center policies regarding DNR, it is possible to institute a DNR order when a research participant is terminally ill, and two attending physicians are in agreement that he is at the end of his life (about 2 weeks life expectancy). In such a case, the family should be informed that the research team is now shifting from the goal of curing the disease to the goal of making the dying process as comfortable as possible, and a DNR is in place. It should be communicated to Mr. Wooten's family that comfort care can be provided within the Clinical Center, but that if they find this unacceptable, the research team can help arrange a transfer to another medical institution.

## Authors' Commentary

This case raised a number of issues that have been debated extensively in the bioethics literature, including what counts as futile care, when doctors may refuse to treat someone, and how scarce resources should be allocated. As a result, our advice in this case was tentative, and we presented the research team with different options that we considered acceptable. It is also worth noting the extent to which our recommendations reflect the interpersonal dimension of the problem. It was considered important not just to lay out which clinical options were permissible but also to suggest ways in which the medical team might present their views to the family.

The circumstances faced by the team requesting this consult involved their being asked both to deny and to provide care against their medical judgment: on the one hand they were asked not to give Mr. Wooten pain medication, and on the other they were asked to give him treatments that were judged to be futile. The consult analysis never explicitly comes back to the question of the pain management (although it is implicit in the ideas of hospice and comfort care). It is not uncommon for family members to want to withhold pain medication because they want their loved ones to be kept as conscious as possible. Unfortunately, this can lead to a great deal of suffering, and, consequently, distress for members of the care team who may feel that they are causing the patient/research participant's suffering. Likewise, there are emotional costs for nurses and doctors who are asked to provide care that they think is futile (and may actually be prolonging suffering). Some medical professionals regard the provision of such care as undermining the integrity of their profession.[7]

One of the other ethical considerations at play in this consult was fairness. Looking back at the report, the paragraph that discusses fairness seems to hint at two arguments, which it may be helpful to distinguish. First, there is an argument concerning how scarce resources should be distributed. When there is not enough of some important good to give to everyone who needs it, some principled approach is needed to decide who should receive it. The consult report suggests that an acceptable way to distribute scarce resources would be to give them only to people who can benefit from them. Second, there is an argument about the treatment of this participant compared with other participants. Like individuals should be treated alike, and the ability of a hospital to ensure that it treats people consistently in this way is enhanced by the presence of institutional guidelines for care.

## ■ CONSULT 6.6: CONFLICT BETWEEN THE RESEARCH TEAM AND FAMILY MEMBERS

### Reason for Consult

Dr. Greta Kircher raised questions during medical rounds regarding a disagreement between a research participant's wife and primary team about the discontinuation of life support. She was referred to the Consultation Service.

### Narrative

Dr. Kircher was prompted to seek ethics support by the case of Jonathan Smith, a 36-year-old man with lung cancer. He was admitted to the Clinical Center several months ago; at that time, he had a DNR order and an advanced directive naming his wife as his primary decision maker placed in his chart. His condition progressively deteriorated. Approximately 2 weeks prior to consultation, he was transferred to the ICU following intestinal bleeding. Mr. Smith developed respiratory failure and was put on a ventilator.

Mr. Smith's wife wished to withdraw life support; she voiced this desire repeatedly. Her decision was based on her husband's previous wishes, his current suffering, and his poor overall prognosis. The research team disagreed with her decision. They held out hope that Mr. Smith could still get some benefit from continued care despite his overall poor prognosis.

A member of the Consultation Service was present during medical rounds in the ICU as recent developments in Jonathan's care were being discussed. Several of the team members expressed their concerns about the disagreement between the wife and the care team. The ethics consultant suggested an ethics consult to address the growing tension surrounding this issue.

The ethics consultant arranged a meeting between the Consultation Service, the family, and the research team. Due to a medical emergency that required the research team's full attention, the consultants met with Mr. Smith's wife in the absence of the team. She explained that she had reached a firm decision to withdraw life support, that she had communicated this decision to the research team, and that she had no desire to meet with the team to discuss the issue again.

## Analysis and Recommendations

Both ethical guidelines and current regulations indicate that a patient has the right to make decisions about his or her own medical treatment and about the withdrawal of life support. When an individual is incapacitated, as Mr. Smith was at the time of the consult, an individual with durable power of attorney (DPA) or the next of kin is an appropriate surrogate decision maker. The decision of a DPA or the next of kin ought to be respected unless there is reason to think that the individual is acting on the basis of conflicting interests. Under Maryland Law a DPA or the next of kin has the power to make medical decisions for an incapacitated patient or research participant, so it is advisable that Mr. Smith's wife's decision be respected.

## Authors' Commentary

In this case the Consultation Service's recommendation was accepted, and life support was withdrawn on the day of the consult. Whereas *Consult 6.5* posed difficult questions about futile care and the rights of individuals to treatment, this consult reports a scenario where the ethical debate has mostly been settled. Just as a competent person should be allowed to refuse life support on the grounds of autonomy, so, too, may a DPA make that refusal on the person's behalf. This case was also simplified by the multiple reasons to respect the DPA's decision: Mr. Smith had stated clear preferences; he had expressly appointed his wife to make decisions for him; he was suffering; and his prognosis was very poor. Had these factors not coincided, the appropriate action might have been less clear. The fact that the ethically appropriate course of action was clear does not mean that ethics consultation was unnecessary or unhelpful, however. In this case, the ethics consultant played a key role in facilitating the wife's wishes being carried out, as an expert who was independent of the research team. It is also possible in this kind of case that the involvement of the Consultation Service is reassuring to members of the research team who are reluctant to assume responsibility for discontinuing treatments or who may feel that a patient's death is a failure on their part.

Members of the Clinical Center Department of Bioethics regularly accompany other staff in the hospital on their clinical rounds. This consult arose because an ethicist saw the team's conflict while on rounds and encouraged Dr. Kircher to call a formal consultation. Such informal routes to ethical consultation are common, and they may be an important way for ethicists to educate and work with researchers who are less familiar with how and why ethics consultation may be useful to them.

## ■ CONSULT 6.7: CONFLICT BETWEEN THE RESEARCH TEAM AND SURROGATE DECISION MAKER

This case involved four separate consultations that unfolded over several months.

### Reason for Consult I

Deborah Chen, a social worker, called to request assistance in determining whether a research participant's advance directive should be reconsidered or rewritten.

### Narrative I

Deborah explained to the Consultation Service that the research participant, Penelope Long, is in the ICU and recently prepared an advance directive designating her nephew as her primary surrogate decision maker. This decision was made with the apparent agreement of Mrs. Long's husband who is present with her in ICU.

According to the clinical team, Mrs. Long's nephew has become difficult to work with, leading some to worry that when the durable power of attorney (DPA) is invoked, he will not make decisions that are in her best interests. Mrs. Long is currently able to make decisions for herself, but it is the opinion of the clinical team that she may lose decision-making capacity in the near future.

### Analysis and Recommendations I

The Consultation Service suggested that it would be reasonable to revisit the advance directive with Mrs. Long, especially as the clinical team believes that she may imminently lose the ability to make decisions for herself.

## Reason for Consult II

Deborah Chen subsequently called the Consultation Service again to request involvement in a care meeting regarding Mrs. Long.

## Narrative II

Mrs. Long has remained an inpatient in the ICU for 2 months. Mrs. Long remains alert and able to make treatment decisions for herself. However, the ICU staff feels that Mrs. Long's nephew, whom she designated as her primary surrogate decision maker in her advanced directive, has at times impeded their ability to provide quality medical care for Mrs. Long by questioning treatment decisions, repeatedly questioning the competence of the ICU staff, and threatening legal action against them.

Deborah Chen, the attending social worker, has spoken on two occasions with Mrs. Long to revisit her decision to have her nephew act as DPA. On each occasion, Mrs. Long reiterated that this is what she wants. Deborah contacted the Consultation Service on behalf of the ICU team to request advice about how to approach Mrs. Long's nephew and to address potential problems with the delivery of care to Mrs. Long.

The Consultation Service led a discussion with members of the ICU team. The discussion focused on whether Mrs. Long's nephew was capable of functioning as a surrogate decision maker: whether he was competent to do so, whether Mrs. Long in fact wanted him to do so, and whether Mrs. Long's nephew will act according to her wishes or in her best interest. The Consultation Service attending noted that a "difficult personality" is not necessarily a poor decision maker. The ICU team felt, however, that the nephew's behavior had and could continue to contribute to suboptimal care for Mrs. Long.

## Analysis and Recommendations II

First, it should be clear to all members of the ICU team and should be reiterated to Mrs. Long's nephew that, at present, Mrs. Long is capable of making treatment decisions for herself. As such, her nephew does not currently have decision-making authority and should not interfere with the ICU staff's ability to carry out interventions consistent with Mrs. Long's wishes. The group agreed that Mrs. Long's nephew would receive a brief description of individual interventions, but for further information, he will be referred to Mrs. Long.

Second, recognizing the uncertain nature of Mrs. Long's prognosis, the instructional component of Mrs. Long's advance directive should be made as explicit as possible. At such time that Mrs. Long is no longer capable of making decisions, treatment decisions will be less uncertain and more difficult to challenge if there has been detailed discussion and documentation of Mrs. Long's preferences.

Third, the team agreed to talk to Mrs. Long about the role she would like her husband to play in decision making regarding her treatment and care and specifically to ask Mrs. Long her feelings on the appropriate course of action if her husband (the alternate decision maker) and her nephew disagree about a treatment decision.

Fourth, in the event of a true medical emergency, appropriate medical care consistent with Mrs. Long's previously stated wishes can be given if the DPA is not available to make decisions.

Finally, the ICU team was advised that when no evidence exists as to the specific treatment preferences of an incapacitated individual, surrogate decision makers are to use the "best interests standard." If the ICU team judges that the surrogate is not making decisions that are in Mrs. Long's best interest (or are inconsistent with the patient's stated wishes), the decision-making authority of the surrogate may be legitimately challenged.

---

## Reason for Consult III

Deborah Chen called again regarding concerns about the decisions and behavior of Mrs. Long's designated surrogate and asked for assistance to evaluate whether he was making treatment decisions that were consistent with her wishes and interests.

## Narrative III

Mrs. Long has been in the ICU for 4 months now. According to a phone conversation with Deborah Chen, Mrs. Long and her family agreed several weeks ago to have a DNR and a do-not-intubate (DNI) order placed on the chart. Roughly a week later, Mrs. Long went to the operating room (OR) to have her pacemaker removed, at which time the DNR/DNI orders were rescinded as part of standard practice. Postoperatively, Mrs. Long has not been sufficiently capacitated to enable further discussion of this issue. The requestors told us that Mrs. Long's nephew has refused to discuss reinstating the DNR and DNI and is sometimes antagonistic with care staff.

The Consultation Service team went to Mrs. Long's room in the ICU to speak with the nephew. Although he spoke to the consultants briefly in Mrs. Long's room, he refused to meet with them outside of her room or to have any discussion related to his role as Mrs. Long's DPA.

## Analysis and Recommendations III

While it is legitimate to question the extent to which the DPA's decisions reflect the research participant's wishes, the ethics consult team saw no compelling reason at this time to challenge the decision-making authority of the DPA. Mrs. Long is currently intubated, and there are no imminent medical decisions that need to be made or would alter the course of her care. Although Mrs. Long's nephew can be difficult to communicate with, there is little evidence that his approach to Mrs. Long's care is inconsistent with her stated wishes.

We believe the best approach at this time is to continue to share information with the DPA about Mrs. Long's clinical situation and to continue to try to communicate with him about treatment options. In the future, when there are treatment decisions that need to be discussed which the DPA will not engage in, his decision-making authority can be challenged and decision-making authority may be transferred to Mrs. Long's designated alternate, her husband.

## Reason for Consult IV

Deborah Chen, the social worker, asked Consultation Service members to participate in a multidisciplinary meeting to discuss Mrs. Long's treatment options and strategies for discussing them with her DPA, whose views are reported to be at odds with those of the clinical team.

## Narrative IV

The ICU doctors now believe that there is little or no chance that Mrs. Long will recover. She is currently receiving extensive and continuous medical support, including a ventilator, feeding tube, antibiotics, and vasopressors (medications to maintain her blood pressure). Periodic acute medical problems, such as hemorrhaging, are being treated aggressively. Doctors report that with continued treatment, Mrs. Long could possibly live for several months. Mrs. Long is sedated for her comfort, and she is not thought to be experiencing any pain. Although members of the ICU team agreed that none of the treatments Mrs. Long is receiving are harmful to her, they believe that they are not offering her any benefit and are simply prolonging her dying. When asked by the ethics consultants, some of the team members expressed concern that the current treatment course is against Mrs. Long's stated wishes and written advance directive.

At the same time, the DPA appointed by Mrs. Long, her nephew, reportedly continues to request full life support, and, in a previous discussion with the ICU staff, disputes the accuracy of Mrs. Long's advance directive, even though it was completed in the presence of the DPA and several witnesses. ICU staff report that the DPA commented previously that he would reconsider his position after Mrs. Long had been intubated for 30 days. He continues declining to speak with ethics consultants about his role as DPA.

## Analysis and Recommendations IV

At the meeting, a number of options were discussed for the future treatment of Mrs. Long. These included transferring Mrs. Long to another ICU, removing her from life support, maintaining her current level of life support but limiting treatment escalations, and continuing to provide all life-extending therapies. Mrs. Long's team reports that she is not stable enough to transfer to another facility, and doctors feel that it is unlikely that another facility would accept her.

Consultation Service team members confirmed that while Mrs. Long's advance directive indicates that she does not want to be on a respirator, a court order would be needed to discontinue life support without the agreement of the DPA, especially because there is some disagreement about the exact meaning of the wishes expressed in the advance directive. It was agreed, however, that the ICU team can consider forgoing diagnostic testing for and treatment of new acute conditions for which treatment would serve neither to improve nor extend the life of Mrs. Long.

Clinical Center policy (Clinical Center Policy and Communications Bulletin "Do Not Resuscitate (DNR) Orders and Limited Treatment Orders" 3(d)) also indicates that the DPA's agreement is not necessarily required should the clinical team decide not to provide CPR in the event that Mrs. Long experiences cardiopulmonary arrest. It may be reasonable to forgo CPR and other escalations in Mrs. Long's current level of care because the goal of improving Mrs. Long's quality of life and enabling her to survive outside of an ICU cannot be achieved. The DPA should be informed of decisions made about treatment and other procedures.

Attendees concluded that it would be best for a small group of ICU team members to discuss concerns about the goals and appropriateness of Mrs. Long's treatment with her designated DPA, her nephew. This group will attempt to be nonconfrontational, minimize conflict, and stress their mutual interest in what is best for Mrs. Long. The group will reiterate that physicians have exhausted all options that could lead to Mrs. Long's recovery, and that there is no reasonable chance that Mrs. Long could survive outside of an ICU. The group will also note that Mrs. Long's condition has not improved in the 30 days that her nephew reportedly said that he would wait before reassessing his decision to request full life support. If the DPA agrees, it would be appropriate to stop Mrs. Long's life-sustaining treatment.

## Authors' Commentary

This lengthy consult illustrates some interesting features of the consultation process. First, this was an iterative process: over a period of time the same problems recurred, sometimes in slightly different forms, and different strategies could be attempted. Second, the recommendations of the consult team changed as the circumstances changed. For example, early in the consult, a great deal of emphasis was placed on engaging the research participant so that she could express her wishes clearly in an advance directive, and in the hope that she would take on board some of the medical team's concerns about her appointed surrogate. Later, when Mrs. Long was unable to communicate her wishes, the emphasis was on the team's engagement with her nephew and their options if he made decisions that they judged were contrary to her wishes. Finally, this consult shows both the importance of communication between everyone involved in an individual's care and the limits to what communication can achieve.

This consult also makes vivid some of the difficulties that can arise when the DPA and the medical team do not see eye to eye. One of the common worries about surrogate decision makers is that they may not make decisions on the right basis. Though there is still some discussion about how surrogates ought to make their decisions, it is generally agreed that a surrogate should choose as the individual would have chosen (the *substituted judgment standard*) or, absent the relevant information about the individual's preferences, the surrogate should choose according to what he or she judges is in the individual's interests (the *best interests standard*).[8] But even well-meaning surrogates may fail to follow these standards. For example, surrogates may make decisions about end-of-life care on the basis of their own values, rather than those of the dying person. Effective communication between individuals and their surrogates and education about what it means to be a surrogate decision maker are necessary to avoid these sorts of problems.

The question of what to do if the decision of the DPA appears to be inconsistent with a person's advance directive has not been resolved. Given the cost, uncertainty of outcome, and potential increase in conflict between family members at an already traumatic time, a legal challenge to a DPA when he is representing someone at the end of her life should probably be contemplated only in rare circumstances.

Of note, this consultation revolves around questions of end-of-life care that may seem removed from issues related to research ethics. The case thus illustrates the reality that some research participants are likely to be terminally ill and hence questions about the ethics of end-of-life care will be part and parcel of the ethical concerns that may arise during their study involvement.

## CONSULT 6.8: RESPECTING MEDICAL BELIEFS

### Reason for Consult

Jackson Feinberg, a nurse, requested an ethics consultation to ensure that the research team with which he was working was aware of a participant's religious concerns that might affect his decision to have invasive surgery.

### Narrative

Jackson explained that he is currently caring for Donald Morrell, a 45-year-old school teacher admitted to the Clinical Center for a partial nephrectomy (removal of part of the kidney). Although Mr. Morrell discussed the operation with his physicians before coming to the NIH Clinical Center, formal informed consent for the research procedure and transfusion was obtained in Jackson's presence. Mr. Morrell subsequently confided to Jackson that he was conflicted about the possibility of receiving a transfusion because it was prohibited by his religious convictions, which are similar to those of a Jehovah's Witness.

Feeling unsettled, Jackson called the Consultation Service. He explained to the ethics consultants that although Mr. Morrell was willing to accept plasma or other partial blood products, he was not willing to accept a transfusion of his own or another's whole blood. Jackson described Mr. Morrell as feeling "forced" into making the decision to sign the transfusion consent form because he was informed that the surgery could not be performed without it. In addition, Jackson told the bioethics consultants that he was concerned the surgeons may not have been fully aware of the strength of Mr. Morrell's wishes to avoid a transfusion.

After speaking with Jackson, members of the Consultation Service went to Mr. Morrell's room and spoke with him. Mr. Morrell told the consultants that he will "feel like someone else" if he receives a transfusion and that his decision to sign the transfusion consent form was a "test of faith" that he "failed." However, Mr. Morrell made it clear to the Consultation Service team that he wanted to live and believed that the nephrectomy was necessary to prevent his death. Mr. Morrell went on to say that he had considered and rejected the possibility of a radical rather than a partial nephrectomy because he believed it is more important to keep a portion of his second kidney than to decrease the chance that he will require a transfusion. Mr. Morrell expressed a desire to confirm that his beliefs were clear to his surgeons.

### Analysis and Recommendations

The surgeons at the Clinical Center have legitimate ethical concerns about engaging in major abdominal surgery without being able to provide blood transfusions they believe may be medically necessary. In light of their belief that it would be inappropriate to operate without transfusion consent, Mr. Morrell is required to make an extremely difficult choice, balancing his religious convictions and his health. The Consultation Service believes that Mr. Morrell is competent to consent to possible transfusions and is well informed about his options. He has clearly thought extensively about his decision.

## Authors' Commentary

This case highlights an important gap in our understanding of the scope of an individual's right to refuse treatment. It is widely agreed that respecting autonomy includes respecting the right of capable individuals to decline treatment, even when that treatment would be in their best medical interests. Many people also agree that under certain circumstances doctors may refuse to perform a procedure for reasons of personal or professional integrity. For example, some doctors maintain a conscientious objection to performing abortions.

In the present case, the surgeons were unwilling to carry out a procedure—abdominal surgery—that a participant wanted, unless they also had the option to use another procedure—blood transfusion—that he did not want. It is the connection between the procedures that made Mr. Morrell's objection to blood transfusion different from simply refusing some sort of treatment: if they were not allowed to transfuse blood, Mr. Morrell's doctors might end up killing someone whom they could have saved. This, they felt, would compromise their moral integrity.

Ultimately, Mr. Morrell opted to proceed with the surgery with a full understanding that it might require a transfusion that contradicts his religious convictions. Prior to his operation, Mr. Morrell's surgeons reassured him that they were aware of and respected his beliefs and would only give him a transfusion if medically necessary.

## ■ NOTES

1. Given the epidemiology service's involvement in the consult, it is indeed possible that these factors were considered and simply not described in the consult report.

2. G. Marks, N. Crepaz, and R. Janssen, "Estimating Sexual Transmission of HIV from Persons Aware and Unaware That They Are Infected with the Virus in the USA," *AIDS* 20 (2006): 1447–1450.

3. B. Armbruster and M. L. Brandeau, "Cost-Effective Control of Chronic Viral Diseases: Finding the Optimal Level of Screening and Contact Tracing," *Mathematical Biosciences* 224, no. 1 (2010): 35–42.

4. The CDC now uses this term instead of "contact tracing" and "partner notification."

5. MMWR, 57(RR09), 1–63, available at: http://www.cdc.gov/mmwr/preview/mmwrhtml/rr5709a1.htm, accessed on April 2, 2010.

6. L. Belsky and H. S. Richardson, "Medical Researchers' Ancillary Clinical Care Responsibilities," *British Medical Journal* 328 (2004): 1494–1496.

7. For more on the question of futility, see P. R. Helft, M. Siegler, and J. Lantos, "The Rise and Fall of the Futility Movement," *New England Journal of Medicine* 343, no. 4 (2000): 293–296.

8. A. E. Buchanan and D. W. Brock, *Deciding for Others: The Ethics of Surrogate Decision Making* (Cambridge, England: Cambridge University Press, 1990).

# 7  Ending Research

The responsible termination of a significant relationship requires care and attention, and research is no exception to this general principle. When researchers end participation for some individuals, when participants choose to withdraw from a study, when a study is terminated prematurely, or even when research naturally comes to a close, many important ethical issues may arise.

Some difficult issues that may arise at the end of a research study stem from the reality that research participants may benefit medically from participation in research and have ongoing health needs. Often, they are participating in a study specifically for their illness; that illness may be chronic or ongoing, and participants may be benefiting from experimental and/or ancillary care interventions received as part of the study. At the same time, many researchers are also clinicians who are familiar with and committed to careful discharge planning to ensure that individuals continue to receive the medical attention they need. Clinical research is different than clinical care in several ethically important ways, however, and there is an inherent tension between the roles of researcher and clinician.[1] Researchers are less likely than clinicians to have long-term ongoing relationships with participants in their care, and they have, at most, limited obligations to provide them with treatment or care, especially after a study is over.[2] The primary obligation of researchers is to conduct ethically sound and scientifically rigorous research. On the other hand, they have responsibilities to ensure the safety of their research participants, some of whom are ill patients, and to transfer them to appropriate caregivers. Research adds a layer of complexity to discharge decisions (decisions that are often already complicated in a clinical care setting). In either setting, discharge decisions may be difficult for a variety of reasons, including differences of opinion between patients/participants, families, and/or providers about the best course of action or because of lack of access to care needed after discharge.[3]

Surprisingly, there has been little ethical guidance about what to do at this critical stage of research until relatively recently. Guidance documents for international research ethics have increasingly begun to address posttrial issues, including whether research participants will have access to the treatment they were receiving during a trial after the trial is over, and whether an intervention being tested will become available to the community hosting the research within a reasonable amount of time after the trial. There has also been some limited discussion of whether and how to share the findings of research with participants and with the relevant community.[4]

The posttrial considerations that have been discussed in the literature and codified in guidelines are far from settled. For instance, since posttrial considerations originated in guidance about international research, it is often unclear how to apply these principles to domestic research. Some researchers we have advised—researchers conducting both domestic and international research—have questioned why they should have any posttrial obligations, taking the view that a researcher's obligations should end when the trial does, and other people or institutions have obligations to help individuals once they are no longer participating in research. There is also dispute about whether ensuring that a research intervention is available to a community after a trial is the best way to meet community needs, or whether other approaches might be better able to protect community interests.[5] It is often unclear how to define the community to which the researcher owes obligations after the trial because there is little consensus on what counts as a community. A community could be understood in a number of ways: the pool of research participants, the host community or communities, people residing in the geographic region where the study was conducted, or even the population of people with the disease under study. One review paper found 94 definitions of community in the sociological literature even as long ago as 1955,[6] and no consensus appears to have emerged since. Moreover, although there is some agreement that researchers should consider issues of posttrial access to treatment for the participants, open and unsettled questions remain about the grounds for any obligation to consider posttrial access, what such an obligation entails, and how long it extends after a study's completion.[7] The cases in this chapter include both issues that have been discussed in the literature and issues that appear to be unaddressed to date.

There has not been much discussion in the literature about whether the decision to terminate one participant's involvement in research has to be fair in light of how other participants are treated. Yet this largely unsettled issue was central to *Consult 7.1*. In this case, two participants had sexual relations in violation of the policies governing the inpatient unit in which they were staying. This was not the first time that these participants had engaged in sexual relations, and they had previously promised the team not to repeat their behavior. The policies had been set in part to maintain a specific therapeutic milieu needed to treat their conditions. The female participant had previously been disruptive demonstrating that her treatment was no longer working, so she was discharged from the study. The male participant was about to become an outpatient, and it was unclear whether he was responding to treatment, so the team was not as certain about discharging him from the study and requested an ethics consult to resolve the issue. This consult raised the interesting question of whether a concern for fairness and for gender equality required that the male participant also be discharged.

*Consult 7.2* focuses on whether it is ethically acceptable to discharge a seriously ill pediatric participant to another country, where the care that the child would receive would likely be inferior to what he would receive at the

National Institutes of Health (NIH). Because the child was seriously ill with leukemia and had not been home in months, the child and his mother appeared to have strong preferences to return home and be with their family. It was not clear whether they understood that the likelihood of receiving adequate treatment at home was low or that even continued care at the NIH did not have a high likelihood of curing him. This was a case where the team was unsure whether the child and the mother had fully reconciled the competing medical and personal interests at stake and needed guidance about whether it was ethically acceptable to comply with the wishes of the mother and child even if it might mean shorter survival.

*Consult 7.3* concerned the scope and limitations of researchers' obligations to continue to treat a research participant beyond the study requirements. In this case, standard treatment was offered as part of the study, but the study was designed to help with research participant recruitment for other studies and the training of fellows (young physician-researchers), the latter being an important mission of the NIH in itself, rather than to answer a particular question about treatment. Therefore, transferring participants to community-based care was compatible with study goals and the goals of the NIH, consistent with what the individual had been told, and relatively easy to arrange. The team was conflicted, however, because transfer was inconsistent with a particular participant's preferences and expectations, and the participant was unwilling to do his part to transition to receiving care outside of the study.

The issues raised by *Consult 7.4* were similar to those in *Consult 7.3* regarding the scope and limitations of researchers' obligations for posttrial treatment needs, yet this consult raised difficult questions about whether or how these obligations change if the study participant lacks health insurance or has limited access to needed care outside of the research. Research staff involved in this case wondered whether these issues should be dealt with at enrollment, such that people without access to posttrial care should be excluded from research as a matter of policy, but all agreed that would be unfair. If those without health care access were included, transitioning them after research participation to care in the community would be complex, resource intensive, and in the end not always satisfactory. These issues would also be challenging for research participants who come to the NIH from other countries, as discussed in *Consult 5.3*, as well as for those in the United States who continue to lack health insurance, although U.S. health care reform passed in 2010 may reduce the number of U.S. citizens without health insurance.

In *Consult 7.5*, investigators wondered what responsibility they had to provide posttrial care if their proposed research intervention was successful at keeping neonates alive in resource-limited settings. In many ways, worrying about care for infants who otherwise would not have survived was a wonderful problem to have, yet this case demonstrates the importance of responsibly considering the consequences of any particular study. Of note, this issue was raised before the study began, which allowed the research ethics consultants and investigators to not only consider the interests of the infants but also to determine how the ethical considerations could have an impact on the study design and research methods and to recommend modifications in advance.

Consult 7.6 also shows the usefulness of early consideration and planning for circumstances that might arise after a study is completed. In this case, a research participant requested withdrawal of her specimens from a stored tissue repository. These researchers had not anticipated that some subjects would want to withdraw their samples, and it would have been very difficult for the researchers to extract and delete the subject's data at the point the request was made. At the time of the consult little guidance existed on research with stored samples, but even subsequently, there has continued to be debate and evolving guidance about issues including consent for future research, storage in databases and repositories, widespread sharing and research use of samples, and mechanisms and limitations on withdrawing samples. In this case, the consultants focused on methods to improve the consent information for subsequent participants so that they would know what their options were.

It is generally accepted that data and safety monitoring boards (DSMBs) can serve a valuable role by monitoring the safety of a trial.[8] An issue that has received little attention is when, if ever, a researcher can challenge a DSMB's decision to stop a trial. *Consult 7.7* came to the Consultation Service from a researcher who was troubled by the expectation that the DSMB overseeing his trial would recommend that the trial be stopped based on interim data. DSMBs are independent committees that research sponsors appoint to monitor the ongoing results from a trial to protect the interests of study participants and the scientific integrity of the study, and they are especially important for trials that pose significant risks. Based on interim findings, DSMBs can recommend stopping a trial early for harm, futility, or benefit.[9] DSMBs typically set rules in advance to decide when to stop the trial; in this consult, the DSMB had set predetermined thresholds of efficacy that they felt were appropriate for this trial. The trial had crossed this predetermined statistical threshold; however, the result was the opposite of what the researcher and clinicians in the field had expected, and the investigator thought that the difference might not hold up with additional participants. The researcher was also concerned that the results were not robust enough to change practice. The researcher anonymously requested a consultation to discuss whether it was ethically acceptable to ask the DSMB to consider keeping the study open, and to explore what options existed if the DSMB recommended closing the study.

Finally, *Consult 7.8* raises an important question that arose at the end of a research project about who merits authorship. More specifically, can the contribution that a participant makes to research be substantial enough to merit authorship under certain circumstances, or is there something about being a participant in research that should preclude that individual from being included as an author? The guidelines for scientific authorship have changed over time, and unlike many other disciplines, the quantity and quality of contribution necessary for authorship of biomedical articles has not always been clear.[10,11] Attributing authorship to someone who did not do the substantive intellectual work to merit authorship is problematic because it may be misleading and unfair to those authors who did the intellectual work. An author included under these circumstances may also have difficulty defending or explaining the work in public settings. On the other hand, there may be studies where a research participant contributes significantly to study planning or data collection, and it seems unfair that the fact of research participation alone should prevent the individual from getting credit for work that might otherwise be rewarded with authorship. The consultants in this case attempted to clarify the guidelines investigators could use for determining authorship, as well as what important downstream effects might result from assigning authorship.

## ■ CONSULT 7.1: STUDY DISCHARGE AFTER VIOLATION OF RULES

### Reason for Consult

Dr. Hal Frankel called for assistance determining what ethical issues arise if one research participant but not another is discharged after both have violated the rules of a particular inpatient therapeutic environment.

### Narrative

The Consultation Service met with Dr. Frankel in his office. He explained that a male and a female research participant—whom he identified as Heather and Tim—were discovered having sex in the male participant's inpatient room in the Clinical Center. Although Heather and Tim were enrolled in two different protocols, both protocols involved psychiatric treatment and required research participants to live in a restrictive inpatient environment for a few months as part of their therapy; therefore, Heather and Tim were admitted to the same inpatient unit governed by the same rules.

According to Dr. Frankel, one of the rules on the unit is that no research participant can be in another research participant's room at any time. The handbook given to all research participants at the time of enrollment, including Heather and Tim, specifies that having sex with other participants is not allowed. These rules and others outlined in the handbook were created in order to protect the research participants, who may experience extremely vulnerable mental states during their hospitalization.

Dr. Frankel explained that the nursing staff had previously discovered that Heather and Tim were having sexual relations and had instructed them not to continue this behavior. When they were discovered again, on the recommendation of leadership within the institute, Heather was discharged from Dr. Frankel's protocol. The decision to discharge her was made because her actions were disruptive and against the rules, and because her behavior demonstrated that the therapeutic environment was not effectively helping her condition. There was separate cause for concern that she had made several suicide attempts in the past year and had stated to Dr. Frankel that she might commit suicide soon, although she had not developed a plan to do so.

Tim was about to become an outpatient, so—even though he too had violated the rules of the therapeutic environment—doubts arose as to whether he should also be discharged from his protocol. As an outpatient, Tim's continued participation in his trial would be less disruptive than Heather's would have been in her trial because she would have been required to continue her inpatient stay. The principal investigator on Tim's study had also expressed concern about discontinuing Tim's research participation because the research team had experienced some difficulty recruiting participants to participate in the trial.

## Analysis and Recommendations

The bioethics consultants supported the research team's decision that dismissing Heather from the protocol was both consistent with therapeutic goals for her and an appropriate consequence for her disruptive behavior. In Tim's case, it was felt that maintaining a sense of fairness—especially for the other participants in the therapeutic milieu and for the staff—argued for dismissing him from the program as well.

The ethics consultant summarized the discussion as follows:

1. The Consultation Service concurs that both participants should be discharged from their respective research protocols.
2. The Consultation Service recommends that neither should be discharged from the Clinical Center until appropriate arrangements are found, the suicidality of the female participant is addressed, and consideration is given to the male participant's continued use of the study drug (unless he is in the placebo arm).

## Authors' Commentary

In a phone conversation with a nurse later that day, the Consultation Service was told that Tim had been discharged from his protocol. Before he left, the blind on his study participation was broken; he had been receiving an active drug that is commercially available. Because his condition appeared to be improving while he was on that drug, Tim was given a supply of the drug and referred to a community health center near his home. Though the center could oversee his ongoing care, it was not clear whether the center would be able to supply the drug.

This consult raises the issue of fairness as to whether research participants who violated the same rule should be treated in the same manner, even when their circumstances differed. The analysis would have been more complicated if treating them similarly occurred at the expense of compromising either the ability to answer the research questions because of difficulties in identifying and enrolling research participants or the benefits a research participant can obtain. Ultimately, because it was believed that allowing the continued inclusion of one participant but not the other would be perceived as unfair and would negatively affect other research participants and the research staff, the ethics consultants and the research team agreed that treating both participants the same was important for the success of the research program. It is interesting to imagine how this case might have been handled differently if the facts were slightly different. What if the participants' genders were switched? Of what if one or both had a rare disease that made replacing them in the research extremely difficult, and discharging them would threaten the successful completion of the research? Finally, the outcome might have been different if either participant was receiving therapeutic benefit from an intervention that was not available outside of the study.

Additionally, although this consult arises from the conduct of a research study, one of its central questions relates to health care ethics. How should clinicians fulfill their obligations of care when discharging individuals who have become dependent on their care? Particularly for inpatients receiving care and attention for psychiatric disorders in a therapeutic milieu, a structured group setting in which the expectations and group activities in the setting are a critical part of the treatment, it would be irresponsible or even harmful to release participants without establishing mechanisms for transitioning their care and making appropriate referrals to meet their other psychosocial needs in the community.[12] Much of the discussion in this consult therefore focused on mitigating the potential harms of discharging these two patient-participants and how to plan for transition of their care. The issue of how to plan for the termination of a significant relationship is enduring and complicated. In the consultations discussed in this chapter, the reader will note that a variety of consults raise a form of this issue that has more recently been applied in the research setting—namely, what posttrial obligations researchers have to participants to help them transition their care.

## CONSULT 7.2: DISCHARGE TO LESS OPTIMAL CARE

### Reason for Consult

Dr. Shen Wu called to discuss whether it would be ethically acceptable to discharge a seriously ill pediatric research participant to a care environment that would likely be inferior to that of the NIH Clinical Center.

### Narrative

Dr. Wu explained to the Consultation Service that Octavio Cabos is an 11-year-old boy admitted to the NIH on a protocol for treatment of leukemia. Octavio and his family live in rural South America where they have limited access to health resources. He is here with his mother who speaks only limited English.

Following bone marrow transplantation, Octavio experienced a series of severe complications, including acute graft-versus-host disease (a common and potentially very serious complication of bone marrow transplantation in which donor immune cells attack recipient cells as "foreign"), respiratory failure requiring a tracheotomy (a tube inserted directly into the trachea or windpipe to create an airway), and a multidrug-resistant infection. In addition, he is suffering from chronic renal function impairment, hypertension, and depression. Although his leukemia is currently in remission, the clinical care team believes that Octavio will require total parenteral nutrition (intravenous infusions of nutrients), supplemental oxygen, antibiotics, and high-dose steroids for the indefinite future. They are willing to treat Octavio at the Clinical Center for as long as he requires care.

Dr. Wu and the attending physician reported to the ethics consultants that Octavio was always reluctant to undergo treatment, but that he has become increasingly upset with standard interventions (e.g., suctioning his tracheotomy) over the last week and has repeatedly expressed the desire to cease treatment and return home. The team reports that Octavio's mother also seems to want to return home. In response to these requests, the team has begun to investigate the feasibility of organizing care for Octavio at an acute care hospital near his hometown. They fear that, given the complexity of Octavio's case, they will not be able to arrange treatment comparable to that which he is receiving at the NIH. They are deeply troubled by their sense that discharging Octavio could hasten his death.

In addition, given the severity and uncertainty of Octavio's current condition and prognosis, the clinical consult team questions whether it is appropriate to reinstate a do-not-resuscitate (DNR) order. Octavio's mother had agreed to a DNR order during her son's stay in the intensive care unit (ICU) earlier this year, saying that she didn't want Octavio to live like a machine. The DNR order was rescinded, however, with parental agreement, when Octavio was transferred out of the ICU because the clinical team did not want to forestall the possibility of providing temporary ventilator support to Octavio in case of an acute respiratory crisis. The clinical team is concerned that if cardiopulmonary resuscitation were performed for Octavio at this point, it would likely increase or prolong his suffering.

The morning after meeting with Dr. Wu and other members of Octavio's interdisciplinary clinical care team, the ethics consultants had an extensive conversation with Octavio's mother via an interpreter. Octavio did not join the conversation because he had been given a medication that was making him confused. A meeting with Octavio was scheduled for another day.

At the beginning of her discussion with the ethics team, Octavio's mother was upset and didn't understand why they were asking questions about returning home. She made it clear that she did not want to give up hope for her son and would not want to return home if she was not comfortable with the level of care that he would receive there. The ethics consultants asked her what Octavio meant when he said he wanted to go home. Octavio's mother expressed her belief that he wants to see his two siblings, only one of whom has been able to visit the NIH. The Consultation Service team did not specifically speak with Octavio's mother about his DNR status, but in the conversation, she offered that she did not want her son "to be a machine" or "to be alive only on machines."

## Analysis and Recommendations

The clinical team requested help in addressing the following two questions:

1) Under what conditions would it be ethical to discharge Octavio to his home country in South America?
2) Should Octavio be returned to a DNR status?

The Consultation Service team recommended that responses to both issues are primarily dependent on Octavio and his family's informed preferences about his future treatment.

### Discharge to a Less Developed Country

Generally, it is ethically acceptable for individuals (or their legally authorized representatives) to choose where they will receive care, even if they are aware that one setting may offer lower quality care than the other. The key question in this case is whether Octavio and his parents understand the full implications of a decision to transfer him. In particular, it is crucial to distinguish what Octavio means when he says he wants to return "home." Does this request emanate from his desire to see his siblings, to discontinue all treatment, to decrease the burden of separation for his family, and/or to return to familiar surroundings? Does Octavio understand that he would go to a hospital rather than to his house?

If comparable care were possible in their home country, Octavio's mother and (she believes) Octavio would want to return for continued treatment there. She said it would be hard to decide to return home if the care were adequate, but marginally less good. If the available care were half as good, she would definitely prefer that her son stay at the Clinical Center. She was awaiting information from the NIH medical team about what was available near their home. From this discussion, we concluded that Octavio's mother is not ready to take her son back home. As more information becomes available, this decision should be revisited.

Because it is possible that she is interpreting the series of discussions about her son's future as part of an effort to convince her and Octavio to leave the Clinical Center, it is important that the clinical team reinforce their willingness to continue treating Octavio at the Clinical Center; their intent to remain in close contact with Octavio's new physicians if he and his mother decide to leave; and their willingness to bring Octavio back to the Clinical Center if he and his mother were to go home and subsequently decide that they would like to return to the NIH.

## Do-Not-Resuscitate Status

Clinical Center Policy states that DNR orders are appropriate under the following circumstances potentially relevant to this case:

- "The patient expresses a preference to forego CPR."
- "The burden of resuscitation from the perspective of the patient or surrogate outweighs its potential benefit."
- "The patient's life would be marked by suffering or would be so limited in its opportunities that the patient would prefer not to survive a cardiopulmonary arrest resuscitation. Quality of life decisions should reflect the patient's perception of 'quality of life.'"

According to the policy, the responsible physician-investigator could follow a specific process to write a DNR order without the parent's consent if he or she feels that CPR would not be effective for Octavio or would only cause him to suffer.

## Authors' Commentary

After additional conversation with the clinical team, Octavio's mother agreed to reinstate a DNR order over the weekend. Sadly, Octavio's condition suddenly deteriorated, and he died a few days later. Although this case ended tragically, this consult raised an important issue about discharge planning and terminating participation in a clinical trial—namely, when can a participant and his family be discharged from research to a place where it can be anticipated they will receive suboptimal care? However, the issue arose not because the team had reason to discharge Octavio or felt some external pressure to do so, but because they thought that Octavio and his mother had a strong preference for being closer to the rest of the family and were therefore willing to accept a different level of care. The first important question to ask was whether the family truly had this desire and understood the consequences. A critical feature of this consult therefore became how to facilitate communication between Octavio, his mother, and the research team about future plans for care.

For clinicians treating pediatric patients at the end of life, communication is an ethically central but complicated component of providing care.[13] One feature of this consult that made the already difficult task of communicating with a parent about a critically ill child even more complicated was the language barrier between the team and the family. A survey of pediatric nurses revealed that language barriers were one of the two greatest obstacles to providing appropriate care at the end of life (along with withdrawing/withholding mechanical ventilation).[14] In a study investigating the perspectives of Chinese and Mexican parents about end-of-life care, parents who did not speak English fluently more frequently lacked information, and some of those parents indicated that they were not even aware that they could access interpreters. The consequences of not receiving information were serious. "Parents who received no information described more anger, distress, and sadness during their child's illness," and parents who were not given adequate information were found to be more likely to experience intense, long-term grief after their child's death.[15] Thus, by helping the team communicate with the family and ensuring that an interpreter was involved in the conversation, the ethics consultants filled a very important role in making sure that the wishes of the family were informed, heard, and respected.

If the family had truly been convinced that Octavio should be taken back to his home country after this discussion occurred, the team would still have been in a difficult position. Parents are generally understood to have legal authority to consent to what is in the best interests of their children. When a decision clearly goes against a younger child's best medical interests, even if the parents have important religious or cultural views that may calibrate that child's interests differently, that parental decision can be legally challenged and overruled in a court of law.[16] Some parents have been convicted of child abuse and murder when their children died as a result of being denied conventional medical treatment, ranging from chemotherapy to insulin to blood transfusions, in favor of spiritual or unproven treatment.[17] Clinicians and researchers may have responsibilities to intervene and refer cases to a local child protective agency when parents decide not to act in a child's best medical interests. This issue becomes even more complicated, however, if conventional medical therapy poses significant risks or a low chance of benefit, or if minors have reached an age where they themselves have adopted the values and beliefs that their parents have.[18] This case introduced further complications—Octavio's poor prognosis, which made it unclear how much benefit he would receive from further treatment anywhere, and the fact that he was enrolled in a research study. In situations like these where it is difficult to determine whether the best interests of the minor would actually be served by receiving treatment, courts are often divided on whether to issue an order authorizing treatment and may take into account other interests that a child has about how to spend the end of his or her life.[19]

## CONSULT 7.3: MANAGING PARTICIPANT'S POST-TRIAL EXPECTATIONS

### Reason for Consult

Dr. Edward Komarov came to the Department of Bioethics seeking help in understanding the extent of treatment obligations for an individual in an evaluation and treatment protocol.

### Narrative

The "Evaluation and Treatment Protocol for Potential Research Participants with Metabolic Diseases" is designed to meet two goals: *(1)* to maintain a pool of possible research participants with metabolic diseases for future studies; *(2)* to provide clinical training for physician-researchers in training. Participants are typically referred by an outside physician who is expected to resume care when participation in the protocol ends. Protocol participants are regularly seen in the NIH outpatient clinic for follow-up, treatment (if needed), and possible enrollment in active research studies. Participation in this protocol is usually terminated when the individual is recruited into another active study.

Outlining the protocol design, Dr. Komarov explained that care for participants in this study can include the use of expensive biologic treatments. Arrangements for receiving care outside the NIH are often made in the interest of maintaining a budget that is able to provide temporary treatment to all participants in the protocol.

Christopher Andrews, a 73-year-old participant, has been treated by infusions of a powerful biologic over the past 18 months and is responding well to treatment. The research team has attempted, over the past 6 months, to arrange for Mr. Andrews to receive the infusions from a nonresearch physician in the community. He has several alternative options for care since he has private insurance and is also eligible for Medicare coverage. However, Mr. Andrews refuses to take the necessary steps to get treated outside the NIH and claims that the research team has an ethical obligation to treat him. Dr. Komarov and other members of the team are unsure whether Mr. Andrews's claim is correct (i.e., whether it is unethical to discontinue the drug) and want to know how they should address the situation.

## Analysis and Recommendations

The discussion with Dr. Komarov focused on four reasons against an ethical obligation to continue Mr. Andrews's treatment with the biologic.

1. The goals of this protocol are recruitment and training, not the provision of all possible clinical care to participants. This was explained to Mr. Andrews in the initial consent to participate in the protocol. Therefore, the physician-investigators did not promise to continue providing the drug.
2. The particular drug in question is part of the standard of care for Mr. Andrews's metabolic disease and is thus available outside the research setting. Mr. Andrews has private insurance that would cover his treatment. Given that he could receive the drug outside of the NIH, there is no obvious practical reason to continue his treatment at the NIH.
3. The institute has limited resources to support treatment of participants in the evaluation and treatment protocol. These resources should be distributed fairly among all protocol participants.
4. The physician-investigators have taken precautions to ensure Mr. Andrews' continued access to this drug. They reexplained Mr. Andrews' need to arrange for care outside of the NIH over the past months, and they have provided support in arranging for this transition (e.g., arranging medical appointments, making contact with his private insurance, helping with his application for Medicare).

The Consultation Service recommends discussing these issues again with Mr. Andrews both in person and in writing and making plans to discontinue infusions of the drug. It was also recommended to involve the Clinical Center patient representative in Mr. Andrews's next outpatient clinic visit. The patient representative serves as an advocate for research participants and helps them to navigate the complexities of research at the Clinical Center. Additionally, the Consultation Service offered to talk to Mr. Andrews if he has the desire to do so.

During the consultation, the ethicist identified another issue of ethical concern. The protocol consent form suggests more extensive treatment of protocol participants than may have been intended. For example, the consent form contains passages that might suggest open-ended treatment ("You will be examined and receive treatment for your disease as needed").

Therefore, the Consultation Service recommends rewording the protocol's consent form to prevent future misunderstanding. These passages should be modified so that the limitations of treatment and services become clearer. The Consultation Service felt comfortable in recommending to discontinue Mr. Andrews's infusions despite the consent form's vagueness because the need for discontinuing his infusions had been discussed with Mr. Andrews over several months and because Mr. Andrews has access to these infusions outside of the NIH.

## Authors' Commentary

Dr. Komarov followed up with the Consultation Service after Mr. Andrews's next clinic visit. According to Dr. Komarov, Mr. Andrews was composed throughout the appointment and accepted the need to receive his infusions outside of the NIH. The research team assisted Mr. Andrews in scheduling an appointment with a physician in the community who would be able to take him as a patient and provide his next scheduled infusion. Dr. Komarov intended to work on a letter to Mr. Andrews explaining the situation and the institute's interest in continuing to follow him in their outpatient clinic.

This consult raises important questions about the limits of research and researchers' obligations, and the differences between clinical research and clinical care.[20] Researchers cannot commit to indefinite treatment of chronic conditions because doing so would divert human and material resources from their primary mission.[21] The NIH mission is to conduct or support research to advance understanding of human health and prevention and treatment of illness. Interestingly, the overall goals of the particular study in which Mr. Andrews enrolled—recruitment and training—are critically related to research, but the study itself was not designed to answer a specific research question. The bioethics consultants did not view continued treatment of Mr. Andrews by the researchers as obligatory because doing so was not contributing to an important scientific question and would have diverted resources away from others in the study. At the same time, continued treatment had not been promised to Mr. Andrews, and in this case, the particular biologic was available outside of the research study, his health insurance would cover it, and he had access to providers who could infuse it.

Nonetheless, this case raises important issues related to research participant expectations and posttrial access to beneficial interventions.[22] Mr. Andrews's metabolic disease was responding to infusions of the biologic, and he was benefiting clinically; therefore, it was in his medical interests to continue to receive infusions if at all possible. Understandably, his expectations might include that he should continue to receive a therapy that is helping him. In this case, the research team had discussed the purpose and limitations of the study with Mr. Andrews on several occasions, but perhaps they needed to be more explicit earlier in the study that they did not plan to continue to treat him indefinitely. In addition, the Consultation Service recommended changes to the consent form and a more explicit discussion of the limits of the study with all participants so that their expectations about treatment might be more realistic. In Mr. Andrews's case, the research team assisted his transition to an outside caregiver. Based on these efforts, the investigators may be seen as having appropriately satisfied their posttrial obligations. These issues are much more complex when an individual does not have insurance or access to reasonable care outside of research, as illustrated by the next consultation.

## CONSULT 7.4: FULFILLING POST-TRIAL OBLIGATIONS TO UNINSURED PARTICIPANTS

### Reason for Consult

Patricia Nantakarn, a social worker, asked for assistance in clarifying the discharge planning and poststudy care obligations that the NIH has to uninsured research participants.

### Narrative

Ms. Nantakarn called to initiate a discussion on care obligations and discharge planning for research participants without health insurance who experience complications. She described a challenging case in which a research participant, Jim Randolph, underwent surgery at an outside hospital and returned to the NIH after experiencing a stroke. Mr. Randolph does not have health insurance.

Members of the Consultation Service attended a preliminary meeting with Ms. Nantakarn and members of Mr. Randolph's interdisciplinary team where Mr. Randolph's medical complications were explained and the problems associated with his long-term care were clarified. A second meeting was scheduled to discuss Mr. Randolph's case and others like it, with more of the research staff for this protocol.

Attendees at the second meeting acknowledged the recent increase in uninsured research participants with needs for long-term care and identified numerous challenges to providing for such care on short notice. Several individuals suggested that insurance status might be used as an eligibility requirement to obviate these concerns. Ms. Nantakarn presented the possibility that social workers could contribute to the care of participants enrolled in this protocol through earlier involvement in their care.

## Analysis and Recommendations

Although the possibility of screening individuals based on insurance status was raised, members of the Consultation Service and others emphasized the importance of including individuals without insurance in research protocols for reasons of fairness. Research is enriched by the inclusion of individuals with various conditions, regardless of their insurance status. The exclusion of uninsured individuals might skew the pool of research participants and reduce the contributions that the NIH is capable of offering to health care through research.

Nevertheless, it is appropriate to consider additional safeguards that may be needed to protect the well-being of the uninsured. By offering support during the enrollment process, social workers can understand the participant's insurance status and begin to identify resources that may be helpful to him or her in the future. The research team agreed to consult the social work department during the screening of participants for this protocol.

Attendees also determined that greater efforts should be made during the informed consent process to clarify the boundaries of NIH obligations for off-protocol medical care. In certain cases when complications related to research participation require extensive measures, the research team may have a commitment to help fund the required procedures.

In summary, the Consultation Service recommended the following:

1. It is worthwhile to understand the insurance status of individuals prior to their enrollment in this protocol. The researchers involved in this protocol will make an effort to involve social work early, when the participants are initially enrolled in the study, so that the social worker can begin to identify resources to meet the participant's anticipated needs at discharge.
2. Efforts should be strengthened to ensure that participants fully understand the boundaries of NIH responsibilities for their care so that they can make informed decisions to enroll.
3. The use of insurance status as an eligibility criterion in the screening process for enrolling participants was rejected as unfair and potentially biasing.

## Authors' Commentary

Participation in clinical research can sometimes offer benefits in terms of treatment and care that might be welcome to people who have limited access to care outside of research. As discussed in Chapter 2: Enrolling Research Participants, participant access to the benefits of research has to be balanced with concern about protecting participants from the burdens of research, and minimizing the possibility of exploiting people with limited access by taking unfair advantage of their willingness to participate in research. The question of how to avoid exploitation while not discriminating against people who are poor or have no insurance often arises at the stage of participant selection and enrollment into research. *Consults 2.1, 5.4,* and *5.5* offer other examples.[23] Important and complex issues also arise at the end of a study. When participation in a research study is complete, individuals may continue to require ongoing care and treatment for their disease.

Although posttrial obligations have been discussed in the literature, the theoretical grounding for these obligations has not been established, and more work needs to be done in this area.[24] Researchers have an obligation to help participants transition to care outside of the study, although as discussed in the previous case, the obligation of researchers to continue to treat people beyond the end of a study is limited by their obligation to conduct research.[25] As noted in the introduction to this chapter, there remains controversy regarding the basis for and extent of researchers' posttrial obligations.

Helping research participants transition from research to ordinary medical care is further complicated by the fact that some individuals do not have health insurance or lack sufficient access to needed medical care. Keeping such individuals out of potentially beneficial research for this reason seems unfair because, in some cases, excluding them may eliminate a welcome option for receiving treatment. Informing research participants about the limits of the researchers' responsibilities and treatment options seems necessary but insufficient. Transitioning to care may be especially hard in cases where researchers have developed significant relationships with participants and participants have become dependent on the research as their primary source for at least some type of medical care (see other examples in *Consults 5.7* and *6.2*).[26] Ethically, it is important to devote institutional resources to help individuals locate outside sources of care or help them apply for health insurance or public assistance. As with all good discharge planning, this requires social workers and others with expertise in this area to become involved early in each person's research participation. It is much less clear what a researcher or research institution should do if, despite their best efforts, they are unable to locate access to care outside the study for an individual. Finding funds to support individuals in this situation is desirable, but not always feasible. Investigators should try all avenues to responsibly transition participants to another source of care while recognizing that there may be times when it is extremely difficult to do so in an unjust and imperfect world.

Although the details are thin regarding the complications that Mr. Randolph suffered from in this case, they appeared to be the result of a surgery that was not part of the research study. The presence of "complications," however, raises another controversial and unsettled issue—that is, compensation for research-related injury.[27] Many have argued that there is a moral obligation to compensate individuals for injuries that they sustain because of their involvement in research. Nonetheless, there is no standard mechanism or requirement in the United States for providing compensation for research-related injuries, and many template consent documents, including some at the NIH, say that short-term medical care will be provided but no compensation or long-term care will be provided. This is in stark contrast to many other countries that have policies requiring that sponsors either compensate participants who are injured as a result of research or take out insurance for this purpose.[28]

## CONSULT 7.5: PLANNING FOR POST-TRIAL CONSEQUENCES OF TRIAL INTERVENTION

### Reason for Consult

Dr. Florence Langley, a researcher, contacted the Consultation Service to evaluate whether there is an ethical obligation to provide neonatal care and/or referral to external care for premature infants in a study in which she is participating.

### Narrative

A research network was created to address major causes of morbidity and mortality in women and children in developing countries, and to build health care and research capacity in resource-limited settings.

Dr. Langley's team is sponsoring a multicountry, randomized, controlled trial investigating the effectiveness of a pharmaceutical intervention in reducing neonatal mortality in preterm infants, without increasing severe maternal infectious morbidity. The study tests methods to facilitate the identification of eligible pregnant women at risk for premature delivery, to increase the availability of the study medication, and to provide training for birth attendants to administer the study medication at all primary health care levels. Many studies conducted in hospitals in developed countries have shown the effectiveness of the study drug in reducing mortality among premature infants, but there are limited data on the effectiveness of this intervention in resource-limited settings that have a high percentage of at-home births and do not have neonatal intensive care units.

Because the study medication is likely to increase survival in some cases, researchers will encounter babies who are born prematurely and survive (including babies who would not have survived but for the study intervention). In the resource-limited settings where the study is being conducted, however, care for premature babies is limited, and survival up to and beyond the first month of life is uncertain. Without adequate care for the premature infants, it is possible that the study interventions would not prevent death but merely delay it.

A study on providing training for neonatal resuscitation for birth asphyxia in rural settings was conducted recently in some of the sites involved in this study.[29] Through that study, resuscitation techniques using bag and mask were taught to local providers in intervention sites, and training in essential newborn care (ENC) was provided at all sites. ENC includes recommendations for thermal regulation through continuous skin-to-skin contact with the mother (or another person) and counseling in initiating breastfeeding, expressing milk, and providing nutrition in other ways if the baby is not yet able to suckle. To be effective, some ENC counseling should be provided and ENC implemented within hours after birth. Another study, an emergency obstetric and neonatal care trial, is about to start at many of the sites. This study is focused on building emergency care capacity, helping providers recognize when mothers and neonates require emergency care, and encouraging communities to develop transportation services for neonates and mothers needing emergency care to the nearest hospitals and clinics (many sites are a good distance from the nearest health care facility).

## Analysis and Recommendations

Developing effective and feasible strategies to reduce neonatal mortality associated with premature birth in resource-poor settings is a laudable goal. If the study medication is effective and feasible in reducing mortality in the first month of life, there still remain many factors that jeopardize the health of these premature infants. Balancing the necessary scientific rigor to isolate the effects of the studied intervention with concern for overall outcomes for the infants can be difficult. Given that the First Breath study demonstrated the feasibility and value of introducing ENC in these settings, that the World Health Organization is expected to soon issue recommendations for ENC as standard of care for premature babies in resource-limited settings, and that the interventions for these children are low cost and potentially lifesaving, the Consultation Service team believes there is an ethical obligation to ensure access to these interventions for the infants in this study. On the other hand, since it is possible that providing rigorous neonatal care could confound the study results, require a larger sample size, and require considerable effort by the study team, the Consultation Service recommends that the study team consider the following steps:

- First, it is important to try to calculate the effect size of providing ENC and referral to the mothers and children to anticipate the difference in sample size needed.
- Second, to minimize confounding the study results, the team should ensure that the standard-of-care package is as consistent as possible for all sites. According to the protocol, health care providers at all study sites attending the mothers or baby will be trained to promote the use of (or promote

mothers to use) a minimum set of evidence-based elements for the care of low birth weight and preterm infants born at home or in health care centers. The selected interventions are as follows: *(1)* thermal regulation through skin-to-skin contact with the mother, *(2)* breastfeeding, and *(3)* referral if needed and possible. This package of interventions should be specified, standardized, and incorporated at all participating sites. Standardizing the care package may be beneficial for reasons of scientific integrity. Without specifying the care package for premature infants, participants may be exposed to very different interventions at various sites. Therefore, providing a standard and rigorous approach to care for all participants is both scientifically and ethically sound. Importantly, this could alter the objectives of the study. With these modifications, the study might be asking whether the study medication can reduce neonatal death in resource-limited settings in conjunction with a standard package of ENC and referral to local hospitals. Given that medication administration alone may merely delay death, rather than reduce it, investigating the effect of the combination of the study medication plus a standard package of ENC and referral may be the most appropriate and relevant question for these communities.

- Third, building on efforts to improve community health capacity and referring participants to local sources of care when appropriate will reduce the burden on investigators and further the goal of building collaborative partnerships with local health officials and the community. Because ENC counseling will need to be provided soon after birth, and the sites may be distant from health care facilities, it would be essential to train study staff to provide counseling about thermal care and newborn feeding during the first few hours after birth. Yet, for more intensive interventions that do not need to be administered soon after birth, referral to local health care facilities may be more appropriate.
- A related issue to consider is whether to follow the participants beyond the 1-month period. Moreover, it is possible that some babies may be so premature that they will not be able to breastfeed for approximately 10 weeks. If this is the case, whether neonates born so prematurely can survive at all in resource-limited settings is an important question for this study to address. One way to address this concern would be to consider extending the follow-up period by adding an additional time point of 60 days or more to the study to assess mortality.

## Authors' Commentary

The investigators of this study, which was designed to test an intervention to reduce neonatal mortality, were faced with the tragic reality that a premature neonate helped to survive past the neonatal period might be especially vulnerable to other common causes of death in resource-poor settings. The investigators could have argued that what happened after the study was someone else's concern, as their research was designed to answer an important question about neonatal mortality; however, these investigators were troubled by the possibility of the study intervention simply delaying death, and they were committed to helping these infants survive. They wondered about their ethical obligation to anticipate the infants' needs for other kinds of care to get them through the fragile early months of life. The Consultation Service ethicists thought that the research team did have some obligation[30] to address these needs resulting from the study intervention and make a reasonable effort to plan strategies intended to enhance the infants' survival beyond the study period. The investigators were familiar with the ENC package and proposed that as an option. Together, the investigators and consultants thought through the implications of making ENC available to infants in the study, and they agreed on methods of incorporating the ENC, standardizing training and components, and extending the follow-up period for the infants, in an effort to serve the interests of the infants while protecting the integrity of the science.

This case shows the ethical importance of considering possible outcomes and planning for the end of the study even before the study begins. In this case, a recommendation to add an intervention led to other important possible modifications in the study design in order to maintain the scientific validity of the research while promoting the interests of the infants. Planning ahead for circumstances that arise at the end of a study is also an issue in the next consult.

## CONSULT 7.6: ADDRESSING A REQUEST FOR WITHDRAWAL OF TISSUE SAMPLES

### Reason for Consult

Quinn Ryan, a research nurse, contacted the Consultation Service to ask what ethical concerns relate to the disposition of tissue samples from a research participant who withdrew from a protocol.

### Narrative

Ms. Ryan is the coordinator for a study that deposits samples in an NIH repository of tissue and blood samples. The NIH repository has been assembled over many years with contributions from clinical investigators at several sites (not just the NIH). Typically, tissues collected as part of various protocols are added to the repository where they may be used for diverse, ongoing research, which may or may not be directly related to the original research for which the samples were collected. Samples may be contributed during or after a tissue donor's research participation.

Ms. Ryan explained that Sophie Schultz is currently a participant in an NIH study. Ms. Shultz has recently expressed her desire to stop her own research participation. Additionally, she requested that the research team remove her samples from the tissue repository to prevent further research with her samples.

## Analysis and Recommendations

The first step was to examine the original consent form signed by Ms. Schultz, the research participant in question. The consent form did not address collection, storage, or withdrawal of samples. The bioethics consultants suggested clarification of Ms. Schultz's preferences by talking to Ms. Schultz and to the relevant primary investigator.

During the consultation, the Consultation Service identified additional ethical issues: namely, *(1)* how to manage samples assembled from multiple sites, and *(2)* how prospectively to introduce the storage and use of tissues in the consent form that participants sign when entering the protocol.

Strategies were discussed for providing information about tissue storage and future use in new consent forms. Integration of information about stored tissues into consent forms may require a stepwise process of educating and convincing principal investigators and institutional review boards (IRBs) of its importance. Along with the information about the intended use of stored samples, a checklist for participants to indicate their preferences about the disposition of their samples might be incorporated. If pursuing such a checklist, it would be necessary to consider the logistics of tracking participants' preferences.

Finally, resources were provided that discuss these issues in depth—specifically, the paper by Clayton et al. from 1995,[31] the NBAC report on the use of human tissues in research (http://bioethics.gov/hbm.pdf), and the Web site for the National Action Plan for Breast Cancer, which includes suggested consent form language regarding stored tissues.

## Authors' Commentary

Human tissue samples have been collected and stored for many years, including collections by single researchers related to a specific disease, collections kept in hospital pathology departments, and large public or private institutional or government sample repositories. Stored biological specimens give researchers an opportunity to study human tissues often correlated with particular clinical information. Repository samples have become more valuable as genetic research and technologies become more available. It has been estimated that there are more than 270 million tissue samples stored in the United States, with an estimated 20 million specimens added each year.[32]

Over the last two decades, there has been considerable attention and notable evolution in norms and policies regarding the ethical research use of stored samples. Important considerations include from whom and under what circumstances samples are collected, the type and extent of informed consent obtained from the sample donor regarding future research use, who has access to the samples, and issues of sample ownership and intellectual property, among others. The consultation called in this case was relatively early in this evolution, and prior to the development of NIH policies, which may be reflected by the fact that the investigators had not thought through how to inform participants about research with stored samples.

In this case, two issues were considered: how to handle Ms. Schultz's particular request to withdraw her sample, and how to inform other participants about the possibility of future research use of their samples and facilitate their decisions about whether their samples could be used for future research. The consultation report is thin on the basis for and the appropriate ethical response to the individual's request. Even in the absence of institutional policies, an individual's request to withdraw her sample from the repository should be honored to the extent practically possible. Practically, however, her samples may have already been used in other research projects or altered in a way (e.g., deidentified) that would have made it impossible to withdraw them. A review of withdrawal policies from across various institutions notes that they offer options that range from anonymization to destruction of samples.[33] The consultation team should have advised the investigator to do whatever he or she could to accommodate the participant's request and to explain the limitations of what was possible.

The consultation team also recommended revising the consent form to ensure that other research participants would be informed in advance about possible future research use of their samples and have options from which to choose. Many commentators at the time recommended using a menu of options for participants to choose whether they wanted their samples used in future research and to specify limits if applicable.[34] Others, worried about the practicality of offering a menu of options and keeping track of participants' preferences, instead recommended a more general consent for future use of specimens.[35] Subsequent to this consultation, institutional policies and guidance were developed regarding collection and use of human tissues for research, as well as regarding informed consent.[36] This institutional guidance and guidance available from the DHHS Office of Human Research Protections[37] remain somewhat vague about withdrawal of samples. Participants should be informed when their sample is collected about the circumstances under which their sample may be used for future research, under what circumstances samples can be withdrawn, and about how they can communicate a subsequent decision to have their samples withdrawn from further research. This information should be clear about the practical limits to withdrawing samples that have been made anonymous or already utilized.

## ■ CONSULT 7.7: QUESTIONS ABOUT DISCONTINUATION OF A TRIAL BY THE DATA SAFETY MONITORING BOARD

### Reason for Consult

An investigator contacted a member of the Department of Bioethics regarding an ongoing trial comparing two therapies. He agreed to participate in a formal consultation but requested to remain anonymous. The investigator asked for assistance in determining whether there are legitimate ethical reasons to ask the DSMB to consider continuing the trial even though the predetermined efficacy boundary had been crossed.

### Narrative

Treatments A and B are currently both used in clinical practice to treat a relatively rare but serious disease X. Although clinicians widely believe A is at least as good as if not superior to B, no randomized controlled trial has directly compared the efficacy of A and B in treating disease X. Treatment A was shown to be superior to B for treating a different disease when a head-to-head comparison was done.

NIH investigators, including Anonymous, designed the current study to test the hypothesis that A is superior to B in treating disease X. To the investigators' surprise, interim analysis revealed that response rates to B at this stage of the study are statistically significantly higher than response rates to A. In fact, this statistical significance has crossed the predetermined stopping boundary that was set for efficacy, though in the opposite direction predicted.

The investigators are fairly confident that even if the study were to continue to full enrollment, it would be improbable that the study could establish the superiority of A over B. However, they note that A is currently used in practice for reasons beyond its relative efficacy to B; for example, A is cheaper, has been shown to be more effective in clinical trials on other diseases, and might have less toxicity. The publication and dissemination of results from a relatively small number of cases or from a study terminated based on an interim analysis may not only fail to demonstrate superiority of B over A but would likely raise more questions about their relative efficacy and would therefore not change practice. More likely, the results would confuse the treating community and leave them unsure what to do in practice.

The interim data are not sufficiently robust at this stage to establish the superiority of B over A. More confidence in the result that the interim data suggest—namely, that B is actually superior to A—might influence practice. According to the investigators, the only published study on A in this disease (a small pilot study) suggested a very high response rate. Therefore, there is a good chance (given the anomalously low rates of response to A on the current protocol) that if data from only a small number of additional randomized participants were collected, the data might show that the two treatments are in fact similar and would no longer trend toward the superiority of B over A.

## Analysis and Recommendations

The question is whether it would be ethical to stop the trial now or to continue enrolling participants.

On the one hand, stopping the trial now and publishing the interim data might merely raise an important question ("Is B superior to A?") without settling it. If this question could be settled by continuing the trial, the value of the study to others and the value of the contributions of the participants to date would be markedly enhanced. However, in order to determine whether it is ethically acceptable to continue the trial, serious consideration should be given to possible harm to future participants who might be enrolled. Since the interim data suggest that B is superior to A, enrolling additional participants might deprive those who are randomized to A of a more effective treatment for their condition. The fact that continuing the study would enhance its social value does not justify harming or failing to prevent unnecessary harm to participants.

The Consultation Service recommended that in order to determine whether continuing the study is ethically justified, several factors should be taken into consideration:

1. The degree and seriousness of harm to participants if they do not respond to a treatment. This might take into account possible harm/toxicity from the intervention itself, as well as harm from not having access to the more effective intervention. The harm from not having access depends on the seriousness of the condition and the clinical significance of response.
2. The size of the apparent difference in the effectiveness of the treatments. Does one appear to be much more effective than another?
3. The strength of the evidence for the apparent difference.

If the degree of harm is negligible or very low, then continuing the study may be justified even if the apparent difference in effectiveness is relatively high and the strength of the evidence supporting this difference is relatively strong. By contrast, if the degree of harmfulness is high, then even weak support for a small difference in effectiveness might make continuation unjustified.

The interim data on toxicity do not suggest that A is more harmful than B in itself, so we can set this issue aside. Interim data on early mortality and long-term survival are currently insufficient to trigger stopping. But the interim data do suggest that patients are considerably less likely to respond to A than to B. So how serious is a failure to respond to treatment? The answer will depend on how serious the disease is and the clinical significance of a response to treatment. Disease X is serious, so if the measured response to treatment leads to significant improvements in condition that endure, then depriving patients of a more effective treatment deprives them of a lot. This is a judgment that should be made by people who have sufficient knowledge of disease X and the meaning of response.

However, even if withholding what appears to be a more effective treatment could deprive patients of a lot, continuation of the study might still be justified if the evidence supports only a slight difference in the effectiveness of A and B or if the evidence favoring B over A is weak AND measures could be put into place to minimize possible harm to patients. As things stand, the interim data indicate that B is considerably more effective than A, but taking into account the totality of the available evidence (e.g., previous data on response to A and to B, the anomalously low rates of response to A in this cohort, and possibly high rates of response to B), one might reasonably remain uncertain whether B is as superior to A as the interim data suggest or even whether B is superior to A at all. Measures such as adding an additional safety monitor to examine closely and regularly participants' clinical outcomes, initiating a shorter time to measure response (e.g., 3 months instead of 6), specifying a "rescue" plan for individuals who do not respond, and others, might serve to adequately mitigate harm to participants to allow the study to continue.

Answering the question of whether the study can justifiably continue to enroll participants calls for judgment informed by consideration of these factors. This judgment should be made by people with expertise regarding the disease and the details of the study (including the statistics). The DSMB is in a good position to evaluate the value of effective treatment to patients and the weight of the evidence supporting one treatment over another. If they deem the risks to future participants to be excessive in light of these factors, their judgment should carry considerable weight since, unlike the investigators, they have no stake in the continuation of the trial.

Members of the Consultation Service thought that since reasonable people can disagree about the point at which risks count as excessive, the investigators should be given a chance to present their case for continuation to the DSMB, but the DSMB should make the decision.

## Authors' Commentary

This consult revolved around the controversial and difficult topic of when a scientific question is still an open question, often described in the context of clinical equipoise. Clinical equipoise requires determining that "in a trial, no arm is known to offer greater harm or benefit than any other arm."[38] There has been a lively debate over whether clinical equipoise is an essential requirement for ethical research[39] or the result of confusion between the ethics of clinical research and the ethics of clinical care.[40] Although equipoise is a controversial issue, it is uncontroversial that participants should not be exposed to risks and burdens in research unless there is a valuable research question to answer.

This consult considered these issues in a somewhat unusual way, raising questions about how much evidence is needed to convince practitioners that equipoise has, in fact, been disturbed. Additionally, if an intervention is significantly cheaper, but thought to be less effective, might it be ethical to continue a trial even in the absence of equipoise? This consult ultimately focused on an issue that is important for the oversight of clinical research and might be legitimately confusing to researchers: Who should decide whether equipoise has been disturbed—should it just be up to the DSMB, or can an investigator play a role in helping the DSMB make this determination?

DSMBs are set up to be independent from the research team so that they can more objectively determine when a study should be stopped in order to protect research participants. To further increase their objectivity, many DSMBs set up predetermined thresholds, or stopping rules, for when a study should be halted in advance; rules that should take into account external factors like precisely what data are needed to inform practice. These protections are very important to resist the pressures to continue a study in hope of obtaining desired results or more publishable data, pressures that may weigh especially heavily on a researcher.

For these reasons, an investigator should not challenge a DSMB's decision to terminate a trial lightly. Ideally, a DSMB's stopping rules would be carefully calibrated to take account of the considerations the investigator was concerned about here, like the worry that a result that showed that B was marginally better than A was very unlikely to change clinical practice. No rule can ever be perfect, however, so a DSMB also should be familiar enough with the field to exercise judgment in deciding whether the stopping rules should be applied to the specific data they are examining.

Yet, from an investigator's perspective, it is not always clear what steps a DSMB has taken and whether they have given adequate consideration to the consequences of stopping the study. Furthermore, a DSMB whose members have the relevant expertise should be strong enough to withstand some outside pressure, from investigators or others, when they know they have reached the correct decision. There may be cases like this one when it makes sense for an investigator to approach a DSMB respectfully and present arguments to the DSMB. In this case, the DSMB was very receptive to the investigator's arguments and ultimately decided to allow the study to continue. When the study was completed, the results demonstrated that A was superior to B.

It is interesting to consider whether this case would have served as an exception to the general rule that investigators not challenge DSMB decisions, if the DSMB had decided to discontinue the study.

A final point to take away from this consult is that the investigator requested an anonymous consult because he felt the situation was sensitive, and he may have been uncertain whether he was overstepping his bounds. This consult is an excellent example of the value of granting a request for anonymous consultation in certain cases, as it appears to have been a meritorious but difficult question, and it is one that the investigator now feels comfortable having published in this book (with details anonymized). When discomfort about a legitimate ethical issue might prevent a consult request from being made, anonymization is an important tool that the ethics consultant can use to respect the wishes of the consult requestor but one that may change the shape of the advice given. The advice given here was not a ruling on the merits of the issue—the consult team did not determine that this investigator was correct. Instead, the consult team helped the investigator to think through the issue, felt that it was appropriate for the investigator to approach the DSMB about the issue and start a dialogue, with the DSMB retaining the authority to make the final decision about the ethics of continuing or stopping the trial.

## CONSULT 7.8: ASSIGNING AUTHORSHIP

### Reason for Consult

Dr. Sachin Dube requested a bioethics consultation to explore whether it would it be ethically appropriate to grant authorship to a research participant.

### Narrative

Dr. Dube is studying families with a heritable condition. One young man, part of a large family that participated in the study, is a medical student. This young man made some contribution to the research, including bringing his family to the attention of the investigators, identifying family members for enrollment, and preparing a genealogy of the family. Now, the young man has written to Dr. Dube requesting to be included as an author on any papers that result from the study. This could be helpful to his future career. Dr. Dube reports that the young man has been in contact with other investigators in the field, and Dr. Dube believes these other investigators may have encouraged the participant to seek authorship.

Dr. Dube feels that the contributions claimed by this young man are somewhat exaggerated, but he is willing to grant authorship, primarily as a gesture of goodwill. Dr. Dube did say that if the man had worked in his lab, the amount of his contribution would likely have been insufficient to merit authorship. Dr. Dube is concerned that if authorship is granted for this student, it will be important to find ways to guarantee other members of the family that their privacy had not been breached.

## Analysis and Recommendations

1. The first question is whether authorship ought to be given to this participant. The Consultation Service felt that authorship for this particular person should be determined in the customary way, based on the individual's contributions and authorship criteria normally applied. The laboratory investigators should judge whether to make the participant a coauthor based upon the usual standards used in their laboratory without regard for extraneous pressures. On this basis, does the contribution of the person warrant authorship status?

One Ethics Committee member serving on the consult team felt strongly that the contributions described did not warrant coauthorship and that the request should not be granted. In light of the varied opinions about authorship, we offered to have Dr. Dube attend an Ethics Committee meeting for further discussion. Additionally, the Consultation Service emphasized that the NIH Ombudsman can act to mediate authorship disputes, and the NIH Committee on Scientific Conduct and Ethics is charged with taking up such matters and also may be accessed by either party.

2. The Consultation Service recommended that if authorship was granted, other considerations are important. First, if the young man is made a coauthor, he should not have access to clinical data about his family members. This should be made clear to him. Other family members may be suspicious that the coauthor family member has access to sensitive medical or genetic information about them. For this reason, all other participants in the study should be notified, in advance of publication, about the coauthorship and the restrictions on the coauthor's access to data.

## Additional Analysis and Recommendations

In light of the varied opinions about authorship among members of the consult team, the case was brought before the full Ethics Committee for discussion. After Dr. Dube presented the case, the Consultation Service attending presented the consultation process and recommendations outlined previously.

Ethics Committee members expressed a variety of views including the following:

- The young man should not be given authorship for the work he has done in facilitating data collection.
- Based on Dr. Dube's description of the participant's letter, the young man's strategy of invoking Dr. Dube's competitors in the field might be viewed as coercive.
- It would not be fair to dismiss the participant's request for authorship without hearing his views.
- The NIH guidelines for authorship require more than this participant appears to have done and writing to him offering this justification should be an acceptable strategy.
- The participant might be offered an acknowledgement and subsequent authorship in future work if he is interested in doing more.

Additionally, the deputy ombudsman commented that while he would not personally recommend authorship, NIH laboratories have variable practices regarding authorship decisions and some might give authorship based on the contribution that the participant claims to have made.

In summary, many—but not all—members of the Ethics Committee thought that the participant did not deserve authorship. However, it was noted that the committee had not heard his perspective in arriving at these views.

## Authors' Commentary

Unlike many of the other consults in this volume, this consult addresses an issue that relates to the ethical concerns that attend the publication of research. Although there are many important ethical issues surrounding the publication of research, the NIH Office of the Ombudsman typically works to resolve these issues. Nevertheless, there are times when an ethics consultation service may be uniquely placed to help think through issues of authorship, particularly if the Consultation Service has had to address similar issues internally, or in unusual cases like this one, where research participants seek authorship.

After the meeting, Dr. Dube reported that he decided to offer authorship following the initial suggestion about fair criteria for authorship and the promise of maintenance of privacy for all family participants. This case provides a nice illustration of the fact that any consult service, whether focused on ethics or cardiology, functions in an advisory role. The consult requestor can choose to follow or not to follow the consultant's advice. Here, the Consultation Service offered an opinion that reflected a majority of the views of the members of the Ethics Committee, but not all of their views, implying that the consult was one about which reasonable people could disagree. The investigator elected to take the approach favored by the minority but also took pains to address the concerns that were raised about granting authorship to a research participant, which seems like a perfectly legitimate response.

One interesting issue raised by this consult is when to bring a consult to the full Ethics Committee for further discussion. The advantages of going to the full committee for further review include the ability to gather more expertise on or experience with a complicated issue, the ability to offer the investigator a diversity of views on an issue or a strong consensus on an issue if everyone happens to agree, and opportunities to train newer Ethics Committee members in ethics consultation. The disadvantages could include that because members of the Ethics Committee may have a diversity of views and different levels of exposure to day-to-day ethics consultation, the advice that the consult requestor receives might be confusing, diluted, or even contradictory.

For some ethical issues, reasonable people can disagree and there may be a range of defensible options from which a researcher can choose, so Ethics Committee involvement may be very helpful to identify the full spectrum of options available to the researcher. For others that merit more definitive ethical judgments, or that have circumstances requiring a quick and firm decision, obtaining the opinions of many consultants may not be advisable. It is unclear what happened in this case, but there may be cases in which involving a full committee would place an undue burden on the requestor or provide the requestor with advice too diverse to be helpful, and it is important for consultants to be mindful of these possibilities.

Interestingly enough, however, the decision made by the investigator and the advice offered by the Consultation Service may not have directly considered the influential Vancouver guidelines on authorship (to which most medical journals subscribe). These guidelines currently specify that data collection alone does not merit authorship, and that each author should meet three conditions: "1) substantial contributions to conception and design, acquisition of data, or analysis and interpretation of data; 2) drafting the article or revising it critically for important intellectual content; and 3) final approval of the version to be published."[41] Nevertheless, it has not been unusual to award authorship on an honorary basis where others have contributed considerably more of the intellectual and logistical work, or for a variety of other reasons. These traditional practices have been criticized for making it difficult to assign responsibility to defend a publication or to give credit where it is due. Nevertheless, it may not be easy for an investigator to elect to follow the rules when the rules are often flouted, and the ethical stakes are relatively low.

Of course, a principal investigator is in a powerful position to determine the extent to which others involved in a research project have the opportunity to contribute in a way that deserves authorship. If the investigator and medical student had had a conversation earlier in the conduct of the study, the student may well have been able to contribute in a manner that indisputably deserved authorship. While the point at which this consult was requested was too late to alter the nature of this particular research participant's involvement, the consulting team could have discussed this possibility with the investigator so that interactions with future research participants might proceed differently. In mentioning such a possibility, a research ethics consultant might enhance the feasibility of more active involvement of a study participant in the research process in unusual cases like this one in which the participant has a medical training or similarly appropriate training and skills.

## NOTES

1. H. Brody and F. Miller, "The Clinician-Investigator: Unavoidable But Manageable Tension," *Kennedy Institute of Ethics Journal* 13, no. 4 (2003): 329–346.

2. National Bioethics Advisory Committee, *Ethical and Policy Issues in International Research: Clinical Trials in Developing Countries* (Rockville MD: U.S. Governmentpublisher, 2001), chap. 4.

3. Swidler, Seastrum, and Shelton, "Difficult Hospital Inpatient Discharge Decisions," *American Journal of Bioethics* 2007.

4. World Medical Association Declaration of Helsinki, *Ethical Principles for Medical Research Involving Human Subjects*, paragraph 33 (2008 revision), available at: http://www.wma.net/en/30publications/10policies/b3/index.html), accessed on May 14, 2010; National Bioethics Advisory Commission (NBAC), Ethical and Policy Issues in International Research: Clinical Trials in Developing Countries 1 (April 2001); Nuffield Council of Bioethics, *The Ethics of Research Related to Health Care in Developing Countries*, at 103 (2004), available at: http://www.nuffieldbioethics.org/go/ourwork/developingcountries/publication_309.html, accessed on July 16, 2008.

5. Moral Standards for Research in Developing Countries: From "Reasonable Availability" to "Fair Benefits," *Hastings Center Report* 34, no. 3 (2004): 17–27.

6. George A. Hillery, Jr., "Definitions of Community: Areas of Agreement," *Rural Sociology* 20 (1955): 111–122.

7. Joseph Millum, "Post-Trial Access to Antiretrovirals: Who Owes What to Whom?" *Bioethics* 25, no 4 (2011; 145–154); Seema Shah, Stacy Elmer, and Christine Grady, "Planning for Posttrial Access to Antiretroviral Treatment for Research Participants in Developing Countries," *American Journal of Public Health* 99, no. 9 (2009): 1556–1562; Christine Pace, Christine Grady, David Wendler, Judith D. Bebchuk, Jorge A. Tavel, Laura A. McNay, Heidi P. Forster, Jack Killen, and Ezekiel J. Emanuel, "Post-trial Access to Tested Interventions: The Views of IRB/REC Chair, Investigators, and Research Participants in a Multinational HIV/AIDS Study," *AIDS Research and Human Retroviruses* 22, no. 9: 837–841.

8. Food and Drug Administration, Department of Health and Human Services, "Guidance for Clinical Trial Sponsors: Establishment and Operation of Clinical Trial Data Monitoring Committees, Non-Binding Recommendations (OMB Control No. 0910-0581)," March 2006, availableat:http://www.fda.gov/downloads/RegulatoryInformation/Guidances/UCM126578.pdf; Holly A. Taylor, Lelia Chaisson, and Jeremy Sugarman, "Enhancing Communication among Data Monitoring Committees and Institutional Review Boards," *Clinical Trials* 5 (2008): 277; J. V. Lavery et al., "In Global Health Research, Is It Legitimate to Stop Clinical Trials Early on Account of Their Opportunity Costs?" *PLoS Medicine* 6, no. 6 (June 2009).

9. T. R. Fleming, S. Ellenberg, and D. L. DeMets, "Monitoring Clinical Trials: Issues and Controversies Regarding Confidentiality," *Statistics in Medicine* 21 (2002): 2843–2851, at 2844.

10. A. Flanagin, L. A. Carey, P. B. Fontanarosa, et al., "Prevalence of Articles with Honorary Authors and Ghost Authors in Peer-Reviewed Medical Journals," *Journal of the American Medical Association* 280 (1998): 222–224.

11. International Committee of Medical Journal Editors, "Uniform Requirements for Manuscripts Submitted to Biomedical Journals:
Ethical Considerations in the Conduct and Reporting of Research: Authorship and Contributorship," available at: http://www.icmje.org/ethical_1author.html (2010).

12. L. Calvocoressi, C. I. McDougle, S. Wasylink, W. K. Goodman, S. J. Trufan, and L. H. Price, "Inpatient Treatment of Patients with Severe Obsessive-Compulsive Disorder," *Hospital and Community Psychiatry* 44, no. 12 (1993): 1150–1154.

13. Institute of Medicine, "When Children Die: Improving Palliative and End-of-Life Care for Children and Their Families" (2003).

14. R. L. Beckstrand, N. L. Rawle, L. Callister, and B. L. Mandleco, "Pediatric Nurses' Perceptions of Obstacles and Supportive Behaviors in End-of-Life Care," *American Journal of Critical Care*, 2010 Nov;19(6):543-52.

15. B. Davies, N. Contro, J. Larson, and K. Widger, "Culturally-Sensitive Information-Sharing in Pediatric Palliative Care," *Pediatrics* 125: 2010 Apr;125(4):e859-65 .

16. Jeffrey D. Hord, Waqas Rehman, Patricia Hannon, Lisa Anderson-Shaw, and Mary Lou Schmidt, "Do Parents Have the Right to Refuse Standard Treatment for Their Child with Favorable-Prognosis Cancer? Ethical and Legal Concerns," *Journal of Clinical Oncology* 24, no. 34 (2006): 5454–5456.

17. Jennifer L. Hartsell, Comment: "Mother May I . . . Live? Parental Refusal of Life-Sustaining Medical Treatment for Children Based on Religious Objections," 66 *Tennessee Law Review* 499 (1999).

18. Jessica A. Penkower, Comment: "The Potential Right of Chronically Ill Adolescents to Refuse Life-Saving Medical Treatment–Fatal Misuse of the Mature Minor Doctrine," 45 *DePaul Law Review* 1165 (1996).

19. Hord, *supra* note 13; C. Dyer, "Trust Decides against Action to Force Girl to Undergo Transplant," *British Medical Journal* 337 (2008): 1132.

20. P. Litton and F. G. Miller, "A Normative Justification for Distinguishing the Ethics of Clinical Research from the Ethics of Medical Care," *Journal of Law, Medicine, and Ethics* 33, no. 3 (2005): 566–574.

21. M. W. Merritt, H. A. Taylor, and L. C, Mullany, "Ancillary Care in Community-Based Public Health Intervention Research," *American Journal of Public Health* 100, no. 2 (2010): 211–216.

22. World Medical Association Declaration of Helsinki, *Ethical Principles for Medical Research Involving Human Subjects*, paragraph 33 (2008 revision).

23. C. Pace, F. Miller, and M. Danis, "Enrolling the Uninsured in Clinical Trials: An Ethical Perspective," *Critical Care Medicine* 31, no. 3 (Suppl. 2003): S121–S125.

24. See S. Shah, S. Elmer, and C. Grady, "Planning for Posttrial Access to Antiretroviral Treatment for Research Participants in Developing Countries," *American Journal of Public Health* 99, no. 9 (2009): 1556–1562; J. Millum, "Post-trial Access to Antiretrovirals: Who Owes What to Whom?" *Bioethics* 25, no. 4 (2011): 145–154.

25. C. Grady. "The Challenge of Assuring Continued Post-trial Access to Beneficial Treatment," *Yale Journal of Health Policy, Law, and Ethics* 5, no. 1 (2005): 425–435; Nuffield Council of Bioethics, "The Ethics of Research Related to Health Care in Developing Countries," 2004, available at: http://www.nuffieldbioethics.org/go/ourwork/developingcountries/publication_308.html.

26. National Bioethics Advisory Commission, *Ethical and Policy Issues in International Research: Clinical Trials in Developing Countries*, published April 1, 2001, available at: http://bioethics.georgetown.edu/nbac/clinical/Vol1.pdf.

27. IOM Responsible Research.

28. *See* Sabina Gainotti and Carlo Petrini, Insurance Policies for Clinical Trials in the United States and in Some European Countries, *Journal of Clinical Research and Bioethics* 1, no. 7 (2010), available at: http://www.omicsonline.org/2155-9627/2155-9627-1-101.pdf; National Bioethics Advisory Commission, "Ethical and Policy Issues in Research Involving Human Participants" 123 (2001), available at: http://bioethics.georgetown.edu/nbac/human/overvol1.pdf.

29. W. A. Carlo, S. S. Goudar, I. Jehan, et al. for the First Breath Study Group, "Newborn-Care Training and Perinatal Mortality in Developing Countries," *New England Journal of Medicine* 362, no. 7 (2010): 614–623.

30. The consultation service believes that this obligation is not unlimited but is currently not well defined.

31. E. Clayton, K. Steinberg, M. Khoury, et al., "Informed Consent for Genetic Research on Stored Tissue Samples," *Journal of the American Medical Association* 274 (1995): 1786–1792.

32. S. Haga and L. Beskow, "Ethical, Legal, and Social Implications of Biobanks for Genetics Research," *Advances in Genetics* 60 (2008): 505–544.

33. Ibid.

34. National Bioethics Advisory Commission (NBAC), "Research Involving Human Biological Materials: Ethical Issues and Policy Guidance (volume 1)," 1999, available at: http://www.georgetown.edu/research/nrcbl/nbac/hbm.pdf; Clayton op cit # 29; American Society of Human Genetics (ASHG) (1996),"Statement on Informed Consent for Genetic Research," *American Journal of Human Genetics* 59: 471–474.

35. D. Wendler, "One-Time General Consent for Research on Biological Samples," *British Medical Journal* 332 (2006): 544–547.

36. "NIH Requirements for the Research Use of Stored Human Specimens and Data," available at: http://ohsr.od.nih.gov/info/sheet14.html

37. Guidance on Research Involving Coded Private Information or Biological Specimens, available at: http://www.hhs.gov/ohrp/humansubjects/guidance/cdebiol.htm

38. Priscilla Alderson, "Equipoise as a Means of Managing Uncertainty: Personal, Communal and Proxy," *Journal of Medical Ethics* 22 (1996): 135–139.

39. P. B. Miller and C. Weijer, "Rehabilitating Equipoise," *Kennedy Institute of Ethics Journal* 13, no. 2 (2003): 93–118.

40. Franklin G. Miller and Howard Brody, "Clinical Equipoise and the Incoherence of Research Ethics," *Journal of Medicine and Philosophy* 32, no. 2 (2007): 151–165.

41. International Committee of Medical Journal Editors, *Uniform Requirements for Manuscripts Submitted to Biomedical Journals*, updated 2009, available at: http://www.icmje.org.

# APPENDICES

## APPENDIX 1. CONSULTATIONS ORGANIZED BY SUBJECT MATTER

| Issue | Cases |
|---|---|
| Ancillary care | 1.5, 4.6, 5.1, 5.2, 5.3, 5.7, 6.4, 7.3, 7.5 |
| Coercion | 2.7 |
| Confidentiality | 2.3, 3.5, 6.1, 7.8 |
| Discharge obligations | 5.3, 6.4, 7.1, 7.2, 7.3 |
| Duty to warn | 3.5, 6.1 |
| Exploitation | 2.1, 5.4 |
| Family dynamics | 3.5, 3.6, 4.2, 4.3, 4.4, 4.5, 4.6, 5.3, 6.1, 6.4, 6.5, 6.6, 6.7 |
| Genetic research | 1.3, 1.5, 1.7, 3.5, 4.5, 7.8 |
| HIV/AIDS | 1.1, 1.5, 5.1, 5.7 |
| Incidental findings | 5.2, 5.4 |
| Inclusion and exclusion from research | 1.3, 1.7, 2.1, 2.2, 2.3, 2.5, 3.2, 3.3, 3.4, 3.6, 5.4, 5.7, 6.2, 6.3, 7.1, 7.3, 7.4 |
| Informed consent | 1.5, 1.6, 2.3, 2.4, 2.6, 2.7, 3.2, 4.3, 4.4, 4.5, 5.2, 6.8, 7.3, 7.4, 7.6 |
| IRBs | 1.3, 1.6, 1.7, 2.4, 3.1, 3.3, 3.4, 7.5 |
| Medical error | 3.4 |
| Noncompliance | 5.7, 6.2, 6.3 |
| Placebo use | 1.4, 1.5, 3.2, 5.6 |
| Recruitment methods | 2.1, 2.4, 2.5, 2.7, 4.5 |
| Research in developing countries | 1.2, 1.5, 5.1, 7.5 |
| Risks | 1.1, 1.2, 1.4, 1.5, 1.6, 1.7, 2.4, 2.5, 3.1, 3.2, 3.3, 3.4, 3.6, 4.1, 5.2, 5.3, 5.5, 5.7, 6.1, 6.2, 6.4, |
| Scientific validity | 1.1, 1.3, 1.4, 1.5, 1.6, 1.7, 2.5, 5.4, 5.5, 6.3, 7.5, 7.7 |
| Social value | 1.1, 1.3, 1.5, 2.4, 2.7, 7.7 |
| Special populations—Pregnant women | 3.3 |
| Special populations—Children and adolescents | 1.4, 1.5, 1.7, 2.1, 3.2, 4.1, 4.2, 5.1, 6.2, 6.3, 7.2, 7.5 |
| Special populations—Cognitively impaired | 4.2, 4.3, 4.4, 6.5, 6.6, 6.7 |
| Special populations—Terminally ill | 1.6, 4.5, 6.5, 6.6 |
| Special populations—Uninsured | 2.1, 4.6, 5.4, 5.5, 7.4 |
| Special populations—Employees | 2.3 |
| Standard of care | 1.5, 1.7, 2.1, 5.4, 5.5, 6.5, 7.3, 7.5 |
| Surrogate decision making | 3.2, 3.4, 4.3, 4.4, 4.5, 6.3, 6.5, 6.6, 6.7, 7.2 |
| Therapeutic misconception | 5.2, 5.5 |
| Trial design | 1.2, 1.4, 1.5, 1.6, 1.7, 3.2, 4.5 |
| Undue inducement | 2.1, 2.5, 2.7, 5.5, 5.7 |

# APPENDIX 2. EVALUATION OF THE CLINCAL CENTER BIOETHICS CONSULTATION SERVICE

Ben Chan, Ph.D., and Marion Danis, M.D.

While this casebook focuses on singular consultations that are worthy of special attention, readers may wonder how the Consultation Service assures the quality of its services in general. This appendix describes the system of evaluation used by the Consultation Service, bearing in mind the prevailing standards for evaluating ethics consultation services and highlighting some challenges in evaluating the quality of ethics consultation.

Standards for research ethics consultation services are less well developed than those for clinical ethics consultations. However, there is a significant push to develop standardized data collection practices to facilitate communication and quality improvement within the community of research ethics consultants.[1] Indeed, this volume was made possible by the fact that the Consultation Service has documented its cases in a standardized database since 1999.

The American Society for Bioethics and Humanities (ASBH) report, "Core Competencies for Healthcare Ethics Consultation," is the current benchmark for evaluating ethics consultations services.[2] While the recommendations in the ASBH report were developed for health care consultation in general, they are relevant to research ethics consultation. The report distinguishes three major dimensions according to which a consultation service should be evaluated: *quality*, *access*, and *efficiency*.

## Evaluating Quality

The ASBH's recommendations emphasize the assessment of a service's *quality*. The report follows Donabedian's model for quality improvement in health care more generally, dividing quality assessment into three parts: structure, process, and outcomes.[3] The "structure" of an ethics consultation service refers to the "enduring characteristics of [the] service," such as its place within the organizational structure of its institution, its membership, finances, and policies. "Process" refers to the actual interactions between the consulting service and those served (e.g., patients, health care workers, medical researchers). "Outcomes" refer, naturally, to the results of the consultation.

### Structure

The ASBH makes two major recommendations on evaluating the structure of a consultation service.[4] First, the ASBH document highlights key questions that institutions should address in their self-assessment, for example: Is there a designated individual who is held accountable through a performance review that explicitly addresses the quality of the facility's ethics consultation activities? At the NIH, the Consultation Service reports to the Clinical Center Ethics

Committee, which in turn reports to the Medical Executive Committee of the Clinical Center. The chief of the Consultation Service is the person designated as responsible. She oversees monthly and annual reports to the Ethics Committee.

The second recommendation is that institutions assess the skills of their ethics consultants, such as their ability to facilitate group decision making and their knowledge of clinical ethics. There are various ways to perform such an assessment (e.g., self-assessment, third-party assessment); the report does not take a stance on which method is preferable. The Clinical Center Department of Bioethics pursues a number of strategies to develop the skills of the fellows who staff the consultation service and to maintain the skills of the attendings. Before taking call for the Consultation Service, fellows participate in numerous educational activities to build their knowledge of research ethics. These include a year-long series of seminars in bioethics, with special attention to research ethics. Fellows also attend NIH IRB and Clinical Center Ethics Committee meetings, and they shadow members of the Consultation Service as they respond to consultation requests. Just prior to beginning their participation on the Consultation Service they undergo orientation to learn about the function of the service and their responsibilities. While we have no formal evaluation of consultation skills, supervision of the fellows by experienced attendings allows for observation, feedback, and improvement of their skills. Clinical Center Ethics Committee members are offered the opportunity to attend intensive bioethics training courses. The attendings are continually updating their knowledge in the course of their interaction with their academic colleagues, participation in conferences and workshops, membership on professional boards, and frequent review of the literature on ethics consultation.

## Process

To evaluate the ethics consultation process, the ASBH recommends that each institution explicitly formulate and implement its own standards regarding such matters as notification of affected parties, documenting consultations, and whether consultants should review the medical record.[5] The Consultation Service has explicit process standards that are articulated in a handbook used by the ethics consultants. For example, with respect to the above issues, the handbook states that consultants must do the following:

- Meet with the requestor, if appropriate, and invite other stakeholders to participate after consultation with the requestor
- Document consultations in the electronic database, using a structured outline that includes the reason for consultation, case background, ethical analysis, and recommendations along with other administrative data required to monitor the service
- Enter the report into the medical record (if applicable) on a case-by-case basis

## Outcomes

The ethical soundness of consultants' recommendations is an outcome of central interest, which might be evaluated by retrospective case evaluation by an ethics committee or (internal or external) peer review.[6] At a minimum, the ASBH recommends that consultation services routinely measure the satisfaction of consultation participants. To this end, after a consultation is completed, those who requested consultations are sent an evaluation form (see Box 1). The feedback from these forms is compiled and presented to the Clinical Center Ethics Committee annually.

---

**BOX 1.** ■ Postconsultation Evaluation Form

1. In my opinion, the consult helped:  *Not at all     As much as possible*

    | | 1 | 2 | 3 | 4 | N/A |
    |---|---|---|---|---|---|
    | a. address my concerns | O | O | O | O | O |
    | b. clarify ethical issues | O | O | O | O | O |
    | c. reduce conflicts among involved persons | O | O | O | O | O |
    | d. provide an opportunity to improve communication | O | O | O | O | O |
    | e. make me feel comfortable with the situation | O | O | O | O | O |
    | f. improve quality of the patient-subject's care | O | O | O | O | O |
    | g. lead to a more ethical decision | O | O | O | O | O |

2. Overall, how satisfied were you with the ethics consult?   O 1   O 2   O 3   O 4   O N/A

3. What was the most helpful about the consultation?

4. Do you have any suggestions for improving the consultation process?

5. Do you have any other comments?

6. What was your role in the consult? (Check as many as applicable)

    [ ] Patient / Research Participant     [ ] Attending Physician
    [ ] Family Member                      [ ] Fellow
    [ ] Principal Investigator             [ ] Requestor of the Consult
    [ ] Nurse                              [ ] Social Worker

---

In addition, the consultation service chief offers a monthly retrospective case review with the Ethics Committee. Each consultation from the previous month is described in brief—the reason for the consult, recommendations, and so on—with one case chosen for more detailed review and discussion. Finally, 4 or 5 consultations a year are presented to the NIH community as a whole at the Clinical Center's Grand Rounds, with an outside (i.e., non-NIH) expert commenting on the case.

## ▪ EVALUATING ACCESS AND EFFICIENCY

With respect to evaluating *access* to a consultation service, the ASBH recommends that each service clearly articulate its target populations and review the sources of consultation requests in order to identify and address gaps in access.[7] The Consultation Service's target population comprises anyone in the NIH Clinical Center research community including patient-participants enrolled in intramural research at the NIH, their families, clinical investigators and other members of research teams, clinical staff such as nurses and social workers, IRB members, and others in the intramural NIH program. The Consultation Service evaluates access by documenting the source of requests—both their role (e.g., research coordinator) and institution (e.g., National Institute for Mental Health)—in its case database. These data are compiled and presented as part of the service's annual review, where potential gaps in access are identified and addressed.

Finally, to evaluate *efficiency*, the ASBH report recommends clearly delineating the range of questions that the service will address, documenting consultations, and tracking workload.[8] The workload of the Consultation Service is tracked in the service's electronic database, where the person-hours spent on each consult are recorded. When combined with other information recorded in the database (e.g., the reason for the consult, the ethical issues identified, the decision-making process), the Consultation Service is able to form an accurate profile of the nature and extent of the work it performs.

## ▪ CHALLENGES IN EVALUATING ETHICS CONSULTATION SERVICES

While we have referred to the ASBH report as the benchmark for evaluating ethics consultations services, we recognize that there are several open questions about how to appropriately measure the effectiveness of ethics consultations.

Determining which outcomes are relevant to evaluating ethics case consultation is a vexing issue with significant disagreement about whether standardized evaluation is desirable.[9] It seems clear that familiar health care quality metrics such as mortality or patient satisfaction are imperfect proxies for ethical decision making, which is a central aim of ethics consultation. Some have suggested that the effectiveness of case consultations might instead be judged according to whether recommendations from consultations reduce discrepancies between medical practice (and by inference, research practice) and consensus medical ethical positions.[10] One difficulty with this suggestion is that, as the cases in this volume illustrate, many cases fall outside of the scope of existing consensus ethical positions—either because there is no consensus concerning the sort of case at issue, or because the existing consensus is inapplicable due to extenuating circumstances.

Another challenge in evaluating consultation services is that it is not yet known how different features of ethics consultations affect outcomes. There are various features that are widely recognized as virtues in the consultation process (e.g., transparent documentation, accessibility, and timeliness). However, there has been little or no systematic investigation as to how these features affect outcomes in ethics consultation.[11] Similarly, there are little data available to confirm or deny the plausible structural worry that ethics consultants' financial dependence on the institutions they serve hinders their ethical objectivity.

Nevertheless, the virtues noted previously—responsiveness to participants, accessibility, institutional oversight, transparency, and so forth—clearly serve another important goal of ethics consultation: creating a space for moral deliberation within the institution.[12] Though unambiguous measures of ethical decision making may be unavailable, the Consultation Service believes that the quality of our service is continually improved by answering to the evolving needs of the community we serve, critically reviewing past cases, keeping apprised of standards in research ethics, and publicizing our activities.

## ■ NOTES

1. M. Kelley, K. Fryer-Edwards, S. Fullerton, T. Gallagher, and B. Wilfond, "Sharing Data and Experience: Using the Clinical and Translational Science Award (CTSA) 'Moral Community' to Improve Research Ethics Consultation," *American Journal of Bioethics* 8, no. 3 (2008): 37–39.

2. American Society for Bioethics and Humanities, *Core Competencies for Health Care Ethics Consultation* (Glenview, IL: American Society for Bioethics and Humanities, 2010).

3. A. Donabedian, *The Definition of Quality and Approaches to Its Assessment* (Ann Arbor, MI: Health Administration Press, 1980).

4. Op. cit., note 2, 38–40.

5. Ibid., 41–42.

6. Ibid., 44.

7. Ibid., 47–48.

8. Ibid., 49–50.

9. Compare, for example, the pessimistic view of standardization in Bishop, J., Fanning, J., and Bliton, M. "Of Goals and Goods and Floundering About: A Dissensus Report on Clinical Ethics Consultation." *HEC Forum* 21, no. 3 (2009): 275–291 with the optimistic view in Dubler, N., Webber, P., Swiderski, D., and the Faculty of the National Working Group for the Clinical Ethics Credentialing Project. "Charting the Future: Credentialing, Privileging, Quality, and Evaluation in Clinical Ethics Consultation." *Hastings Center Report* 39, no. 6 (2009): 23–33.

10. Op. cit., note 2, 44.

11 Lo, B., "Answers and Questions about Ethics Consultations," *The Journal of the American Medical Association* 290, no. 9 (2003): 1208–1210..

12. Walker, M.,"Keeping Moral Space Open," *The Hastings Center Report* 23, no. 2 (1993): 33–41.

## APPENDIX 3. CLINICAL CENTER POLICY M77-2: INFORMED CONSENT

### Background

Ethical considerations and Federal regulations (codified in Title 45, Code of Federal Regulations, Part 46 [45 CFR 46], "Protection of Human Subjects") require that investigators obtain the subject's informed consent or permission from the subject's legally authorized representative (LAR) before any research procedures are initiated. This requirement is articulated in the National Institutes of Health's Assurance of Compliance (Multiple Project Assurance [MPA]) and is consistent with DHHS Regulations for the Protection of Human Subjects (45 CFR 46), and it is also found in M93-1 "Research Involving Human Subjects at the Clinical Center."

The ethical principle of respect for persons requires that individuals with decision-making capacity decide whether they want to participate in research. This is accomplished through a process of informed consent. Informed consent requires the following: *(1)* disclosure of relevant information about the research to prospective subjects; *(2)* their comprehension of the information, and *(3)* their voluntary agreement, free of coercion and undue influence, to participate in research. Typically, consent is documented by the signature of the consenting subject or LAR and the investigator on an approved informed consent document. As new information of relevance to a subject's participation becomes available, it should also be provided as appropriate.

### Definitions

- An **adult** is anyone 18 years of age or older. For purposes of providing consent, a minor who is married or a parent may also be considered an adult at the Clinical Center.
- **Informed consent** is an affirmative agreement to participate in research given by a person who:
    - Has the legal capacity to give consent
    - Exercises free power of choice
    - Has sufficient knowledge and understanding of the nature of the proposed research, the anticipated risks, potential benefits, alternatives, and the requirements of the research as to be able to make an informed decision.
- **Research** means a systematic investigation, including research development, testing, and evaluation, designed to develop or contribute to generalizable knowledge (45 CFR 46.102 (d).).

- **Human subject** means a living individual about whom an investigator (whether professional or student) conducting research obtains one of the following:
  - Data through intervention or interaction with the individual
  - Identifiable private information (45 CFR 46.102 (f).)
- **A decisionally capacitated** adult is an adult that has sufficient mental capacity to understand the information that is provided, to appreciate how that information is relevant to his or her circumstances, and to make a reasoned decision whether to participate in the study.
- **Legally authorized representative** means an individual or judicial or other body authorized under applicable law to consent on behalf of a prospective subject to the subject's participation in the procedure(s) involved in research (45CFR.46.102(c)).
- **Surrogate** means an individual authorized under applicable law to consent to noninvestigational procedures, that is, procedures that are clinically indicated and not performed as part of the research study.

## Policy

- In order-to participate in research activities at the Clinical Center of the National Institutes of Health (NIH) (hereafter referred to as the Clinical Center), each adult person, or his or her legally authorized representative, shall provide informed consent prior to beginning study participation by signing a "Consent to Participate in a Clinical Research Study" (NIH-2514-1). For screening procedures performed to determine eligibility for research participation, consent shall be documented on NIH-2514-1. In some cases, the General Admission Consent form (NIH-1225-1) may be used for screening procedures that are no more than minimal risk and when approved by the IRB. The signed consent documents will be maintained in the patient's medical record under divider "Protocol Consent." In rare cases, the IRB may approve a modification or waiver of informed consent consistent with 45 CFR.46.116(c).
- Investigators are responsible for informing potential research subjects of the nature of the study, the risks and benefits of, and alternatives to participation, and all other information necessary for the subjects to make a considered decision whether or not to participate. Investigators are responsible for assessing that subjects understand the information provided and that individuals give voluntary consent, free of coercion or undue influence.
- *Minors.* For a minor to participate in research, permission must be obtained from parent(s), legal guardian(s), or other LAR and assent obtained from

the child (if capable of giving assent as determined by the IRB) and documented on "Minor Patient's Assent to Participate in a Clinical Research Study" (NIH-2514-2). Investigators are responsible for informing parent(s) or guardian(s) about the research as well as assessing their understanding and voluntariness as described in this policy. Refer to MAS 92-5, "Research Involving Children and Children's Assent to Research," for additional requirements and procedures for research with children.

- For minimal risk research or research involving greater than minimal risk but a prospect of direct benefit to the individual child, the permission and signature of one parent is generally sufficient, if approved by the IRB.
- For other IRB approved research with children (i.e., greater than minimal risk with no prospect of direct benefit), the permission and signature of both parents is required unless one parent is deceased, unknown, legally incompetent, or not reasonably available, or when only one parent has legal responsibility for the care and custody of the child (45 CFR.46.408(b)).

- *Adults Incapable of Providing Consent.* For research involving adults who are unable to provide their own consent, permission for research participation must be obtained from an LAR. Individuals designated as durable power of attorney for health care via the NIH-200 Advance Directive or other valid advance directive, or court-appointed guardians are acceptable as LARs. Investigators are responsible for informing the LAR about the research as well as assessing his or her understanding and voluntariness as described in this policy. Subjects deemed unable to provide their own consent should be so informed. Refer to MAS 87-4, "Research Involving Adults Who Are or May Be Unable to Consent," for requirements regarding adults with limited capacity to consent.

## Procedures

### I. The Process of Informed Consent

A. Informed consent in research is a process that shall include the following:

- Presentation and discussion of information about the study in language understandable to the subject or LAR by the principal investigator (PI) and other members of the research team as appropriate assessment of the subject's capacity to understand and the subject's or LAR's understanding of the study information provided; sufficient time and

opportunity for the subject or LAR to consider, free of coercion or undue influence, whether to participate
- Signing the written informed consent document (oral consent is allowed under certain circumstances, see Section IV of this policy)
- Ongoing discussion with the subject or LAR and education about the study after the informed consent document is signed.

B. Informed consent begins when an individual initiates discussions with a member of the NIH Staff about participation in an NIH Intramural Research Program (IRP) protocol and continues until the individual completes study participation, withdraws consent, or is withdrawn from the study.

## II. The Written Informed Consent Document

- NIH Consent document Form 2514-1, "Consent to Participate in a Clinical Research Study," is used for all research conducted at the Clinical Center. Form 2514-1 is available from IRB coordinators, electronically from the Clinical Center's Homepage (http://www.cc.nih.gov/), or from the Protocol Coordination Service Center.
- The consent form shall include all elements required by 45 CFR 46.116 and any other information needed for an individual to be fully informed about study participation.
- Consent documents shall be written, in non-technical language that can be understood by the layperson, commensurate with the educational level of the intended subjects, and shall include at least the elements listed in Appendix 1.
- NIH form 2514-1 also includes information in the boilerplate on the first and last pages. For consent documents used at the Clinical Center, changes to the boilerplate language should only be made with approval of the IRB, as well as the Office of Human Subjects Research (OHSR) or the Office of General Counsel (OGC). Different boilerplate language is sometimes used at NIH intramural research programs in other locations.
- The consent process and document shall not include language waiving or appearing to waive any legal rights of the subject or releasing or appearing to release the investigators, sponsor, or institution from liability.

## III. Approval of Informed Consent

- Written consent documents shall be approved by the IRB along with the written research protocols. Amendments or other changes in the approved

protocol that may affect informed consent shall be incorporated into a revised consent document and approved by the IRB prior to use. Minor changes may sometimes be approved by expedited review. The consent document shall be reviewed and approved by the IRB at least once a year.
- Consent documents and protocols involving the research use of ionizing radiation shall also be reviewed by the Radiation Safety Committee and, if indicated, by the Radioactive Drug Research Committee. See Medical Administrative Series MAS 93-1, "Research Involving Human Subjects at the Clinical Center: Structure and Process."
- In certain circumstances prescribed by the Federal regulations (45 CFR 46), an IRB may waive the requirement to obtain informed consent or may approve a consent process which alters or does not include some of the elements above. For more information see NIH Multiple Project Assurance F.3 or 45 CFR 46.117 (b) and (c).
- The IRB has the authority to have IRB members observe or monitor the consent process or to require that an impartial third party observe the consent process.
- Subsequent to final approval by an IRB (as indicated by the signature of the IRB chair on the NIH-1195) but before use by the investigator, the protocol and consent form are sent for review by the Protocol Coordination Service Center (PCSC) as well as review and approval by the Associate Director for Clinical Research, Clinical Center. PCSC then adds consent and assent forms to the Intranet for access by NIH staff. Dates of approved usage are included on these forms.
- Copies of the approved consent form for a protocol will also be kept in the IRB files and the files of the Clinical Center Medical Record Department, Protocol Coordination Service Center. Protocol consent documents are time limited and must be signed and dated by the subject, parent(s), or LAR within the date identified on the last page of the document.

## IV. Oral Informed Consent: Content and Documentation

In certain circumstances (e.g., illiterate research subjects, blind research subjects), an IRB may approve an oral consent process (see 45 CFR 46.117(b)(2), and 21 CFR 50.27(b)(2), for FDA regulated research). This process requires that the IRB review and approve the following:

- **A written summary** of what the PI (or person authorized to obtain consent) will say to the subject or his or her legally authorized representative. The summary must be signed by the person obtaining consent and a witness to the oral presentation.

- **A short written consent form** stating that the required elements of consent as required by 45 CFR 46.116 were presented orally to the subject by the PI (or his designate). This short written consent form must be signed by the subject and a witness who observed the presentation of information. In the case of illiterate subjects, "making their mark" is adequate. The short written consent form may be obtained by calling Protocol Services or on the Clinical Center Web site under "Staff Information" (see "Short Written Consent Forms for English and Non-English Speaking Research Subjects").

Copies of both documents are given to subjects or their representatives and filed in the Clinical Center medical record. Whenever possible, information in these documents should be provided to the subject or authorized representative in the way that she/he can review and understand (e.g., a tape recording, a Braille document).

## V. Non-English-speaking subjects

- *Expected enrollment of non-English speaking subjects*: In some protocols, the PI expects non-English-speaking subjects to enroll because, for example, the protocol is studying a disease or condition that is likely to attract them or the PI is actively recruiting them. When the study subject population includes non-English-speaking people or the PI and/or the IRB anticipates that *consent discussions will be conducted in a language other than English*, the IRB shall require a translated consent document to be prepared. To assure itself that the translation is accurate, the IRB may choose to have a back translation or review of the document by an IRB member or other person who is fluent in that language. When non-English-speaking subjects enroll, they are given a copy of the translated consent document.
- *Unexpected enrollment of a non-English-speaking subject*: If a non-English-speaking subject is unexpectedly eligible for protocol enrollment, there may not be an extant IRB-approved written translation of the consent document. Investigators should carefully consider the ethical and legal ramifications of enrolling subjects when a language barrier exists. If the subject does not clearly understand the information presented at the signing of the consent document or in subsequent discussions, his or her consent may not be informed and therefore not effective.

If a PI decides to enroll a subject into a protocol for which there is not an extant IRB-approved informed consent document in the prospective subject's language, the PI must receive IRB approval following the procedures described in section IV, above (Oral Informed Consent). The English version of the informed consent document may be used as **the written summary** (see IV(a) above). The Clinical Center standard **short written consent form** translated into the most common languages used in the Clinical Center may be obtained by contacting Protocol Services or on the Clinical Center Web site under "Staff Information" (for translations and back translations, see "Short Written Consent Forms for English and Non-English Speaking Research Subjects"). For all other languages the PI is responsible for obtaining translation(s) of the short written consent form.* When these documents are submitted to the IRB, the Chair will determine whether or not expedited procedures may be used.

- *Use of interpreters in the consent process*: Unless the PI is fluent in the prospective subject's language, an interpreter will be necessary to facilitate the conversation. Preferably someone who is independent of the subject (i.e., not a family member) shall assist in presenting information and obtaining consent. Interpreters can be located through the Department of Social Work (301-496-2792). Whenever possible, interpreters should be provided copies of the relevant consent documents well before the consent conversation with the subject (24 to 48 hours if possible).

The interpreter may sign the consent document as the witness (see IV, above) and should note "Interpreter" under the signature line.

The PI (or authorized person) must document this process in the progress notes of the subject's medical record, including the name of the interpreter.

## VI. Responsibility for Obtaining Informed Consent

- It is the responsibility of the principal investigator (PI) to ensure that informed consent is obtained. This includes ensuring that the subject is decisionally capacitated and that the potential risks and benefits of the research have been adequately explained. In some cases, the IRB may require an independent capacity assessment.
- Written consent must be obtained by the PI or by a PI-designated member of the research team who is knowledgeable about the protocol. Whenever consent is to be obtained by someone other than the PI or an associate investigator on the study, this must be approved by the IRB.
- Any member of the health care or research team who has concerns about the process of informed consent or questions about the decision-making capacity of the prospective subject or LAR is obligated to take appropriate further steps, including discussing concerns with the PI and consulting with appropriate resources. Procedures contained in policy MAS 87-4,

---

* Translation of the short written consent form may be obtained by contacting the NIH Library.

"Research Involving Adults Who Are or May Be Unable to Consent," are to be followed for an adult subject unable to provide his or her own consent.

- The consent document must be signed and dated by (a) the subject or his or her LAR, (b) the PI or designee obtaining the consent, and (c) a witness who attests only to the validity of the signature (i.e., that the research subject actually signed the consent), not to the validity or quality of consent. Any adult other than the person obtaining or providing consent may be a witness to the signature.
- Each page of the consent document shall be labeled with the subject's name and hospital number. The subject shall be given a copy of the signed consent document. The original signed consent document is filed in the subject's medical record under section "Protocol Consent."

## VII. Additional Informed Consent for Surgical or Invasive Procedures

- For **surgical procedures and other single invasive procedures**, NIH-2626 "Request for Administration of Anesthesia and for Performance of Operations and Other Procedures" should be completed within 30 days prior to the procedure. Any procedure previously consented to but not initiated within 30 days of signing the consent form shall not be performed until a new consent is obtained. The time and date of the consent shall be recorded on the consent document.

  For all surgical patients, the NIH-2626 shall be completed prior to the administration of preoperative medication. Patients should give and sign consent before leaving the nursing unit (inpatients) or during the surgical clinic visit (outpatients).

  The attending clinician who will perform the invasive procedure is responsible for the consent process for any procedures, which require completion of NIH-2626. The responsible physician or his or her designee who is knowledgeable about the procedure shall explain in detail the nature, purpose, risks and benefits, and alternatives of the procedure. This explanation will be in language that the subject understands.

  A detailed summary of the informed consent discussion must be documented in the progress notes of the patient's record or in the relevant sections of NIH-2626.

  The Medical Staff Handbook should be consulted for a current list of procedures requiring the completion of NIH-2626.

- In special circumstances, for **noninvestigational procedures indicated to meet the clinical needs of a subject who cannot provide his or her own consent**, and for whom a surrogate is not present, telephone consent from a surrogate may be obtained. When consent is obtained by telephone, a third party shall monitor the conversation. The circumstances and manner of obtaining consent and the name of the person providing consent shall be documented in a progress note in the medical record.

## VIII. Use of Additional Consent Forms for Specific Procedures

Separate written informed consent, in addition to protocol consent or NIH form 2626, shall be obtained in certain circumstances, regardless of whether procedures are a direct part of the research protocol. (Examples of other consent forms listed here in the policy document have been deleted for brevity).

## IX. Consent for Postmortem Examination

At the Clinical Center, postmortem examination (autopsy) and disposition of a subject's body shall be permitted upon written consent of the responsible individual in accordance with applicable law. If the responsible individual is not at the Clinical Center, consent may be obtained via facsimile or telegram, according to instructions provided by the Clinical Center Admissions Office (301-496-3315). The following forms should be utilized for these purposes:

SF-523 Authorization for Autopsy
NIH-1286 Relative's Instructions Regarding Disposition of Body

There may be protocols in which postmortem examination is desired for scientific reasons. In such cases, protocol consent discussions should include consideration of autopsy. Where appropriate, consent documents should provide the subject an opportunity to indicate preferences about postmortem examination (e.g., a checkoff item). Consent for postmortem examination, however, shall be obtained from the legally responsible individual.

Consent for organ or tissue donation shall be obtained from the legally responsible individual according to the procedures outlined in policy MAS 94-6 "Organ and Tissue Donation."

## X. Obtaining Consent from Someone Not at the Clinical Center

For **research protocols** or any procedures performed for the purposes of research that involve obtaining consent via technology and/or electronic process, rather than in person, the procedures for obtaining consent, including how information will be transmitted and documented and by whom, shall be detailed in the written protocol. Review and approval must first be obtained from the Institute Clinical Director and the relevant IRB.

## XI. Consent for Emergency Procedures

In the case of an emergency, consent should be obtained from the subject for any medically indicated interventions or procedures that normally require consent. If the subject is unable to provide consent for **medically indicated emergency procedures,** permission shall be sought from a surrogate. When permission is obtained by telephone, a third party shall monitor the conversation. An explanation of the circumstances and manner of obtaining permission and the name of the person providing it shall be documented in a progress note in the medical record, and signed and dated. In the event that no one is available to provide consent in a clinical emergency, treatment may be given in accordance with standard clinical practice.

**Investigational emergency procedures** must be part of a protocol that has been reviewed and approved by the relevant IRB, in accordance with federal regulations.

## Information to be Included in the Consent Document

1. A statement that the study involves research
2. An explanation of the purpose of the research, an invitation to participate and explanation of why the subject was selected, and the expected duration of the subject's participation
3. A description of procedures to be followed and identification of which procedures are investigational and which might be provided as standard care to the subject in another setting. Use of research methods such as randomization and placebo controls should be explained
4. A description of any foreseeable risks or discomforts to the subject, an estimate of their probability and magnitude, and a description of what steps will be taken to prevent or minimize them; as well as acknowledgment of potentially unforeseeable risks
5. A description of any benefits to the subject or to others that may reasonably be expected from the research, and an estimate of their likelihood
6. A disclosure of any appropriate alternative procedures or courses of treatment that might be advantageous to the subject
7. A statement describing to what extent records will be kept confidential, including examples of who may have access to research records such as hospital personnel, the FDA, and drug sponsors
8. For research involving more than minimal risk, an explanation and description of any compensation and any medical treatments that are available if subjects are injured through participation; where further information can be obtained, and whom to contact in the event of research-related injury
9. An explanation of whom to contact for answers to questions about the research and the research subject's rights (include the name and phone number of the principal investigator [PI] and the phone number of the Clinical Center's Patient Representative)
10. A statement that research is voluntary and that refusal to participate or a decision to withdraw at any time will involve no penalty or loss of benefits to which the subject is otherwise entitled
11. A concluding statement indicating that the subject is making a decision whether to participate, and that his or her signature indicates that he or she has decided to participate having read and discussed the information presented

**When appropriate, or when required by the IRB, one or more of the following elements of information will also be included in the consent document:**

1. If the subject is or may become pregnant, a statement that the particular treatment or procedure may involve risks, foreseeable or currently unforeseeable, to the subject, or to the embryo or fetus
2. A description of circumstances in which the subject's participation may be terminated by the investigator without the subject's consent
3. Any costs to the subject that may result from participation in the research
4. The possible consequences of a subject's decision to withdraw from the research and procedures for orderly termination of participation
5. A statement that the PI will notify subjects of any significant new findings developed during the course of the study that may affect them and influence their willingness to continue participation
6. The approximate number of subjects involved in the study
7. If the investigator is not planning to return results to the subjects, a statement should be included that explains the reason for planned nondisclosure and recognizes the subject's right to that information under the Privacy Act. The following language has been recommended by NIH legal counsel:

The investigators conducting this study do not plan to provide you with the results of any medical tests or evaluations or other information pertaining to you, or other research data or results because *[the results will be preliminary] [the results will require further analysis] [the results may reveal unwanted information about family relationships] [further research may be necessary before the results are meaningful]. [If meaningful information is developed from this study that may be important for your health, you will be informed when it becomes available.]*

"By agreeing to participate in this study, you do not waive any rights that you may have regarding access to and disclosure of your records. For further information on those rights, please contact Dr. _____ (PI).

# APPENDIX 4. CLINICAL CENTER POLICY M92-7: ADVANCE DIRECTIVES

## Background

People's preferences concerning their health care, research participation, and the manner in which they die are issues of great importance. Too often, when patients cannot speak for themselves, critical health care and end of life decisions are made without sufficient knowledge of their preferences. Health care professionals have a responsibility to discuss these issues with their patients so that clinical care can be provided in accord with what their patients would have wanted. At the Clinical Center, investigators have the additional responsibility of exploring and honoring their subjects' preferences regarding research participation.

## Purpose

The purpose of this policy is to delineate staff responsibilities and procedures for informing research subjects about advance directives, to assist them in articulating their preferences regarding health care and research participation, and to honor those preferences. This policy satisfies the 1990 federal legislation, "Patient Self-Determination Act," which requires that health care institutions inform patients of their right to participate in, and direct, their health care by implementing advance directives. This policy complements Medical Administrative Series policies M87-4, "Research Involving Adults Who Are or May Be Unable to Consent" and M91-7, "Do Not Resuscitate (DNR) Orders and Limited Treatment Orders."

## Definitions

### A. Adult Research Subject

An adult is a person who *(1)* is 18 years or older, or *(2)* is married, or *(3)* has a child. The term "research subject" in this policy refers to adult patients and clinical research volunteers seen at the Clinical Center.

### B. Advance Directives

Advance directives are written documents that allow individuals to specify in advance their preferences concerning their health care and/or research participation. Advance directives go into effect when individuals are unable to make or communicate their own decisions. NIH advance directives (see section C below) and non-NIH advance directives can be changed at any time and remain in effect unless changed or canceled by the research subject.

The two principal kinds of advance directives are the "Durable Power of Attorney for Health Care" and the "Living Will." A Durable Power of Attorney for Health Care is an advance directive in which individuals appoint an agent to make health care decisions for them in the event that they become incapable of doing so. A Living Will is an advance directive in which individuals specify which medical interventions they would want instituted, continued, withheld, or withdrawn in the event that they are in a persistent vegetative state or diagnosed with a terminal illness and are incapable of making these decisions.

### C. The NIH Advance Directive for Health Care and Medical Research Participation (form NIH 200)

The NIH Advance Directive for Health Care and Medical Research Participation form combines the essential components of a living will and a durable power of attorney for health care and research participation. Part I of the form allows research subjects to appoint a substitute decision maker (agent). Part II allows research subjects to document specific preferences they have concerning their medical research participation. Part III allows research subjects to document specific preferences they have concerning health care; this section is similar to a living will. In contrast to living wills, however, form NIH-200 is not restricted to individuals who are terminal or in a persistent vegetative state. The NIH Advance Directive for Health Care and Medical Research Participation is designed for use only at the Clinical Center. It may, however, provide guidance as to a person's preferences when they leave the Clinical Center. This form and directions for its use may be obtained from the Clinical Center Department of Bioethics, 301-496-2429.

## *Policy*

A. All adult research subjects will receive written information on advance directives at the time of their initial admission to the Clinical Center.
B. All adult inpatient research subjects will be asked about their advance directive status during each nursing admission assessment.
C. In light of the unique research environment of the NIH, research subjects without an advance directive or with a non-NIH advance directive will be encouraged to execute an NIH Advance Directive for Health Care and Medical Research Participation (form NIH 200) to address both their research and health care preferences.
D. Research participation and the provision of care at the Clinical Center are not dependent upon the execution of an advance directive, except for certain protocols as stipulated by an Institutional Review Board or as required by Medical Administrative Series policy M87-4, "Research Involving Adults Who Are or May Be Unable to Consent."

E. Advance directives (NIH and non-NIH) will be kept in the subject's chart in the Advance Directive section while on an inpatient unit and subsequently in the medical record after discharge.
F. Health care providers will be familiar with the advance directives of research subjects under their care.
G. The medically responsible physician will discuss with their research subjects the implications of their advance directives, and will honor these preferences.
H. Bioethics consultation will be obtained whenever there is disagreement, uncertainty or conflict regarding a subject's advance directive.

## Procedure

### A. Admission to the Clinical Center

1. Initial Admission

The admitting clerk, at the initial admission, will provide an admissions packet to research subjects. This packet contains written information on subjects' right to make decisions concerning their health care, including the right to execute an advance directive.

2. Assessment

   a. The inpatient admitting nurse, as part of each admission assessment, will ask research subjects if they have an advance directive and, if so, whether they want it to continue in effect at the Clinical Center.

   1) If the research subject has an advance directive on hand and wants it to continue in effect, a copy of the advance directive is placed in the Advance Directive section of the inpatient chart by the admitting nurse. The patient will be encouraged to complete the NIH Advance Directive for Health Care and Medical Research Participation (Form NIH 200). A social work referral will be made in the Clinical Research Information System (CRIS), if the advance directive is not in the medical record by the end of the admitting nurse's shift.

   2) If the research subject's advance directive is in the medical record, it will be removed from the chart, verified with the patient, and placed in the current inpatient chart. If the advance directive is not in the medical record, clinical staff will assist the research subject in obtaining the advance directive. In the meantime, the patient will be encouraged to complete the NIH Advance Directive for Health Care and Medical Research Participation (form NIH 200). A social work referral will be made in CRIS if the advance directive is not in the medical record by the end of the admitting nurse's shift.

3) If the research subject does not have an advance directive but wants more information or assistance in executing one, clinical staff can assist them or they will be referred to the social worker if not resolved by the end of the admitting nurse's shift.
4) If the subject does not have a written advance directive in the inpatient chart but makes a statement to their medically responsible physician designating his or her decision maker or preferences, this statement must be witnessed by a third party. This information will be documented by the physician and signed by the witness, recorded on the Continuation page of the NIH Advance Directive for Health Care and Medical Research Participation (form NIH 200-1). This statement should include the heading "Oral Advance Directive" and the document should be filed in the Advance Directive section of the inpatient chart. This Continuation page may be filed alone, without NIH 200.
5) If the research subject does not have an advance directive and does not wish to execute one, and further, does not wish to orally designate his or her decision maker or preferences, no further action except documentation of this is necessary.

b. The social worker and members of the bioethics department are available to assist clinical staff in advising research subjects about advance directives and assisting them in obtaining and executing advance directives.
c. The individual who obtains the advance directive will ensure that the care team is notified of the existence of the research subject's advance directive.

3. Reassessment

The advance directive status of all research subjects will be reassessed whenever there is a significant change in the research subject's clinical status.

## B. Documentation

1. At each admission, the admitting nurse will document each research subject's advance directive status in CRIS or on an approved medical record form. In addition, nurse and/or social worker will document changes in the research subject's advance directive status as they occur.
2. Upon completion of the NIH Advance Directive for Health Care and Medical Research Participation (form NIH 200), the top copy will be filed in the Advance Directive section of the active medical record. Copies will be distributed as designated on the form. The Medical Record Department will maintain the advance directive in the Advance Directive section of the medical record after discharge.

3. Non-NIH advance directives will also be filed in the Advance Directive section of the chart during the admission and maintained in the medical record after discharge.
4. If a research subject indicates that he or she would like to modify his or her current advance directive, the subject should be asked to execute a new NIH advance directive. In the rare situation where the subject is not able to execute a new NIH advance directive, he or she may give an oral advance directive to the physician as outlined above. The new advance directive should replace the old one in the subject's chart. If a research subject who has a valid advance directive decides that he or she no longer wants any advance directive to remain in effect, this should be explicitly documented. Clinical Center staff will assist that subject in indicating and dating this change on the NIH Advance Directive Continuation page.

### C. Special Concerns

The advance directive process may raise ethical or legal issues that require more in-depth consideration. These may include questions about the interpretation and application of advance directives already in existence or the cognitive ability of the research subject to execute an advance directive. In addition, health care providers should be aware that individuals unable to execute an advance directive for cognitive reasons may also be unable to consent to research participation (see Medical Administrative Series policy M87-4). Consultation on these issues is available through the Department of Clinical Bioethics.

## *Education*

### A. Clinical Personnel

The Clinical Center, through the Department of Clinical Bioethics, will provide formal training, educational materials, and on-going instruction and support for Clinical staff.

### B. Community Education

At the direction of the Medical Executive Committee, the Clinical Center Ethics Committee, Clinical Center Communications Office, and other appropriate departments will coordinate community outreach educational activities on advance directives.

## *Supervision*

Responsibility for this policy's implementation and evaluation rests with the Medical Executive Committee, with the assistance of its various subcommittees, most notably the Clinical Center Ethics Committee.

## APPENDIX 5.

## NIH ADVANCE DIRECTIVE FOR HEALTH CARE AND MEDICAL RESEARCH PARTICIPATION

### INSTRUCTIONS

The NIH is committed to respecting your health care and medical research participation wishes. As long as you are able to make decisions for yourself, we will determine what you want by speaking with you. However, it is possible that you may lose the ability to make your own decisions. At that point, it could be difficult for us to determine what kind of care you want. The NIH advance directive addresses this difficulty by allowing you to indicate in advance your health care and medical research wishes. This form goes into effect only if you lose the ability to make your own decisions. If you are completing this form, and have a non-NIH Advance Directive that you would like to remain in effect during your stay at the NIH, a copy of the non-NIH Advance Directive must be attached to this form.

The NIH advance directive is designed for use at the NIH Clinical Center. In addition, it can provide evidence of your wishes outside the Clinical Center. You can change this form at any time. You may fill out as much or as little as you want. This form must be signed and witnessed. You should keep the gold copy and give the pink copy to the person you name in part 1, if any. You should then give the remaining copies to your nurse or doctor. If you have any questions, or would like additional information, please speak with the members of your medical team, or contact the Department of Clinical Bioethics (301-496-2429).

PART 1 YOUR CHOICE FOR A SUBSTITUTE DECISION MAKER: This section is similar to a **Durable Power of Attorney** (DPA) for health care. It allows you to name someone to make medical research and health care decisions for you if you ever become unable to make these decisions for yourself. To ensure that the person you name can make the decisions you want, you should discuss your health care and medical research wishes with the person you name.

PART 2 YOUR WISHES ABOUT MEDICAL RESEARCH PARTICIPATION: This section allows you to indicate any wishes you have about your medical research participation in the event you become unable to make your own decisions. Some issues you may want to consider are listed on the back of this form. You should discuss your medical research wishes with your research team.

PART 3 YOUR WISHES FOR HEALTH CARE: This section is similar to a **Living Will**. It allows you to indicate any wishes you have for your health care in the event you become unable to make your own decisions. Some issues you may want to consider are listed on the back of this form. You should discuss your health care wishes with the doctor taking care of you.

## Issues for Consideration and Discussion

Think about the things that are most important to you (your core values). Use these core values to decide which treatments you would or wouldn't want, and what types of research, if any, that you would be willing to participate in, if you lost the ability to make your own decisions. For instance, some people value certain abilities (such as the ability to communicate) so much that they would not want to be kept alive if they lost these abilities. In contrast, some people value life itself so much that they would want treatments to keep them alive no matter what their circumstances. Below are some additional issues that you may want to consider in thinking about, and discussing, your preferences with your doctor, substitute decision maker and family.

### MEDICAL CONDITIONS RELEVANT TO END OF LIFE DECISION MAKING

Terminal Condition: A medical condition from which, in the opinion of the patient's doctors, there is no reasonable chance of recovery and the use of life-sustaining treatments would only prolong the dying process.

Permanent Coma: A complete loss of consciousness that the patient's doctors believe is not reversible.

Loss of the capacity for communication: The inability to communicate and interact with others.

Loss of the capacity for self care: The inability to perform the activities of daily living such as bathing, eating, and dressing without substantial assistance from others.

Intractable Pain: Persistent and significant pain that continues despite maximum pain relief efforts.

### TREATMENT OPTIONS

Emergency resuscitation: The attempt to restart a person's breathing and/or heartbeat. Resuscitation efforts may include Cardiopulmonary Resuscitation (CPR) which involves pushing on the patient's chest or inserting a breathing tube in the patient's throat. Resuscitation efforts may also include the use of drugs or electric shock.

Do Not Resuscitate (DNR) order: When patients do not want emergency resuscitation attempted in the event their breathing or heart stops, instructions are written not to attempt resuscitation. This is called a DNR order.

Ventilatory Support: A ventilator is a machine that helps patients' breath when their lungs fail. Ventilator support often involves a breathing tube being placed in the patient's throat.

Artificial Nutrition and Hydration: Nourishment and fluids provided by tubes into the stomach or veins or by other artificial means.

Comfort Measures: Treatments, such as pain killers, that are intended to keep patients comfortable.

### KINDS OF RESEARCH

Research with the potential for direct medical benefit: Research that offers the chance of improving the subject's medical condition.

Research with no potential for direct medical benefit: Research that does not offer the chance of improving the subject's medical condition, but will help doctors learn more about the disease under study and thus may help others with that disease.

In general, clinical research is divided into two categories of risk: minimal risk and greater than minimal risk of harm. Minimal risk means that the likelihood and degree of harm that you might experience in the research are no greater than those encountered in everyday life such as routine physical examinations and blood tests.

| MEDICAL RECORD | NIH Advance Directive for Health Care and Medical Research Participation |
|---|---|

**PART 1: Your Choice for a Substitute Decision Maker**

I authorize the person(s) named below to make decisions for me concerning my health care and participation in medical research in the event that I become unable to make these decisions for myself:

| Primary Substitute Decision Maker | Alternate (Used if Primary Substitute Decision Maker is Unavailable) |
|---|---|
| Name: | Name: |
| Address: | Address: |
| Telephone # | Telephone # |

**PART 2: Your Wishes About Medical Research Participation**

A. If you lose the ability to make decisions, you may continue in your present study or be enrolled in a new study if your substitute decision maker agrees. You may also initial the following statements that reflect your wishes.

    If I lose the ability to make my own decisions:
        ___ I do NOT want to participate in any medical research.
        ___ I am willing to participate in medical research that might help me.
        ___ I am willing to participate in medical research that will not help me medically, but might help others and involves minimal risk of harm to me.
        ___ I am willing to participate in medical research that will not help me medically, but might help others and involves greater than minimal risk of harm to me.

B. You can use this space to indicate any values, goals, or limitations you would like to guide your participation in medical research. For more space use the NIH-200-1 Continuation form.

_____
_____

**PART 3: Your Wishes for Health Care**

A. You may initial the statements below that reflect your wishes. Your doctors can then make medical decisions for you based on your wishes and specific situation. If you have any questions about the situations you might face in the future, please speak with your medical team.

        ___ I want all effective treatments for keeping me alive, no matter what my condition.
    OR
    I do NOT want life-sustaining treatments if:
        ___ I have a condition that cannot be cured and will soon lead to my death, and life-sustaining treatment will only prolong the process of dying.
        ___ I am in a permanent coma.
        ___ I am awake, but have permanently lost the ability to communicate and interact with others.

B. You can use this space to indicate any values, goals, or limitations you would like to guide your healthcare. For more space use the NIH-200-1 Continuation form.

_____
_____

| Patient Signature | | Witness Signature | |
|---|---|---|---|
| Print Name | Date | Print Name | Date |
| Patient Identification | | NIH Advance Directive for Health Care and Medical Research Participation<br>NIH-200 (10-00)<br>P.A. 09-25-0099<br>File in Section 4: Advance Directives | |

WHITE-Medical Record     GOLD-Patient     PINK-Substitute Decision Maker

## APPENDIX 6. CLINICAL CENTER POLICY M87-4: RESEARCH INVOLVING ADULTS WHO ARE OR MAY BE UNABLE TO CONSENT

### Purpose

To set forth Clinical Center policy for nonemergency research involving adults who are or who may be unable to provide initial or ongoing informed consent.

### Policy

Adults are presumed capable of giving informed consent. When questions arise regarding an adult's ability to provide initial or ongoing consent, the individual should be evaluated. Adults who are unable to provide initial or ongoing consent may participate in research only when the IRB has approved the research for adults who cannot consent, and an appropriate surrogate provides permission (unless the IRB waives the requirement for informed consent). Assent (i.e., affirmative agreement) should be obtained from individuals who are capable of providing it. Individuals' objections (dissent) should be respected.

### Procedures

1. Principal Investigator Responsibilities
    a. All research protocols should state whether adults who are unable to provide initial informed consent are excluded or are eligible to enroll, and the conditions, if any, under which adults who lose the ability to provide ongoing consent subsequent to giving initial consent, may continue to participate.
    b. If adults who are unable to consent are eligible for enrollment and/or continued participation, the protocol will describe the following:
        i. The justification for their inclusion
        ii. How adults' ability to provide initial and ongoing consent will be assessed
        iii. That the permission of an appropriate surrogate will be obtained per this policy
        iv. The risks of the research and likelihood of benefit (if any) for adults unable to consent
        v. The procedures for obtaining assent and the procedures for respecting dissent
        vi. Any additional safeguards that will be used (e.g., consent monitoring)
    c. Investigators should encourage adults who are at risk for losing the ability to consent to complete a research advance directive.

2. IRB Responsibilities

    a. If the investigator proposes to include adults who cannot provide initial consent and/or adults who cannot provide ongoing consent, the IRB will do the following:

        i. Ensure there is a compelling justification for including adults who cannot consent (e.g. the research question cannot be answered by enrolling only adults who can consent; participation offers the potential for important clinical benefit)
        ii. Ensure that the procedures for assessing adults' ability to provide initial and ongoing consent are appropriate
        iii. Stipulate that the permission of an appropriate surrogate will be obtained for adults who cannot consent
        iv. Document the risks and likelihood of benefit (if any) for adults unable to consent
        v. Ensure that the procedures for obtaining assent and respecting dissent are appropriate
        vi. Determine whether any additional safeguards will be used (e.g., consent monitoring)

    b. IRBs may approve inclusion of adults unable to consent in the following categories only:

        i. *Research not involving greater than minimal risk.* Minimal risk means that the probability and magnitude of harm or discomfort anticipated in the research are not greater in and of themselves than those ordinarily encountered in daily life or during the performance of routine physical or psychological examinations or tests.
        ii. *Research involving greater than minimal risk but presenting the prospect of direct benefit to the individual subjects.* Inclusion of adults who cannot consent may be approved in this category only when the prospect of benefit to the subjects justifies the risks and burdens to them and the risk-benefit profile of the research is at least as favorable for the subjects as the risk-benefit profile of available alternatives.
        iii. *Research involving a minor increase over minimal risk and no prospect of direct benefit to individual subjects.* Adults who cannot consent may participate in research in this category only after Bioethics consultation finds the legal guardian or holder of the durable power of attorney (DPA) is appropriate and provides permission in accordance with this policy (see section 3).
        iv. *Research involving more than a minor increase over minimal risk and no prospect of direct benefit to individual subjects.* Research in this

category must be approved by the IRB and subsequently approved by the NIH Deputy Director for Intramural Research following review by a panel of independent experts. The Deputy Director for Intramural Research can approve studies in this category only when the IRB and the independent experts find that the knowledge to be obtained is of vital importance, cannot reasonably be obtained by studying adults who can consent, and cannot be obtained in a way that poses less risk. Additionally, adults who cannot consent may be enrolled in research in this category only after Bioethics consultation determines that the surrogate is appropriate (see section 3) and there is compelling evidence (e.g., written research advance directive and no clear conflicting evidence) that participation in the study is consistent with the individual's preferences and values.

3. Identification of an Appropriate Surrogate

   a. Adults who cannot consent and have a court-appointed guardian or a durable power of attorney (DPA) for health care and/or research participation.
      The court-appointed guardian or holder of the DPA may authorize the research participation of an adult who cannot consent provided the surrogate is appropriate, including that the surrogate *(1)* understands the study involves research; *(2)* understands the risks, potential benefits and alternatives to the study; and *(3)* has sufficient reason to believe participation in the study is consistent with the individual's preferences and values. This evaluation may be conducted by the principal investigator (or designee) or by Bioethics. For research that does not offer a prospect of direct benefit and poses greater than minimal risk (section 2B, categories III and IV), this evaluation must be performed by Bioethics.
   b. Adults who cannot consent and who do not have a DPA or court-appointed guardian, but who are capable of understanding the DPA process.
      Adults who cannot provide informed consent and do not have a guardian or a DPA may retain the ability to assign a surrogate. This determination must be made by Bioethics. If the individual is capable and assigns a surrogate, the assigned surrogate may authorize the individual's research participation provided Bioethics finds the surrogate is appropriate, including that the surrogate *(1)* understands the study involves research; *(2)* understands the risks, potential benefits and alternatives to the study; and *(3)* has sufficient reason to believe participation in the study is consistent with the individual's preferences and values.

c. Adults who cannot consent, who do not have a DPA or court-appointed guardian, and who are not able to understand the DPA process.

A person at the highest level on the following list may serve as surrogate for these individuals: *(1)* spouse or domestic partner,* *(2)* adult child, *(3)* parent, *(4)* sibling, *(5)* other close relative.

The selected surrogate may authorize the individual's participation only in research which the IRB has approved as minimal risk or prospect of direct benefit (section 2B, categories I and II). Consultation with Bioethics is required to ensure the surrogate is appropriate, including that the surrogate *(1)* understands the study involves research; *(2)* understands the risks, potential benefits, and alternatives to the study; and *(3)* has sufficient reason to believe participation in the study is consistent with the individual's preferences and values.

4. Consultation

Consultation regarding this policy may be obtained by contacting Bioethics at 301-496-2429. Consultation regarding whether an individual is able to provide consent may be obtained by contacting the NIH Ability to Consent Assessment Team (301-496-9675 or 301-496-2429), which is a group trained to evaluate individuals' ability to consent and includes members from Psychiatry, Bioethics, and other disciplines.

---

*A domestic partnership is defined as a relationship between two individuals who *(1)* are at least 18 years old, *(2)* are not related to each other by blood or marriage within four degrees of consanguinity under civil law rule, *(3)* are not married or in a civil union or domestic partnership with any others, and *(4)* have agreed to be and continue to be in a relationship of mutual interdependence in which each individual contributes to the maintenance and support of the other individual and the relationship, even if both individuals are not required to contribute equally to the relationship.

## APPENDIX 7. SELECTED PUBLICATIONS INSPIRED OR INFORMED BY THE WORK OF THE BIOETHICS CONSULTATION SERVICE

Abdoler, E., Taylor, H., and Wendler, D. "The Ethics of Phase 0 Oncology Trials." *Clinical Cancer Research* 14 (2008): 3692–3697.

Applbaum, A. I., Tilburt, J. C., Collins, M. T., and Wendler, D. "A Family's Request for Complementary Medicine after Patient Brain Death." *Journal of the American Medical Association* 299, no. 18 (2008): 2188–2193.

Beskow, L., Grady, C., Iltis, A., Sadler, J., and Wilfond, B. "Points to Consider: The Research Ethics Consultation Service and the IRB." *IRB: Ethics & Research* 31, no. 6 (2009): 1–9.

Brown, A., Wendler, D., Camphausen, K., Miller, F., and Citrin, D. "Performing Non-diagnostic Research Biopsies in Irradiated Tissue: A Review of Scientific, Clinical, and Ethical Considerations." *Journal of Clinical Oncology* 26 (2008): 3987–3994.

Danis, M., Farrar, A., Grady, C., et al. "Does Fear of Retaliation Deter Requests for Ethics Consultation?" *Medicine, Health Care and Philosophy* 11, no. 1 (2008): 27–34.

Denny, C., Wilfond, B. S., Peters, J. A., Giri, N., and Alter, B. "All in the Family: Disclosure of 'Unwanted' Information to an Adolescent to Benefit a Relative." *American Journal of Medical Genetics Part A* 146A, no. 21 (2008): 2719–2724.

Dickert, N., and Grady, C. "What's the Price of a Research Subject? Approaches to Payment for Research Participation." *New England Journal of Medicine* 341, no. 3 (1999): 198–203.

Dickert, N., and Wendler, D. "Ancillary Care Obligations of Medical Researchers." *Journal of the American Medical Association* 302, no. 4 (2009): 424–428.

DuVal, G., Gensler, G., and Danis, M. "Ethical Dilemmas Encountered by Clinical Researchers." *Journal of Clinical Ethics* 16, no. 3 (2005): 267–276.

Grady, C., Horstmann, E., Sussman, J., and Hull, S. "The Limits of Disclosure: What Research Subjects Want to Know about Investigator Financial Interests." *Journal of Law, Medicine, and Ethics* 34, no. 3 (2006): 592–599.

Hardy, N. M., Grady, C., Pentz, R., Stetler-Stevenson, M., Raffeld, M., Fontaine, L. S., Babb, R., Bishop, M. R., Caporaso, N., and Marti, G. E. "Bioethical Considerations of Monoclonal B Cell Lymphocytosis: Haematologic Stem Cell Donation." *British Journal of Haemotology* 9, no. 5 (2007): 824–831.

Hull, S., Glanz, K., Steffen, A., and Wilfond, B. S. "Recruitment Approaches for Family Studies: Attitudes of Index Patients and Their Relatives." *International Review Board* 26, no. 4 (2004): 12–17.

Loud, J. T., Weissman, N. E., Peters, J. A., et al. "Deliberate Deceit of Family Members: A Challenge to Providers of Clinical Genetics Services." *Journal of Clinical Oncology* 24, no. 10 (2006): 1643–1646.

Miller, F., and Grady, C. "The Ethical Challenge of Infection-Inducing Challenge Studies." *Clinical Infectious Diseases* 33 (2001): 1028–1033.

Pace, C., Miller, F., and Danis, M. "Enrolling the Uninsured in Clinical Trials: An Ethical Perspective." *Critical Care Medicine* 31, no. 3 (2003, Suppl): S121–125.

Persad, G. C., Little, R. F., and Grady, C. "Including Persons with HIV Infection in Cancer Clinical Trials." *Journal of Clinical Oncology* 26, no. 7 (2008): 1027–1032.

Shah, S., and Wendler, D. "Interpretation of the Subjects' Condition Requirement: A Legal Perspective." *Journal of Law, Medicine, & Ethics* 38, no. 2 (2010): 365–373.

Varma, S., and Wendler, D. "Research Involving Wards of the State: Protecting Particularly Vulnerable Children." *Journal of Pediatrics* 152 (2008): 9–14.

Wendler, D. "Minimal Risk in Pediatric Research as a Function of Age." *Archives of Pediatric and Adolescent Medicine* 163 (2009): 115–118.

Wendler, D., and Grady, C. "What Should Research Participants Understand to Understand They Are Participants in Research?" *Bioethics* 22, no. 4 (2008): 203–208.

Wendler, D., Rackoff, J., Emanuel, E., and Grady, C. "The Ethics of Paying for Children's Research Participation." *Journal of Pediatrics* 141 (2002): 166–171.

Wendler, D., Shah, S., Whittle, A., and Wilfond, B. S. "Non-beneficial Research with Individuals Who Cannot Consent: Is It Ethically Better to Enroll Healthy or Affected Individuals?" *Institutional Review Board* 25 (2003): 1–4.

Wilfond, B. S., and Candotti, F. "When Eligibility Criteria Clash with Personal Treatment Choice: A Dilemma of Clinical Research." In *Ethics and Research with Children: A Case-Based Approach*, ed. E. Kodish (Oxford: Oxford University Press, 2005): 310–322.

Wolitz, R., Emanuel, E., and Shah, S. "Rethinking the Responsiveness Requirement for International Research. *The Lancet* 374, no. 9692 (2009): 847–849.

# INDEX

*Abigail Alliance*, court case, 125, 147
Ability to Consent Assessment Team (ACAT), participants, 104
access, evaluating, 223
acquired immunodeficiency syndrome (AIDS). *See also* human immunodeficiency virus (HIV)
 smallpox vaccine study, 25
adult, definition, 225
adults incapable of providing consent, 227
advance directives
 Clinical Center policy, 237–241
 definitions, 237–238
 education, 241
 NIH Advance Directive for Health Care and Medical Research Participation, 238, 242–244
 policy, 238–239
 procedure, 239–241
 purpose, 237
 supervision, 241
alcoholism, discharging at-risk participant, 159, 168–171
Alzheimer's disease, depression protocol and early signs of, 124, 138–141
American Society for Bioethics and Humanities (ASBH), report, 220–222
ancillary care, obligations, 123, 125–128
anesthesia, magnetic resonance imaging (MRI) in children, 24, 44–45
anonymous consultations, handling requests for, 14
aplastic anemia, determining participant inclusion or exclusion, 49–50, 53–57
attention-deficit/hyperactivity disorder (ADHD), transcranial magnetic stimulation (TMS), 102, 105–107
authorship, assigning, for research, 188–189, 212–216
autoimmune disorder, evaluating evolving risks, 79, 83–87

behavior problems, excluding noncompliant participant, 158, 164–165
Belmont Report, ethical principles, 2, 100
best interests standard, surrogate, 181
bioethics, National Institutes of Health (NIH), 4–6
biologic treatments, participant posttrial expectations, 196–199
bioterrorism
 concerns, 27
 smallpox attack, 24, 26
blind participants, informed consent, 70
blood samples, participant requesting withdrawal of, 188, 205–208
blood stem cells, donation of, 135
bone marrow harvest, medical care to donor, 135–136
bone marrow transplantation, children with aplastic anemia, 50, 53–57
brain tumors, research with terminally ill, 102–103, 116–118
breast cancer gene, confidentiality vs. duty to warn, 80, 92–97

cancer gene, confidentiality vs. duty to warn, 80, 92–97
cancer patients
 cancer Phase I trials, 50, 57–59
 postoperative, and discharge of at-risk participant, 168–171
 research with terminally ill, 102–103, 116–118
candidate vaccines, malaria, 28–29
capacity assessment
 compliance, 149
 research participants, 103–104
cardiac medications, evolving risks in pediatric participant, 83–87
case review process, Consultation Service, 10–11
cell-based toxicology testing, public policy, 33–34

251

252 ■ Index

Centers for Disease Control (CDC), infectious diseases, 163–164
cerebral palsy, evaluating body mechanics, 166–167
children
 anesthesia during magnetic resonance imaging (MRI), 24, 44–45
 dependence of, 102
 informing minor, of diagnoses, 102, 107–109
 pediatric leukemia patient, 192–196
 risk without direct benefit, 101–102, 105–107
 transcranial magnetic stimulation and ADHD, 102, 105–107
chronic granulomatous disease (CGD), excluding noncompliant participant, 164–165
Clinical and Translational Science Awards (CTSA) program, 3
clinical care
 access to experimental drugs outside protocol, 145–147
 balancing clinical research and, 122–125
 disclosure of incidental findings, 123, 129–134
 meeting needs without compromising scientific validity, 124–125, 141–145
 noncompliance, 147–153
 obligations to medical care of donors, 123–124, 134–138
 obligation to treat STI symptoms, 123, 125–128
 withholding, for scientific validity, 124, 138–141
Clinical Center Bioethics Consultation Service. *See also* Consultation Service
 admission to, 239–240
 Department of Bioethics, 6
 documentation, 240–241
 education, 241
 National Institutes of Health (NIH), 5–6
 policy M77-2 (informed consent), 225–234
 policy M87-4 (adults unable to consent), 245–248
 policy M92-7 (advance directives), 237–241

Clinical Laboratory Improvement Amendments (CLIA), requirements, 33
clinical research
 balancing clinical care and, 17
 motivation, 2–4
 process, 16–18
clinical research ethics consultation, definition, 1
Clinical Research Information System (CRIS), NIH protocols, 67
clinical trials, phases and types of, 5t
coercion
 assessing study procedures, 72–76
 enrolling and recruiting, 52–53
 free hysterectomy, 53, 72, 73–74
cognitively impaired participant, surrogate decision makers, 102, 110–112
community, posttrial obligations, 185–186
comorbidity, participant exclusion, 50, 57–59
compensation, multiple protocols, 66–67
compliance, poor, and noncompliance, 125, 147–153
confidentiality
 consultations, 16
 preventing harm and protecting, 160–164
 reconciling, and duty to warn, 80, 92–97
conflict
 regulations and analysis, 13–14
 research team and family members, 159, 174–176
 research team and surrogate decision maker, 160, 176–181
consent. *See also* informed consent
 confidentiality, 157–158
 consultations, 16
 oral process, 114
 participant posttrial expectations, 197–198
 research in emergency, 113–116
 surrogate, 102, 110–112
consultants, Consultation Service, 8–9
consultations
 consent and confidentiality, 16
 organization of book, 16–18
 organized by subject matter, 219
 reports in book, 15–18

Consultation Service
  American Society for Bioethics and
    Humanities (ASBH) report,
    220–222
  authorship, 213–214, 215
  case review process, 10–11
  challenges, 3–4, 223–224
  consultants, 8–9
  criteria for ethical screening, 42, 43
  defining scope of consultation
    question, 12–13
  disclosure of incidental findings,
    130–132
  evaluation, 12, 220–222
  handling anonymous consultations, 14
  handling conflicts between regulations
    and analysis, 13–14
  insurance status, 200
  intake, 10
  neonatal care, 203–205
  philosophy, 6–7
  poor compliance and
    noncompliance, 147–153
  process, 10–12
  publications inspired or informed
    by, 249–250
  quality, 220–222
  report preparation and
    dissemination, 11–12
  risk and donation, 136–138
  role, 7–8
  skills and knowledge, 9
  study participant inclusion, 14–15
Cooperative Research and Development
  Agreement (CRADA), hysterectomy
  study, 73–74
cosmetic surgery, research
  risks, 78–79, 81–83

data safety monitoring board (DSMB)
  developing situations, 84, 85, 87
  discontinuation of
    trial, 188, 208–212
  pulmonary hypertension treatment, 142
decisionally capacitated adult, 226
Declaration of Helsinki
  ancillary care, 128
  medical research, 29
  research ethics, 2
  social value and research, 31

Department of Bioethics. *See also*
    Consultation Service
  ancillary care, 128
  Clinical Center, 6
  responsibility, 6
depression protocol, participants with early
    signs of Alzheimer's disease, 124,
    138–141
device manufacturers, payment for
    hysterectomies, 74–75
diagnostic trials, definition, 5t
distortion of results, multiple protocols, 67
donepezil hydrochloride, depression and
    Alzheimer's disease, 124, 138–141
donor, stem cell, and medical care,
    123–124, 134–138
do-not-intubate (DNI) order,
    surrogate, 178
do-not-resuscitate (DNR) order
  end-of-life care, 173, 174
  pediatric leukemia patient, 192–194
double-blind, placebo-controlled trial,
    experimental drugs, 125, 145–147
drugs. *See* experimental drugs
durable power of attorney (DPA)
  end-of-life care, 175
  surrogate decision maker, 176–181
duty to warn, reconciling confidentiality
    and, 80, 92–97

economically disadvantaged,
    caring for, 103, 118–120
efficiency, evaluating, 223
emergency, consent for research
    in, 102, 113–116, 234
encephalitis, research in
    emergency, 102, 113–116
ending research
  assigning authorship, 188–189, 212–216
  data safety monitoring board
    (DSMB), 188, 208–212
  discharging to less optimal
    care, 186–187, 192–196
  managing posttrial expectations
    of participant, 187, 196–199
  posttrial consequences of trial
    intervention, 187–188, 202–205
  posttrial considerations, 185–186
  posttrial obligations to uninsured
    participants, 187, 199–202

ending research (Cont'd)
  request for withdrawal of tissue samples, 188, 205–208
  responsible termination, 185
  trial termination, 17
  violation of rules, 186, 189–191
end-of-life care
  futile care, 159, 171–174
  pediatric leukemia patient, 192–196
  protocol, 117
essential newborn care (ENC), recommendations, 203–205
ethical challenges, clinical research, 1
ethical screening process, design of, 23, 41–43
Ethics Grand Rounds, responsibility, 6, 99
evaluation
  access and efficiency, 223
  Consultation Service, 12, 220–222
  postconsultation evaluation form, 222
experimental drugs
  access to, outside study protocol, 145–147
  addressing medical errors, 79, 90–92
exploitation, withholding care, 140–141

Fair Benefits, framework, 40
fairness
  enrolling research participants, 49, 56
  testing journalist's cells, 32, 34
familial Mediterranean fever, economically disadvantaged participant, 103, 118–120
family members, conflict with research team, 159, 174–176
Federal Privacy Act, confidentiality vs. duty to warn, 94, 97, 162, 236
First Breath study, infant care, 203
Fragile X, surrogate for male with, 110–112

gene mutation, confidentiality vs. duty to warn, 80, 92–97
general anesthesia and endotracheal intubation (GETA), reconciling multiple institutional review boards, 24, 44–46
Genetic Information Non-Discrimination Act of 2008 (GINA), passage, 96
genetic mutations

testing, 35
toxic exposures, 32–33
glioma patients, research with terminally ill, 102–103, 116–118
Grand Rounds. See Ethics Grand Rounds
guinea-pigging, making a living, 69

health insurance
  participant posttrial expectations, 187, 196–197
  posttrial obligations to uninsured participants, 187, 199–202
hepatitis B virus infection, confidentiality, 160–162
human immunodeficiency virus (HIV)
  ancillary care of STI symptoms, 126
  level of compliance of participant, 148
  smallpox vaccination, 21, 24–28
  testing in Uganda, 37, 38–39
human leukocyte antigen (HLA)
  excluding noncompliant participant, 164–165
  stem cell transplant, 134
human papilloma virus (HPV), infection, 163
human subject, 226
human T-lymphatic virus type 1 (HTVL-1), confidentiality, 160–162
Huntington disease (HD), designing ethical screening process, 41–43
hysterectomy
  coercive to offer free, 53, 72, 73–74
  U.S. taxpayers paying for, 74–75

illiterate participant, informed consent, 69–70
imaging study, National Institutes of Health (NIH), 51
immune systems, smallpox vaccine for HIV, 24–28
incidental findings, disclosure of, 123, 129–134
infant care
  essential newborn care (ENC), 203–205
  posttrial consequences, 187–188, 202–205
infectious diseases
  preventing harm and protecting confidentiality, 158, 160–164

Uganda, 38
informed consent. *See also* consent
  approval of, 228–229
  definitions, 225–226
  elements, 52, 71
  emergency procedures, 234
  inability of participants, 69–72
  information for document, 235–236
  languages, 52, 72
  non-English-speaking subjects, 230–231
  obtaining from someone not at center, 233
  oral, 229–230
  policy, 226–227
  policy for adults unable to consent, 245–248
  postmortem examination, 233
  procedures, 227–234
  process of, 227–228
  protecting participants, 78
  responsibility for obtaining, 231–232
  surgical or invasive procedures, 232–233
  surrogate decision makers, 102, 110–112
  written forms, 72, 228
institutional review boards (IRBs)
  ethics, 1
  information for consent documents, 236
  preparing protocol for submission to, 51
  reconciling judgments from multiple, 24, 44–46
  recruitments with public records, 63–64
  responsibility, 6, 8
insurance. *See* health insurance
intake process, Consultation Service, 10
International Ethical Guidelines for Biomedical Research Involving Human Subjects, research ethics, 2
international research
  sickle cell disease and pulmonary hypertension in Uganda, 37–41
  Uganda, 23
interpersonal difficulties
  conflicts with surrogate decision maker, 176–181
  discharging at-risk participants, 158–159, 168–171
  end-of-life care decisions, 159, 171–174
  excluding noncompliant participants, 158, 164–165, 166–167
  life support decisions, 174–176
  medical beliefs, 160, 182–183
  navigating, 17, 157–160
  preventing harm and protecting confidentiality, 158, 160–164
  religious convictions, 160, 182–183
interpreters, consent process, 231
intravenous immunoglobulin G (IVIG), consent in emergency, 113–116
invalidation of results, multiple protocols, 67
invasive procedures, informed consent, 232–233
investigational emergency procedures, 234

journalist, genetic testing, 22, 32–35
justification, research risks, 78–79, 81–83

knowledge, Consultation Service, 9

LaFora's disease, informing minor children, 107–109
language, informed consent, 52, 72
legally authorized representative, 226
leukemia
  discharge to less optimal care, 192–196
  futile care for dying, 159, 171–174
life support, withdrawing, 159, 174–176
lung cancer, life support withdrawal, 159, 174–176

magnetic resonance imaging (MRI)
  anesthesia during, in children, 24, 44–45
  disclosure of incidental findings, 123, 129–134
malaria vaccine
  assessing social value, 28–32
  responsiveness, 21–22
Mali, malaria vaccine participants, 30–31
medical beliefs, respecting, 160, 182–183
medical care, obligations to donors, 134–138
medical errors, addressing, 79, 90–92

medically indicated emergency
   procedures, 234
methicillin-resistant staphylococcus
   aureus (MRSA) infection,
   discharging at-risk participant, 159,
   168–171
Ministry of Health (MoH), syndromic
   management protocol, 126–127
minors, 226–227
"miracle drug," placebo-controlled trial,
   125, 146–147
morality, recruitment method, 64, 65
motor vehicle accident, participants
   through public records, 62–66
multiple protocols
   problems of participation in, 66–68
   research participant enrollment, 52,
   66–69

National Action Plan for Breast Cancer, 206
National Cancer Institute, participant
   enrollment, 51
National Institutes of Health (NIH). *See
   also* Clinical Center
   authorship and NIH
      Ombudsman, 213, 214
   bioethics at, 4–6
   Clinical and Translational Science
      Awards (CTSA) program, 3
   Clinical Center, 5–6, 226–227
   consent forms, 157–158
   imaging study, 51
   institutes and centers of, 4t
   NIH Advance Directive for Health Care
      and Medical Research Participation,
      238, 242–244
   Public-Private Partnership Program, 76
natural history trials, definition, 5t
neonates, posttrial consequences, 187–188,
   202–205
New Zealand, automobile crash
   injuries, 65
NIH Advance Directive for Health Care
   and Medical Research Participation,
   238, 242–244
noncompliance
   excluding participant for behavior
      problems, 158, 164–165
   excluding participant without prospect
      of benefit, 158, 166–167

participants and clinical care, 125,
   147–153
non-English-speaking subjects, informed
   consent, 230–231
Nuremberg Code, research ethics, 2

obesity study, multiple protocols, 66
obligations
   ancillary care, 123, 125–128
   medical care of donors, 123–124,
      134–138
   obtaining informed consent, 231–232
   posttrial, to community, 185–186
   posttrial, to uninsured participants,
      199–202
   preventing harm and protecting
      confidentiality, 160–164
Office of Human Research Protections,
   guidance, 207
opt-out option, research participants, 130
oral informed consent, 229–230

participants. *See* research participants
pathophysiology trials, definition, 5t
pediatric participant, autoimmune disorder
   and cardiac issues, 79, 83–87
Phase I trials
   cancer study, 50, 57–59
   definition, 5t
   malaria vaccine, 28–32
   proof of concept study, 73
Phase II trials
   definition, 5t
   proof of concept study, 73
Phase III trials, definition, 5t
Phase IV trials, definition, 5t
philosophy, Consultation Service, 6–7
placebo-controlled trials
   ethical study design, 22–23
   experimental drugs, 125, 145–147
   sham intravenous (IV) and saline
      infusion, 35–36
police records, recruiting, 62–66
policies, conflicts with analysis, 13–14
populations, malaria vaccine trial in local,
   28–32
postconsultation evaluation form, 222
postmortem examination, consent, 233
postoperative cancer survivors, discharge of
   at-risk participant, 159, 168–171

Index ■ 257

posttrial expectations,
  participants, 187, 196–199
posttrial obligations
  community, 185–186
  uninsured participants, 199–202
pregnancy, balancing risk and participant
  choice, 79, 87–89
premature infants, posttrial
  consequences, 187–188, 202–205
prevention trials, definition, 5t
prisoners, vulnerable population, 101
privacy. *See also* confidentiality
  recruitment method, 63
protection of research
  participants, 17, 78–80
  balancing risks and respecting
    choice, 79, 87–89
  confidentiality and duty to
    warn, 80, 92–97
  evaluation of evolving risks, 79, 83–87
  justification of research risks, 78, 81–83
  medical errors, 79, 90–92
  risks to third parties, 80, 97–99
psychiatric disorders, exclusion for
  comorbidity, 50, 57–59
psychiatric treatment, violation
  of rules, 186, 189–191
public policy, cell-based toxicology
  testing, 33–34
public-private partnerships,
  coordination, 76
public records, individuals from motor
  vehicle accident (MVA), 62–66
publications, Bioethics
  Consultation Service, 249–250
pulmonary hypertension
  SCD (sickle cell disease)
    patients, 124–125, 141–145
  SCD and, in Uganda, 37–41

quality, Consultation Service, 220–222
quality of life trials, definition, 5t

radiation exposure, multiple protocols, 67
reconstructive surgery, research risks,
  78–79, 81–83
recruitment
  participants through public
    records, 52, 62–66
  recommendations for terminally ill, 117

Reed, Walter, Yellow Fever Board, 61
regulations, conflicts with analysis, 13–14
religious convictions, respecting medical
  beliefs, 160, 182–183
reporting process, Consultation
  Service, 11–12
research
  definition, 225
  social value, 21–22
research participants. *See also*
  protection of research participants
  aplastic anemia treatment, 50, 53–57
  capacity assessment
    procedures, 103–104
  discharge for violating rules, 189–191
  discharging at-risk, 168–171
  disclosure of incidental
    findings, 123, 129–134
  economically disadvantaged, 103,
    118–120
  enrolling, 17, 49–53
  exclusion for behavior
    problems, 164–165
  exclusion of noncompliant, 164–165,
    166–167
  expectations, 131
  inclusion in consultations, 14–15
  malaria vaccine, in Mali, 30–31
  malaria vaccine, in United States, 29–30
  managing posttrial
    expectations, 187, 196–199
  meriting authorship, 188–189, 212–216
  multiple protocols, 52, 66–69
  opt-out option, 130
  poor compliance and noncompliance,
    125, 147–153
  posttrial obligations to
    uninsured, 199–202
  protecting, 17
  requesting withdrawal of tissue
    samples, 188, 205–208
  staff member enrollment, 50–51, 59–62
  terminally ill, 102–103, 116–118
  undue inducements, 56–57
research protocols, consent, 233
research risks
  addressing medical errors, 79, 90–92
  balancing risk and participant
    choice, 79, 87–89
  children, 101–102, 105–107

research risks (*Cont'd*)
  confidentiality vs. duty to
    warn, 80, 92–97
  evaluation of evolving, 83–87
  justification of, 78–79, 81–83
  third parties, 80, 97–99
research team
  conflict with family
    members, 159, 174–176
  conflict with surrogate decision maker,
    160, 176–181
responsibility. *See* obligations
  obtaining informed consent, 231–232
responsiveness
  host community, 21–22
  target population, 30
result invalidation, multiple protocols, 67
risk-benefit ratio, balancing risk and
    participant choice, 79, 87–89
risk in procedures, multiple protocols, 67

safeguards, staff member enrollment, 61
safety. *See* data safety monitoring
    board (DSMB)
saline infusion, placebo-controlled
    trials, 35–36
scientific validity
  assessment of, 22, 32–35
  meeting needs without
    compromising, 124–125, 141–145
  withholding clinical care, 124, 138–141
screening trials, definition, 5t
sexually transmitted infections (STIs),
    obligation to treat, 123, 125–128
sexual relations, violation of trial
    policies, 186, 189–191
sham intravenous (IV), placebo-controlled
    trials, 22–23, 35–36
short written consent form, oral, 230
sickle cell disease (SCD)
  pulmonary hypertension
    and, 124–125, 141–145
  pulmonary hypertension and,
    in Uganda, 37–41
skills, Consultation Service, 9
smallpox vaccine
  bioterrorism threat of smallpox, 27–28
  ethical arguments against
    research, 26–27
  ethical arguments favoring
    research, 25–26
  human immunodeficiency
    virus (HIV), 21, 24–28
social value
  ethics against research, 26–27
  ethics favoring research, 25–26
  malaria vaccine trials, 21–22, 28–32
  smallpox vaccine for human
    immunodeficiency virus
    (HIV), 21, 24–28
  World Medical Association
    requiring, for research, 31
South America, discharge of leukemia
    patient and return to, 192–196
staff members
  clinical study
    enrollment, 50–51, 59–62
  reasons not to enroll, 60–61
  reasons to enroll, 60
  safeguards, 61
standard of care
  futile care for terminally ill, 172–174
  placebo-controlled trials, 22–23
stem cell transplants, obligations to medical
    care of donors, 123–124, 134–138
study designs
  ethical screening process, 23, 41–43
  placebo-controlled trials, 22–23
study participants. *See* research participants
study procedures, assessing coercive or
    undue influence, 72–76
substituted judgment standard,
    surrogate, 181
suicidal risk, discharging at-risk
    participant, 168–169
surgery
  procedures for informed
    consent, 232–233
  religious concerns, 160, 182–183
  research risks, 78–79, 81–83
surrogate, 226
surrogate decision makers
  cognitively impaired
    participant, 102, 110–112
  conflict with research
    team, 160, 176–181
  consent in emergency, 102, 113–116
  identification of appropriate, 247–248

taxpayers, hysterectomies, 74–75
terminally ill
    futile care, 159, 171–174
    research with, 102–103, 116–118
termination. *See* ending research
third parties, research risks to, 80, 97–99
tissue samples, participant
    requesting withdrawal
    of, 188, 205–208
toxic exposures, genetic mutations, 32–33
toxicology testing, cell-based, 33–34
transcranial magnetic stimulation (TMS),
    children and ADHD, 102, 105–107
treatment types, definition, 5t

Uganda
    international research, 23
    sickle cell disease and pulmonary
        hypertension, 37–41
undue inducement
    influencing compliance, 149–150
    research participation, 56–57, 69
    uninsured and access to health care,
        144–145
undue influence
    assessing study procedures, 72–76
    recruiting and enrolling, 52–53
unfairness, withholding care, 140–141
United States, malaria vaccine
    participants, 29–30
U.S. Common Rule, multisite study, 45

vaccine studies, staff members enrolling in,
    50–51, 59–62
vulnerability
    definition, 100
    ethical issues, 100–103
vulnerable populations
    Ability to Consent Assessment Team
        (ACAT), 104
    capacity assessment procedures,
        103–104
    children, 101–102, 105–107, 107–109
    coercion, 52–53
    conducting research with, 17
    economically disadvantaged, 103,
        118–120
    guidelines 45 CFR 46, 100
    inclusion of historically excluded, 55
    research participants, 50–51
    terminally ill, 102–103, 116–118

women, assessing hysterectomy study,
    72–76
World Medical Association, social value and
    research, 31
www.guineapigzero.com, jobzine, 69

Yellow Fever Board, staff members, 61

written document, informed consent, 228
written summary, oral informed
    consent, 229

www.ingramcontent.com/pod-product-compliance
Ingram Content Group UK Ltd.
Pitfield, Milton Keynes, MK11 3LW, UK
UKHW041259180426
11947UKWH00008B/570